Experimental Psychopharmacology

Contemporary Neuroscience

Experimental Psychopharmacology

Edited by

Andrew J. Greenshaw and **Colin T. Dourish**

Humana Press   •   **Clifton, New Jersey**

Library of Congress Cataloging in Publication Data

Main entry under title:

© 1987 The Humana Press Inc.
Crescent Manor
PO Box 2148
Clifton, NJ 07015

Printed in the United States of America

Library of Congress Cataloging-in-Publication Data

Methods in experimental psychopharmacology.

  (Contempoary neuroscient)
  Includes bibliographies and index.
  1. Experimental psychopharmacology. I. Greenshaw,
Andrew J. II. Dourish, Colin T. III. Series.
RM315.M44   1987   615′.78   86-18630
ISBN 0-89603-095-4

Preface

Psychopharmacology may be defined as the study of the effects of drugs on behavior. As an established scientific discipline, this is a relatively new area of research. Despite its short history, however, psychopharmacology has achieved a considerable degree of sophistication in the variety of experimental approaches that are currently employed. Consequently, the interpretation of data accumulated through the use of various experimental laboratory techniques has become increasingly difficult and complex.

Numerous excellent texts and review articles are available that serve to outline recent progress in psychopharmacology (particularly the *Handbook of Psychopharmacology* series, edited by L. L. Iversen, S. D. Iversen, and S. H. Synder). Volumes such as these serve to usefully review the available literature without attempting a critical appraisal of the utility and limitations of methods and the difficulties of interpreting empirical data. Such conceptual and methodological problems are now an issue of paramount importance in studying the behavioral effects of drugs.

The present volume can be regarded as a "conceptual cookbook" that examines the utility and limitations of various experimental approaches commonly taken in psychopharmacology. This practically oriented text should prove particularly useful for pharmacologists and neurochemists who have no formal training in behavioral research and require an introduction to the actual laboratory practice of the field. In addition, the useful and informative treatment of current issues in psychopharmacology will undoubtedly appeal to the majority of active researchers.

The research topics covered in this volume have been chosen to encompass the major areas of interest in contemporary experimental psychopharmacology. The scope of the volume is consequently fairly broad, ranging from the interpretation of the effects of drugs on spontaneous motor activity to a consideration of the application of signal detection theory in the analysis of sensory effects of drugs.

In planning this book we have attempted to strike a balance permitting both access by the nonspecialist and useful analysis for active researchers in the broad area of psychopharmacology. The book is organized so that each part is self-contained, and the reader may thus concentrate on selected chapters without needing to read each part of the book sequentially. It is clear, however, that some areas of the subject are more accessible to the nonspecialist than others. To those readers who are unfamiliar with techniques in psychopharmacology, we recommend an exploratory approach to the book.

The text is nonetheless well integrated and each chapter refers occasionally to other areas of the book. The material encompassed in the chapters by Dourish, Miczek and Winslow, and Cooper and Turkish is somewhat less dependent on an understanding of techniques involving classical and operant conditioning. These areas of the book may be more readily accessible to readers lacking familiarity with the analysis of animal learning. The chapters by Dantzer, Greenshaw and Wishart, Järbe, and Dykstra and Genovese provide a conceptual appraisal of those research areas that primarily emphasize the analysis of patterns of learned responses, and a basic understanding of animal learning is advantageous when reading them. Nevertheless, the chapters by Goudie and by Sanger provide access to some basic issues, as well as providing useful analyses of major areas of research.

We felt that the provision of an overview of research in psychopharmacology would help to integrate the material in the book, and the chapter by Blackman provides such an overview. This contribution is clearly related to the main theme of the text and is, of necessity, dependent on a degree of familiarity with some aspects of experimentation and the analysis of behavior. Thus, although Blackman's chapter is an appropriate and perhaps pleasantly contentious beginning for the book, an initial exploration of some of the other articles is recommended for those who may be unfamiliar with psychopharmacology.

This volume will prove useful to researchers in neuroscience, which of course encompasses psychology, psychiatry, pharmacology, and biochemistry. Graduate students in these disciplines will find that the contents provide an invaluable introduction to current concepts and methods in research on drug action and behavior. We hope we have achieved a significant balance in the collective presentations of this book.

We thank the contributing authors for providing interesting and thought-provoking chapters and would like to acknowledge the invaluable comments and advice of many of our colleagues. The efficient and patient secretarial assistance of Rosalee James is also particularly appreciated.

The advice and encouragement of Professor Alan A. Boulton and Dr. Steven J. Cooper were invaluable in the planning of this text, particularly in the early stages of its organization; to them we owe special thanks.

Andrew J. Greenshaw
Colin T. Dourish

Contents

Effects of Drugs on Spontaneous Motor Activity
Colin T. Dourish

Effects of Drugs on Schedule-Controlled Behavior
David J. Sanger

Behavioral Analysis of Anxiolytic Drug Action
Robert Dantzer

Effects of Drugs on Reward Processes
Andrew J. Greenshaw and Thomas B. Wishart

Aversive Stimulus Properties of Drugs
The Conditioned Taste Aversion Paradigm
Andrew J. Goudie

Measurement of Drug Effects on Stimulus Control
Linda A. Dykstra and Raymond F. Genovese

Drug Discrimination Learning
Cue Properties of Drugs
Torbjörn U. C. Järbe

Contributors

DEREK E. BLACKMAN • *Department of Psychology, University College, Cardiff, UK*

STEVEN J. COOPER • *Department of Psychology, University of Birmingham, Birmingham, UK*

ROBERT DANTZER • *Neurobiologies des Comportments, Université de Bordeaux II, Bordeaux, France*

LINDA A. DYKSTRA • *Department of Psychology, University of North Carolina, Chapel Hill, North Carolina*

COLIN T. DOURISH • *Psychiatric Research Division, University of Saskatchewan, Saskatoon, Saskatchewan, Canada. Present address: Merck, Sharpe, & Dohme Research Laboratories, Neuroscience Centre, Harlow, UK*

RAYMOND F. GENOVESE • *Department of Psychology, University of North Carolina, Chapel Hill, North Carolina*

ANDREW J. GOUDIE • *Department of Psychology, The University of Liverpool, Liverpool, UK*

ANDREW J. GREENSHAW • *Psychiatric Research Division, University of Saskatchewan, Saskatoon, Saskatchewan, Canada*

TORBJÖRN U. C. JÄRBE • *Department of Psychology, University of Uppsala, Uppsala, Sweden*

KLAUS A. MICZEK • *Department of Psychology, Tufts University, Medford, Massachusetts*

DAVID J. SANGER • *Laboratoires d'Etudes et de Recherches Synthélabo, Bagneux, France*

SUZANNE TURKISH • *Department of Psychology, University of Birmingham, Birmingham, UK*

JAMES T. WINSLOW • *Department of Psychology, Tufts University, Medford, Massachusetts*

THOMAS B. WISHART • *Department of Psychology, University of Saskatchewan, Saskatoon, Saskatchewan, Canada*

Experimental Psychopharmacology

PAST, PRESENT, AND FUTURE

Derek E. Blackman

1. Historical Background

A teasing aphorism claims that psychology has a long past but a short history. If this is so, the past of psychopharmacology is almost as long, but its formal history is even shorter. This chapter provides a brief general review of the development of this interdisciplinary science. It attempts to provide a context for the contemporary research that is reviewed and evaluated in subsequent chapters. It ends with a short consideration of the prognosis for experimental psychopharmacology.

The past of the preemergent science of psychology is of course to be found in the inherent fascination of "what makes people tick" and in the informal ability developed in human cultures to allow for differences between people. Such ability existed long before psychological studies were formally instituted. Psychopharmacology's past is to be found in the many cultures in which people had for long taken drugs that they knew could change their moods, perceptions, or abilities. In our own cultural context it is easy to see both from documentary evidence and from more creative writings the prominence accorded to the use of alcohol to ease misery and to facilitate social interaction. The critical analogy between religion for the masses and opium reveals some knowledge of the possible psychological effects of opiates, which was easy to garner informally from the widespread use of such substances in Victorian England. A fascinating case study in the prehistory of psychopharmacology is provided by the Victorian novelist Wilkie Collins. Collins was in the habit of taking regular and large doses of laudanum, initially to relieve the pain of gout, and eventually came to write in such a state of dissociated consciousness that he claimed to not recognize his own narrative and was unable to take it up again unless he first returned to the drugged condition in which he had previously written. The phenomenon of drug dissociation provides the central feature of the plot in his novel *The Moonstone* (Collins, 1868), in which a man who had hidden a gem after being given laudanum was unable to remember where he had put it until he was subsequently given the drug again (in a larger dose). This novel therefore contains incidents that reveal Collins' familiarity with concepts of state-dependency and drug dissociation, and of the development and retention of tolerance to repeated drug administration. Such phenomena form prominent parts of contemporary psychopharmacology (Siegel, 1983).

In his brief history, Pickens (1977) traces the development of psychopharmacology (*see* Fig. 1). Although he places the beginning of formal research into the effects of drugs on behavior in the early part of this century (including pioneering studies carried out in Pavlov's laboratory), it can be seen that the critical point of take-off occurred in the period 1940–1955, as a result of two significant events: the discovery of the antipsychotic effects of chlorpromazine and a surge of interest in the United States in the recreational use of drugs, especially those described as psychedelic, hallucinogenic, or "consciousness-expanding." The revolutionary impact of chlorpromazine on psychiatry and mental health set the stage for an increasingly dedicated and successful search for other drugs with psychological effects that might be used therapeutically in the fields of mental health and mental hygiene (e.g., antidepressants, tranquilizers, anxiolytics, and so forth). The

recreational use of psychoactive drugs has of course continued to increase, with an ever-wider range of drugs being used
or abused and a concomitant rise in problems of addiction.
Pickens shows (Fig. 1) that these two major strands feed into
the core of the contemporary interdisciplinary science of
behavioral pharmacology and its search for organizing principles to summarize the effects of drugs on behavior, and for
behavioral mechanisms of drug action. Note however that
Pickens' figure is classified by him as depicting the history of
"behavioral pharmacology," whereas this chapter begins with
general comments about "psychopharmacology": the significance of this different terminology is explored in the next
section.

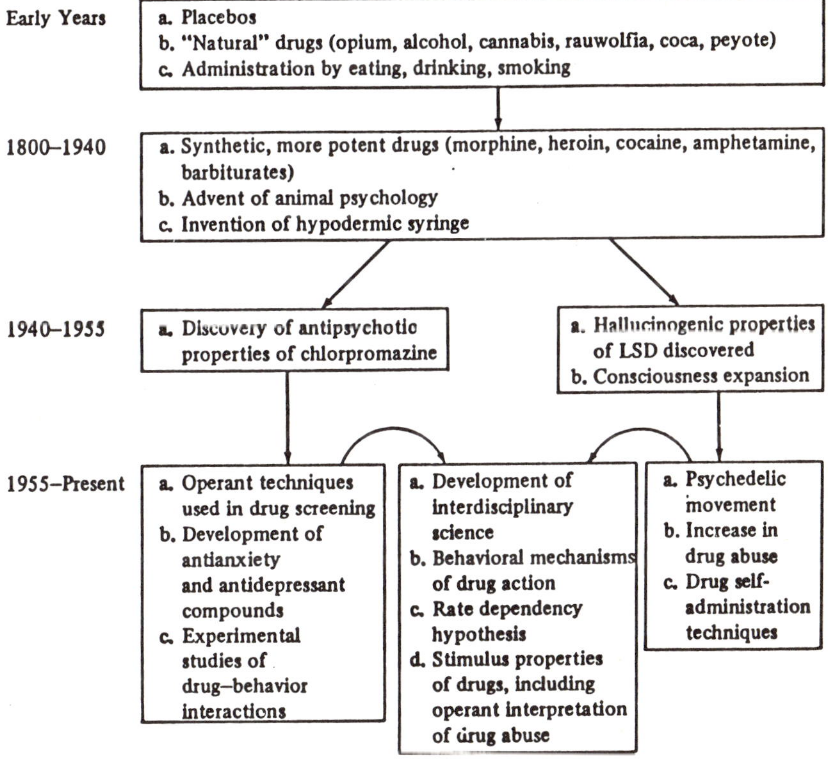

Fig. 1. A brief history of behavioral pharmacology (from Pickens, 1977, with permission).

2. Experimental Psychopharmacology and Behavioral Pharmacology

Both pharmacology and psychology trace their history as formal and self-contained disciplines from the last part of the nineteenth century. Psychopharmacology has a shorter history as the overlapping interests of the two parent disciplines were recognized and developed as studies in their own right.

In general, pharmacology can be conceptualized as the scientific study of the effects of drugs on living organisms or their constituent parts. The subject is securely placed within the domain of experimental biology, and like other sciences in this category it relies heavily (but not entirely) on the use of animals as comparative models. For ethical as well as practical reasons, there are considerable constraints on conducting experiments with people, and so pharmacology has provided a base for its spectacular progress on a major commitment to controlled experimentation with laboratory animals, often rats. Such studies offer gains in scientific rigor, allowing for the control of extraneous variables and thus the elucidation of specific effects that can be unambiguously attributed to the drugs whose properties are being investigated. The general program is systematic and cumulative in nature, as is shown by the emphasis on the development of reliable experimental methods, including the use of different routes of administration to intact animals. The plotting of dose–response curves, rather than of the effects of idiosyncratic or arbitrarily chosen doses, the study of the time course of action of a drug, and the exploration of drug antagonisms and synergisms are examples of the systematic approach in the development of a database for pharmacology and in the search for organizing principles and mechanisms of action.

Many hypotheses and explanations in contemporary pharmacology are based on a reductionist scientific model, with particular emphases on physiological, chemical, and endocrinological mechanisms. Of course the scientific study of the effects of drugs on animals is not carried out principally as an end in itself, and a major goal of pharmacologists is to extrapolate their experimental findings with animals to humans with due caution, particularly when they may appear relevant to possible therapeutic innovation. Such extrapolations can be confined to the theoretical level or, especially when there is potential clinical relevance, by means of carefully regulated experimental studies with selected human subjects. An interest in the applied relevance of the basic experimental science of experimental pharmacology is one of its main justifications, and it has led to the current expectation on the part of many patients that the use of drugs provides an easy remedy to many ills. Clinical pharmacology also feeds back the results of its controlled studies to the core or basic science.

In short, pharmacology is today a secure member of the biological sciences with a substantial commitment to basic or fundamental experimentation with animals and to the extrapolation of the findings of such work to fields of clinical relevance.

A review of the methods and status of contemporary pharmacology is offered here in order to provide a contrast with the situation that exists with psychology, in which there are some signs of considerable tension. This is indeed to be found in the very definition of the subject: The late nineteenth century aspirations to a science of mental life quickly gave way to the recognition that there are major problems in securing a database that is open in the normal scientific manner to public, objective, and reliable inspection. Although we cannot deny that people will tell psychologists about their private and inner experiences, we can deny that these accounts are necessarily accurate or meaningful. Introspection is often surprisingly vague and inarticulate, and it is also strongly conformist in nature. Self-reports may reflect ignorance of private and inner workings, and they may even be (accidentally or even deliberately) inaccurate. In the light of such a fundamental problem, psychology was faced early with a choice of two basic routes. Either it should retain its original focus on mental life and thereby accept that the traditional methods of objective science are not wholly appropriate, or it should become scientific by directing its principal efforts to studying behavior rather than mental life, since behavior is open to public and potentially reliable inspection, as is the case with the data of other sciences. Characteristically perhaps, psychology appears to have decided to follow both paths, but only the latter will be discussed.

The experimental study of behavior can readily be placed within the traditions of experimental biology. For reasons similar to those that apply in pharmacology, this approach to psychology relies heavily, but not exclusively, on controlled experimental studies with animals, again often rats. Experimental psychologists in this field have applied themselves to developing reliable methods that allow the collection of valid empirical data, and they have sought to manipulate in a systematic manner those variables that might affect behavior. In laboratory conditions it has been shown that a major determinant of the behavior of animals is provided by the environmental conditions to which they are or have been exposed. The effects of such variables are subtle and of infinite variety, but they are orderly and reliable, and a very large part of the experimental analysis of behavior has been devoted to exploring them. Other influences on behavior include those resulting from genetic variation, which can be manipulated experimentally by means of selective breeding programs within the framework of contemporary biometrical genetics, and those resulting from the physiological state of the animal, which can be manipulated by means of surgical, microelectrical, or chemical interventions. As is shown in the other chapters of this book, the administration of drugs to animals in controlled experiments can also result in reliable and systematic effects on behavior. Thus the experimental analysis of behavior has developed a wide variety of experimental techniques that allow the determinants of behavior to be explored reliably, systematically, and in a cumulative program.

As with other sciences, the data that emerge from these studies are subjected to a search for general organizing principles and mechanisms of action. Experimental psychology aims in this way to develop theoretical accounts that allow data to be interpreted within an integrative framework, and thus to be explained and understood. The nature of explanation in psychology is more contentious than is the case in pharmacology: there continues to be lively debate in contemporary experimental psychology about the levels of explanation appropriate for dealing with behavior in general and the behavior of animals in particular. Some favor reductionist accounts couched in terms of underlying physiological or cognitive processes that may be presumed to mediate overt behavior. Others, e.g., Skinner (1950), feel that it is sometimes too easy to develop quasiexplanations of behavior by translating that which is observed in the behavioral domain into being merely an appendage to variables or processes at other levels that have not been observed and perhaps are not even observable. In general terms, however, and as with pharmacology, experimental studies of the behavior of animals in laboratory conditions are not usually seen as ends in themselves. Careful extrapolation to the behavior of humans is attempted, though again this appears to be more contentious in principle within psychology than in other biological sciences. An interest in gaining a better understanding of human behavior is of course central to any attempt to ameliorate in a systematic manner behavioral or psychological problems that may be found in clinical practice, and indeed in everyday life. A clearer understanding of the determinants of human behavior can be used of course to facilitate potential in behavioral development, as well as to relieve suffering.

Thus, within contemporary psychology there is an approach that uses the conceptual and empirical apparatus of other biological sciences such as pharmacology. Behavior is seen as a naturally occurring biological phenomenon that can be studied experimentally in its own right, often with animals and with a view to identifying basic mechanisms. The findings of this experimental and conceptual program are extrapolated cautiously to human behavior. It is this approach within psychology, naturally enough, that has contributed most prominently to attempts to develop an interdisciplinary science of psychopharmacology. Its emphasis on the effects of drugs on behavior gives rise to use of the term "behavioral pharmacology" rather than "psychopharmacology," as is favored by Pickens' diagrammatic representation of the development of this interdisciplinary study (1977, *see* Fig.1). The terms experimental psychopharmacology and behavioral pharmacology, though having different nuances of meaning to *cognoscenti,* can be considered as synonyms for the present purpose.

3. Experimental Strategies in Experimental Psychopharmacology

Behavioral pharmacology or experimental psychopharmacology represents, then, the coming together of two aspects of experimental biology in order to explore the effects of drugs on behavior. The following chapters in this book illustrate many of the areas of particular interest within this field. It would be spurious to attempt any form of summary of their contents in this introductory chapter. Instead, an attempt will be made to identify some general themes that may be detected within the more detailed contributions, in the hope of capturing some of the broad principles of contemporary research.

All of the contributions to this book may be said to fit the general definition of the subject offered above: They each report the results of experiments carried out with animals, and they each consider the relevant scientific literature with a view to organizing the material within an interpretative framework. They thus contribute to what has been described above as a systematic and cumulative science addressed to understanding and explaining the effects of drugs on behavior. Traditional pharmacological parameters are emphasized, such as the route of drug-administration, the varying of drug-dosage in order to develop dose–response curves, and the investigation of the effects of different classes of drugs, often including the interacting effects of drugs given together. Traditional psychological or behavioral parameters also find repeated emphasis, in particular the varying of the environmental conditions in which behavior is studied and of which it is therefore a function. This allows for an attempt to develop more understanding of drug effects when they are administered against different behavioral baselines. Variation in environmental conditions is achieved particularly by means of schedules of reinforcement, and thus many studies report the modulating effects of such schedules on the behavioral action of psychoactive drugs. Within this broad approach, different stimuli, especially those such as food, water, or mild electric shock, can be delivered to the animal subjects, and may serve to maintain the behavior to which they are related as reinforcers in a response-dependent manner. Other stimuli that are varied are those that set the occasion for behavior to be reinforced and thus come to exert stimulus or discriminative control over behavior. Physiological or motivational states are also often manipulated in the experiments reported throughout the present book.

All of the chapters included here therefore provide reviews of empirical data in their field, and all attempt to set these data in an interpretative or theoretical context (though such organizing principles of interpretation at present arise more readily from some fields of experimental psychopharmacology than from others). In general therefore, the chapters herein review the current status of what might be described as basic science in different aspects of interdisciplinary research. Few of the chapters spell out in specific detail the potential contribution of this research to applied problems or to therapeutic contexts, or indeed its relevance to human behavior in general. Thus, this book fits into the approach favored generally in experimental biological science, namely an attempt to establish basic principles in comparative experimentation in the hope that a more sophisticated understanding of basic phenomena will be of intellectual interest in itself and, no doubt, ultimately of potential relevance in more applied contexts.

Although the chapters share these general characteristics, it is also possible to identify differences of emphasis or approach between them. One that perhaps deserves some consideration here arises from the nature of the general experimental strategy favored in different areas of contemporary experimental psychopharmacology. In some cases data are obtained from conventional comparisons between different experimental and control groups of subjects, and inferential statistics are used to evaluate any differences in the data that they produce. In other cases a strategy is favored that exerts strict experimental control over the behavior of individual subjects serving as their own controls in balanced repeated-measures designs. The adoption of either strategy is not a necessary or simple consequence of the specific field of study, and some chapters interweave data obtained in both ways. In general terms, however, the between-groups design is appropriate when a pattern of behavior is being investigated for which the environmental variables exercising precise control over behavior cannot be explicitly identified. It is also appropriate when there may be reasons to suppose that exposure of individual animals to one condition may have an effect on their behavior in any subsequent exposure to another, i.e., that sequence effects may contaminate data. In either case, the contaminating effects of unrecognized or uncontrolled independent variables can be avoided to some extent by exposing groups of animals to one set of conditions. Differences between animals *within* each group can be handled by means of statistical methods, and any significant differences *between* the groups as summarized in this form can themselves be identified by means of inferential statistics.

When brief profiles of the experimental sciences of pharmacology and psychology were offered in the previous section, some emphasis was placed on the need for *systematic* studies in which the effects of an experimental variable can be studied within a range of values of that variable. The pharmacologist's dose–response curve, for example, is based on the effects of a number of different doses of a drug. If such parametric investigation is important in the parent sciences, it is surely also important in their fusion in psychopharmacology. However, the requirement to vary experimental parameters in two dimensions can quickly give rise to pragmatic problems, and it can become irksome when a between-groups design is being used. For example, if a dose–response curve is to be based on the study of, say, four doses (with an appropriate control group of course) and if the environmental determinants of behavior are to be explored through, say, no more than three variations of the basic condition, then the experimental design finds itself based on 15 (5 × 3) groups, each perhaps comprising eight subjects.

The analysis of data obtained from such an experimental design poses no special problems with techniques such as analysis of variance. However, the practical problems of having to run some 120 animals should not be minimized, especially if it is necessary to run them over a fairly extended period of time in order to establish some form of environmental control over their behavior. It is therefore perhaps not surprising that relatively few studies in experimental psychopharmacology achieve such a balanced design. It is also hardly surprising that parametric variation is more likely to be retained for a pharmacological variable than for a psychological variable: in truth, many psychopharmacological studies take the form of plotting a dose–response curve for the effects of a drug on a pattern of behavior that is established experimentally in what may appear to be a relatively arbitrary manner. Such a model of psychopharmacology inevitably gives the lion's share of analytical power to pharmacology and there may be a real danger that this power is applied to an exemplar of behavior from which generalizations cannot effectively or safely be made.

The alternative experimental strategy is associated in experimental pyschology with studies of operant conditioning. The use of the techniques of operant conditioning and a single-subject research design has made a very important impact on behavioral pharmacology, as is again attested in the following chapters of this book. Indeed, the argument can be made that the advent of this approach has helped to make experimental psychopharmacology a more truly *inter*disciplinary science and has led to a greater approximation of balanced inputs from the two parent disciplines.

The general use of single-subject research designs has nowhere been more cogently evaluated than in Sidman's early exposition (1960), but their specific application in behavioral pharmacology has been described clearly and in detail by Thompson and Schuster (1968). Using the techniques of operant conditioning, animals can be exposed to daily sessions in which environmental procedures are carefully controlled until their behavior becomes orderly and predictable from session to session. Such an unusual degree of experimental control over "spontaneous" (as opposed to elicited) behavior leads to the possibility of "probing" that behavioral baseline with repeated administration of a drug. This might be done using a single dose or with a range of doses given in a random or counterbalanced sequence. Drug-probe sessions are normally interspersed at random or in a structured way with control or saline sessions in which the behavioral control is sustained. Using a dependent variable, such as operant response rate, it is possible, by means of an inductive process, to infer the effects of the drug (or of different doses of the drug) on the behavioral baseline. In this way, orderly dose–response curves can be obtained from individual animals acting as their own controls, and in this book there are many illustrations of data obtained with this kind of experimental design. The generality of findings, however orderly, obtained from single subjects can be explored by running further individual animals in the same procedure, though perhaps with a different sequence of doses, and by seeking consistencies in the data that emerge (not by collapsing individuals' data into statistical averages or the like).

The possibility arises from such an experimental design to strengthen the impact of behavioral or psychological variables in psychopharmacological studies. It is well understood empirically that different schedules of reinforcement in operant conditioning experiments establish and maintain predictable but very different patterns or rates of operant responding. It has also now become abundantly clear that such patterns are differentially affected by many psychoactive drugs (*see* chapter by Sanger for review). Using single-subject research designs, it is possible to expose individual subjects to different schedules of reinforcement. This can be done in a number of ways: seriatim in a reversal design, simultaneously by means of concurrent schedules, or intercurrently by means of multiple or mixed schedules that present short but repeated periods of single schedules at different times within one experimental session. When this is done, different behavioral baselines can be obtained from individual subjects, and these can then enter into an investigation of the effects of different doses of a drug (or of different drugs) on more than one pattern of behavior, and thus can be described as truly interdisciplinary, yet this is achieved by means of the intensive study of a few individual animals.

In addition to prompting the study of schedule-dependent effects of drugs on behavior, the power of operant conditioning techniques with either single-subject designs or indeed with between-groups designs, can be used as a tool in other areas of behavioral pharmacology, making it possible to investigate the effects of drugs on further variables of interest, for example on behavior maintained by different kinds of reinforcer (chapter by Greenshaw and Wishart), or on the ways in which behavior is modulated by environmental stimuli within a discriminative context (chapter by Dykstra and Genovese). The stimulus properties that drugs themselves may have when administered to animals can also be investigated (chapter by Järbe), as can the effects of a class of drugs such as anxiolytics (chapter by Dantzer).

There is a further general difference in research strategies used in experimental psychopharmacology that is amply illustrated in other chapters of the present book. This relates to the *nature* of the behavior that is studied. Operant conditioning techniques provide good behavioral baselines for psychopharmacological studies by allowing essentially arbitrary patterns of behavior to adjust to carefully controlled environmental conditions. Typically the form of the behavior studied is the pressing of a lever by a rat, and this is occasionally followed by reinforcement. Just as rats are taken as convenient models of behaving organisms within the tradition of comparative experimental biology, so lever-pressing is taken as a convenient model of behavior. The act is chosen largely because of its tractability in experimental work: Animals may emit this behavior at high, low, or intermediate frequencies, the pressing of a lever is a discrete act that can be easily and reliably quantified in terms of response rates or response probabilities, the occurrence of the act is easily detected experimentally, and it can be easily recorded and handled with respect to programming contingencies of reinforcement. Pressing levers is surely not a prominent component of the "natural" behavioral repertoire of albino rats, but the frequency of its occurrence adjusts to changing environmental conditions in an orderly and reliable manner. It thereby provides a model of how "behavior" adjusts to environmental circumstances and, in psychopharmacology, of how "behavior" is affected by psychoactive drugs. Other interests in experimental psychopharmacology, however, have focused on categories of behavior that are defined in terms that have more immediate functional significance from a biological point of view, e.g., eating and drinking (chapters by Cooper and Turkish and by Goudie), locomotor activity (chapter by Dourish), and agonistic or aggressive behavior (chapter by Miczek and Winslow). Here the task is to develop objective and reliable methods for recording the occurrence of such "natural" behaviors. Of course these patterns of behavior may in turn be affected by precise environmental circumstances, but they have also been widely investigated in terms of other influences, such as physiological or endocrinological substrates. It has been noted above that mechanisms of action in pharmacology are often expressed in such terms, and so psychopharmacological studies of these patterns of behavior have tended to be more sophisticated with respect to these biological phenomena than with respect to environmental analyses (but *see* Miczek and Winslow, section 3). In comparison with the arbitrary acts studied in operant conditioning, these patterns of behavior are *relatively* insensitive to control by environmental circumstances, and this tends to make psychopharmacological studies in this area more dependent on between-groups designs and statistical inference.

4. The Future for Experimental Psychopharmacology

Although the formal history of experimental psychopharmacology may be short, there is currently a great deal of scientific effort being expended on the analysis of the behavioral effects of drugs, as the chapters in this book show. One might therefore expect the future of this interdisciplinary field to be secure and full of promise. Some observers, however, although not denigrating current research efforts, have expressed some reservations about the conceptual status of contemporary behavioral pharmacology and have suggested that it may not bode well for the future. In a recent review, Branch (1984), for example, has claimed that, "Behavioral pharmacology as a unique, identifiable entity seems to be disappearing" (p. 511). The problems that Branch sees are in fact those that have been alluded to earlier in this chapter. As Branch puts it, "Pharmacology is a more well-developed science than is psychology," and whereas its "principles provide an organized, logical framework from which experimental ideas can be interpreted, behavioral prinicples, by contrast, are not as widely accepted and they tend to provide a weaker interpretive base" (p. 518). Thus Branch argues that most research in contemporary behavioral pharmacology is designed to explore pharmacological rather than behavioral questions.

It should be emphasized here that Branch's strictures are related by him to the orientation of behavioral pharmacology that relies almost completely on the model provided by operant conditioning techniques and single-subject research strategies. But if they have relevance in this context, it is only too easy to see how they might be extended to other aspects of a more broadly defined experimental psychopharmacology. It certainly seems fair to say that there is in general an imbalance in the technical, empirical, and analytical or conceptual contributions to experimental psychopharmacology currently emanating from its parent disciplines of psychology and pharmacology. In order to explore this imbalance further, it may be useful to step back from an attempted *inter*disciplinary perspective in order to ask explicitly what each discipline can offer the other.

Behavior can be used as a tool for studying the effects of different drugs, and psychology is in a position to provide pharmacology with techniques and skills with which this tool can be exploited. With such an approach the empirical base of *pharmacology* can be broadened, and its general organizing principles and explanatory models extended to a new domain. For example, behavioral techniques might offer pharmacologists further data for classifying drugs. It is clear that such a model is attractive and widely used. By way of illustration one may cite the way the development and screening of some new drugs already relies quite heavily, both in basic research and in commercial research and development, on an overt "boot-strapping" operation. To illustrate (and caricature) this, if (i) drug A is a neuroleptic, anxiolytic, or analgesic, and if (ii) drug B produces similar effects to those produced by drug A when tested against behavior (*any* behavior, not necessarily only those behaviors that appear to have some face-validity with respect to mental illness, anxiety, or analgesia), then (iii) this provides some evidence for classifying drug B along with drug A as a neuroleptic, anxiolytic, or analgesic. Clearly, such an approach depends hardly at all on *understanding* behavior: it merely (but often it seems, effectively) adds measures of behavior to the array of techniques available to pharmacologists in their efforts to classify drugs. In this sense there can be no doubt that psychology has something to offer pharmacology (*see* chapter by Dantzer in relation to anxiolytic drugs).

On the other hand, drugs can be used as tools for studying different aspects of behavior. Pharmacology may therefore have something to offer psychology in a unidirectional sense. Although this is certainly true in principle, in practice it is much more difficult to find successful examples of this process. An oversimplified "boot-strapping" argument might be presented as follows: if (i) behavior A is affected by a drug (any drug) differently from behavior B, then (ii) the two types of behavior are empirically distinguishable and psychological theories should seek to incorporate this. Although such a generalization may appear promising, the truth is, as mentioned by Branch, that psychological theorizing is less developed and more tentative than is the case in pharmacology. This may be illustrated by a specific case. It has been shown (Branch et al., 1977) that pentobarbital increases operant behavior that is suppressed by mild electric shock punishment but does not have a similar effect on behavior suppressed by punishment in the form of time-out from positive reinforcement. This finding at least makes it possible to assert that positive and negative punishment procedures are distinguishable in functional as well as procedural terms. The problem for psychology, however, is in taking such an insight and building it into a convincing integrative scheme in the way that, for example, chemical analyses of drug action allow pharmacology to integrate the gains of their "boot-strapping" in behavioral fields.

In comparison with pharmacology, psychology could be said to lack cogent and universally accepted organizing principles. Its disadvantage in this respect is accentuated by the fact that psychology's past (as opposed to its formal history) gives us all very strong interpretative schemes based on common sense. These are usually couched in global or macroscopic terms that arise from the hurly-burly of everyday life rather than from controlled and cumulative experimentation. They may be wrong, and the relative lack of systematic understanding of what might be termed the microstructure of behavior leads in turn to an inability or reluctance to vary psychological/behavioral parameters. This of course further unbalances the contributions of the parent disciplines to psychopharmacology.

A striking example of this situation is to be found in the currently burgeoning study of the stimulus properties of drugs (*see* chapter by Järbe). From the prehistorical past illustrated by Wilkie Collins' experience and writings, it has been shown experimentally that animals can be readily trained by means of operant conditioning techniques reliably to emit one response when given a drug and another response when given saline. In variations of this procedure, two different training doses may be given, or the animal may be trained with two different drugs. The administration of drugs can therefore lead to the development of discriminative control over behavior. Once such discriminative control has been established, it is possible to probe with other doses or drugs to examine the extent to which the control exerted by a drug used in training will generalize to other test doses or drugs.

The interoceptive stimulus properties of drugs can thus be investigated experimentally using animals as subjects.

From a unidirectional perspective, this finding may be exploited in two ways. In psychology, the drug discrimination paradigm may be used to explore the parameters of interoceptive stimulus control, a fascinating but notoriously difficult area to investigate in a controlled way, but one that has great theoretical importance and may well have major implications for the analysis and treatment of some psychological or behavioral problems. Such a research orientation would lead to investigations of the effects of different procedures on the stimulus control exerted by specific drugs, a program that would complement studies of the way in which exteroceptive control is affected by environmental and other contingencies.

In pharmacology, the drug-discrimination paradigm may be exploited because it offers, for example, a further way of exploring and classifying the effects of drugs of different classes. Thus a "boot-strapping" operation can be used to develop profiles of new substances. To oversimplify this process also, if (i) drug A can be classified from a pharmacological point of view as an opiate, and if (ii) animals trained with drug A generalize to other opiates, but not to nonopiate substances, and if (iii) animals trained with drug A generalize to drug B, then (iv) drug B may be an opiate.

A glance at the literature on drug discrimination, e.g., Colpaert and Slangen (1982), readily confirms that it is the latter of the above two possibilities that has been by far the more exploited, to such an extent that the drug discrimination paradigm has now evolved into a common pharmacological screening technique. This of course gives rise to pressure from a pharmacological point of view to standardize the procedure in order to reduce any unwanted variation in the effects of drugs. As Branch (1984) has pointed out, "Drug-discrimination procedures have assumed the status of basic pharmacological preparations and are used mainly to investigate strictly pharmacological questions." As Branch (1984) and others have also pointed out, this emphasis on using drug discrimination as a tool for pharmacological analysis has been greatly accentuated by contemporaneous and spectacular advances in research on the binding of drugs to specific receptors. The identification of receptors for drugs that have different profiles has provided a very powerful integrative framework for interpreting data obtained from the drug discrimination procedure. Thus, drugs that show similar discriminative properties may be assumed to bind to the same receptor, and, as Branch has succinctly put it, "neuropharmacology has provided a reductionistic theoretical base for interpreting a drug's behavioral effects" (Branch, 1984). No integrative scheme has emerged with such force from the body of psychology to balance the impact of these neuropharmacological analyses of drug discrimination.

Schuster and Balster (1977) have given a clear indication of behavioral principles that should be explored in this field. As is also suggested above, they note that the research paradigm has much to offer to the behavioral analysis of stimulus control in general, and they plead the need for systematic explorations of the behavioral as well as the pharmacological parameters of the phenomenon. As also noted above, however, this argument has done little to correct the imbalance that can so readily be seen in the current literature.

The above should not be taken to imply that no organizing principles in psychology have emerged from psychopharmacological research. One of the most striking examples of such a principle is that of rate-dependence. It has been shown that in many circumstances the effects of some psychoactive drugs on operant behavior depend on the rate of responding in control conditions. For example, amphetamines tend to increase low rates of responding and to decrease high rates (*see* Sanger and Blackman, 1976). Control response rate can in fact be more important in determining a drug's effects than the nature of the reinforcer that maintains the behavior (Kellerher and Morse, 1964). The principle was largely prompted by psychopharmacological investigations, but it is not limited to the effects of drugs (*see* Blackman, 1977, for example). Although, as Branch (1984) points out, further behavioral analysis has shown that the principle of rate-dependence is not ubiquitous or all-embracing, the concept of rate-dependence as an organizing principle has been important and constructive, and provides an illustration of how psychopharmacological research can contribute to the conceptual as well as the empirical base of psychology.

Organizing principles do not in themselves identify behavioral mechanisms of action that might parallel those of contemporary pharmacology. For example, operant behavior (as expressed by response rate or other measures) may be controlled by a number of variables, such as deprivational state, the schedule of reinforcement to which an animal is exposed, variations in the strength of discriminative control, and so on. If the behavioral mechanisms of action of drugs are to be elucidated, psychopharmacologists will need to address the question of how drugs affect these variables or mechanisms.

One area of experimental psychopharmacology that is currently vibrant, and which Branch expects to remain so (1984), is the study of the self-administration of drugs by animals, described alternatively as the study of the reinforcing effects of drugs. In his recent review of this field, Thompson (1984) provides a lucid exposition of how behavioral mechanisms of action should be sought through studies of the reinforcing effects of drugs. There is no chapter specifically devoted to drug self-administration in the present book (although, *see* chapter by Greenshaw and Wishart), and Thompson's paper therefore provides a useful context for the present considerations and for recognizing their general relevance.

Thompson (1984, p. 3) considers a mechanism as "a description of a given phenomenon in terms of more general principles." He points out that the mechanisms predominantly favored in pharmacology are reductionistic in their conceptual status; that is, the effects of drugs are largely interpreted in terms of biochemistry and/or physiology. However, Thompson argues, the level of analysis that might most readily lead to identifying *behavioral* mechanisms of action need not necessarily be reductionistic in this sense and might in fact be more likely found in terms of "a more general set of *environmental* principles regulating behavior," p. 5 (emphasis added). Thompson goes on to identify three classes of *antecedent* behavioral mechanisms in the context of drug dependence: (i) environmental history (e.g., the way in which past experience, including experience with drugs, can modulate the reinforcing effects of a drug), (ii) deprivation conditions (status with respect to access to reinforcers in general, but particularly, in the case of drug-dependence, access to the drug), and (iii) aversive stimulation (that might relate to the way in which a reinforcing effect of a drug may be modulated by its leading to a decrease in the aversive stimulation arising, for example, from withdrawal symptoms). Thompson next considers mechanisms of *stimulus control* (the ways in which discriminative control over behavior can modulate or be modulated by the administration of a drug: For example, in the context of drug self-administration the drug may have a reinforcing effect on behavior by changing the impact of other discriminative stimuli). The next class of behavioral mechanisms is described as relating to the *behavioral locus* of drug action (for example, rate-dependencies show that different patterns of behavior may be differentially affected by drugs, and topographically different patterns of behavior may similarly be differentially affected). Finally Thompson (1984) considers those mechanisms that relate to the nature of the relationship between behavior and its consequence (in the case of the self-administration of drugs, the infusion of the pharmacological substance): to borrow an ugly phrase, these mechanisms relate to the *consequation* of behavior, and they provide a forum for evaluating the effects of different relationships between behavior and different kinds of consequences, such as positive or negative reinforcers, punishing stimuli, conditioned reinforcers, delayed reinforcement, and so forth.

As stated above, Thompson's exposition is offered with special reference to the behavioral analysis of the self-administration of drugs, but it has general relevance to experimental psychopharmacology. Only by seeking to organize the data of drug-behavior interactions in this way will psychopharmacology move toward a more truly interdisciplinary science that can make synergistic contributions to both parent disciplines, as well as develop within its own sphere of interest. In general, as Branch (1984) has bemoaned, the relative strengths of the integrative schemes used in pharmacology have seduced researchers into adopting a position that increasingly makes behavior merely another variable in the domain of pharmacology. Yet, as noted earlier, generalizations from behavioral findings won in an *ad-hoc* or nonsystematic manner may be limited or even ultimately misleading.

It should be emphasized here that behavioral analyses *are* to be found in the chapters of the present book. The above argument addresses the question of the *balance* of analytic power arising from pharmacological and psychological theory. This balance differs from one area of psychopharmacology to another, but, it is claimed here, it is generally distorted toward the analyses of pharmacology.

In this context, the review of conditioned taste aversions given is particularly interesting (*see* chapter by Goudie), for it illustrates well the symbiosis that is possible when due consideration is given to both pharmacological and psychological principles of analysis. The point emerges with special force in this area of research, perhaps, because of some still-puzzling complexities in the conditioned taste aversion paradigm. Put at its simplest, there is a paradox: Drugs that will prove to be positively reinforcing when their delivery is made dependent on operant behavior may also prove to be aversive in that animals will drink less of a liquid that has a novel taste and that has been associated with administration of the drug. The enigma arises perhaps from too-ready an assumption that we have an adequate grasp of the underlying mechanisms both of conditioned taste aversion and of the reinforcing effects of drugs. Taste aversions are too easily assumed to reflect nausea, malaise, or discomfort arising from a drug or toxin associated with the taste; the reinforcing effects of drugs are too easily assumed to reflect positive hedonic qualities of those drugs, the pleasant feelings that may be associated with taking them. Investigations of drug-induced conditioned aversions to tastes challenge both of these common sense interpretations—both, let it be noted, drawn from the domain of psychology rather than that of pharmacology. Even more important in the light of the conceptual imbalance in psychopharmacology, however, are the clear conclusions to be drawn from Goudie's chapter *both* that the use of drugs as tools will help us to understand better the underlying behavioral mechanisms in the conditioned taste aversion procedure, *and* that the use of this behavioral paradigm will help us to understand better the pharmacological actions of drugs.

5. Conclusion

In this introductory chapter an attempt has been made to provide a context for the more detailed contributions that form the rest of this book. It is exciting to find so much research activity in a field that represents the fusion of two biological sciences, but which has such a relatively short formal history. The following chapters illustrate the breadth and subtlety of current experimental psychopharmacology as well as its vigor.

Experimental reseach has already done much to establish psychopharmacology as an experimental science in its own right. However, pharmacology has offered more to, and has gained more from, the interdisciplinary approach than has psychology. In part this is a reflection of the fact that relevant organizing principles and mechanisms of action have been more fully elaborated in pharmacology than in psychology, both as a whole and in the areas of psychology that are most germane to an interdisciplinary and experimental study of the behavioral effects of drugs. Branch (1984) has suggested that "behavioral pharmacology has evolved largely into a subdiscipline within pharmacology wherein drug similarity is examined with intact organisms." Yet the case can surely be made that the data of experimental psychopharmacology such as those reviewed in the subsequent chapters offer interesting and potentially productive challenges to the organizing principles of psychology.

The present chapter has not attempted to present more data than are to be found in other chapters, nor has it attempted to summarize those data. It has offered no novel form of theoretical analysis based on the content of other chapters. It has emphasized, however, the need for greater theoretical sophistication within psychology if psychopharmacology is to be truly interdisciplinary, a view advocated by others (Branch, 1984). It may be appropriate to conclude by stating that the chapter has been written by a psychologist rather than by a pharmacologist, so perhaps it is not surprising if its main thrust is that an interdisciplinary science of psychopharmacology will flourish only if it emerges from the creative endeavours of two equal partners, *psychology and pharmacology*, working in balanced harmony.

References

Blackman D. E. (1977) Conditioned Suppression and the Effects of Classical Conditioning on Operant Behavior, in *Handbook of Operant Behavior* (Honig W. K. and Staddon J. E. R., eds.), Prentice-Hall, New Jersey.

Branch M. N. (1984) Rate dependency, behavioral mechanisms, and behavioral pharmacology. *J. Exp. Anal. Behav.* **42**, 511–522.

Branch M. N., Nicholson G., and Dworkin S. I. (1977) Punishment-specific effects of pentobarbital: Dependency on the type of punisher. *J. Exp. Anal. Behav.* **28**, 285–293.

Collins W. (1868) *The Moonstone: a Romance.* Tinsley, London.

Colpaert F. C. and Slangen J. F. (eds.) (1982) *Drug Discrimination: Applications in CNS Pharmacology.* Elsevier, Amsterdam.

Kelleher R. T. and Morse W. H. (1964) Escape behavior and punished behavior. *Fed. Proc.* **23**, 808–817.

Pickens R. (1977) Behavioral Pharmacology: A Brief History, in *Advances in Behavioral Pharmacology Vol. 1* (Thompson, T. and Dews P. B., eds.), Academic, New York.

Sanger D. J. and Blackman D. E. (1976) Rate-dependent effects of drugs: A review of the literature. *Pharmacol. Biochem. Behav.* **4**, 73–83.

Schuster C. R. and Balster R. L. (1977) The Discriminative Stimulus Properties of Drugs, in *Advances in Behavioral Pharmacology,* Volume 1 (Thompson T. and Dews P. B., eds.), Academic, New York.

Sidman M. (1960) *Tactics of Scientific Research.* Basic, New York.

Siegel S. (1983) Wilkie Collins: Victorian novelist as psychopharmacologist. *J. Hist. Med. Allied Sci.* **38,** 161–175.

Skinner B. F. (1950) Are theories of learning necessary? *Psych. Rev.* **57,** 193–216.

Thompson T. (1984) Behavioral Mechanisms of Drug Dependence, in *Advances in Behavioral Pharmacology,* Volume 4 (Thompson T., Dews P. B., and Barrett J. E., eds.), Academic, New York.

Thompson T. and Schuster C. R. (1968) *Behavioral Pharmacology.* Prentice-Hall, New Jersey.

Psychopharmacological Research on Aggressive Behavior

Klaus A. Miczek
and James T. Winslow

1. Objectives of the Behavioral Neurosciences

Psychopharmacological methods for studying aggressive behavior follow two directions. One approach uses drugs as tools to delineate characteristics of neural processes that mediate aggressive behaviors. A second type of investigation uses aggression tests to learn about the functional state of a specific neurotransmitter (*see,* for example, apomorphine-induced aggression, section 2.3).

Early efforts attempted to associate drug-induced changes in synaptic neurotransmission of a particular biogenic amine with a specific behavioral change, sometimes referred to as "neurotransmitter phrenology." In retrospect, one may view the early proposals of neurochemical coding (Miller, 1965), such as portraying hypothalamic acetylcholine as part of an "innate system for killing" behavior (Smith et al., 1970) or "aggressive monoamines" (Eichelman and Thoa, 1973) or brain serotonin as a "civilizing neurohumor" (Everett, 1975), as being overly optimistic.

During the 1970s the view of neurotransmitter mechanisms of aggression broadened from single neurotransmitter codes to "neurochemical dualism." The neurophysiological phenomena of excitation and inhibition were transposed from the cellular level to the integrated behavior of an organism. For example, neuropharmacological manipulations and direct neurochemical measurements of the catecholamines attempted to assign either dopamine or norepinephrine a critical role in the initiation ("excitation") of aggressive behavior, and an opposing role for serotonin ("inhibition"). This view expanded into ever growing neurotransmitter profiles of aggression, as summarized by several reviews (e.g., Reis, 1974; Pradhan, 1975; Daruna, 1978; Eichelman, 1979; Karczmar et al., 1978). The mismatch between the complexity of behavioral processes, such as aggressive interactions, and currently available indices of neurotransmitter activity is apparent. In recent years, primarily as a result of biochemical advances in identifying different classes of receptors for drugs and endogeneous substances, simplistic notions linking the activity at a specific receptor to a complex behavior or disease have been advanced. So far, this new "receptorology" has yet to prove its value for enhancing our insights into the neuro-chemical mechanisms of aggressive behavior patterns.

2. Traditional Laboratory Methods for the Study of Aggression

Traditionally, the methods for inducing aggressive behavior in animals under controlled conditions have included (1) environmental manipulations, such as isolated housing or the exposure to aversive electric shock pulses; (2) neurological manipulations, such as neural ablations or electrical stimulation of discrete brain loci; or (3) pharmacological manipulations, such as the delivery of neurotoxins or large doses of psychotropic drugs. These methodological traditions emerged from divergent views on the causative factors for aggressive behavior, placing the cause either within or outside the organism.

2.1. Aggression Resulting From Environmental Manipulations

The approach of experimental psychology to aggression research is the major source for techniques and protocols that manipulate environmental stimuli. These manipulations range from the delivery of specific unconditioned stimuli, such as noxious, painful electric shock, noise or airblasts, or the omission of scheduled positive reinforcement ("frustrative nonreward") to pervasive manipulations, such as crowding, isolated housing, or food deprivation. We have selected the three most often used research methods from this tradition for description and discussion.

2.1.1. Isolation-Induced Aggression

The most often used method in psychopharmacological research on aggression relies on socially isolating male mice for several weeks, and thereafter observing their aggressive behavior toward an opponent during a short test. After a period of individual housing, adult male mice, like many other mammals, exhibit a range of aggressive or, alternatively, defensive and flight behaviors when confronted with another mouse (Ginsburg and Allee, 1942). Generally, the proportion of animals exhibiting aggressive behavior and the intensity of this behavior increases as a function of the length of isolated housing (Valzelli, 1969). Yen et al. (1959) first used pharmacological manipulations of isolated mice in an effort to alter their "abnormal" aggressive behavior. Since that time pharmacological studies of isolation-induced aggression have been conducted using a variety of different test parameters (Malick, 1979); these include variations in (1) test locale, either the home cage of one of the mice or, alternatively, a novel test cage unfamiliar to all combatants; (2) the number of mice per test, ranging from pairs to 30; or (3) the number of mice in a test that are administered a drug, either all or one focal animal. In fact, the result of prolonged individual housing can be varied (Krsiak, 1974, 1975); a certain proportion of mice exhibits aggressive behavior, additional mice display defensive and flight responses when interacting with a nonaggressive partner, and a further proportion investigates and grooms a partner without any aggressive or defensive responses.

There are divergent views on whether isolation-induced aggressive behavior represents an "abnormal," "compulsive" behavior as a result of the presumed stress of isolation or, alternatively, whether such behavior resembles the behavior pattern of a territorial mouse that lives behaviorally isolated from other males (e.g., Valzelli, 1973; Brain, 1975). When compared to group-housed mice, isolated mice show distinctively different behavioral, physiological, and neurochemical profiles (Garattini et al., 1967; Welch and Welch, 1969), from which the term "isolation syndrome" was coined (Valzelli, 1973). When compared to mice with a history of aggressive behavior, isolated mice hardly differ physiologically or behaviorally from their counterparts outside of the laboratory (Scott, 1966; Brain, 1975). The acts, postures, and movements of aggressive behavior in mice have been described in detail (e.g., Grant and Mackintosh, 1963; Crowcroft, 1966; Brain and Poole, 1974; Brain and Nowell, 1970).

The way in which isolation-induced aggression is measured reflects different theoretical approaches to this class of behavior. Single measures, such as a score of aggressiveness, fighting duration, latency to fight, or proportion of animals exhibiting aggressive behavior, suggest a unitary view of the behavior and its underlying mechanisms (e.g., Valzelli et al., 1967; Welch and Welch, 1969; Thurmond, 1975). The ethological tradition has provided a considerably more detailed assessment of isolation-induced aggression. The salient acts and postures of the aggressive animal and the elements of flight and defensive behavior by the opponent are recorded in terms of latency, frequency, and duration (Brain and Nowell, 1970; Krsiak, 1975, 1979; Miczek and O'Donnell, 1978; Poshivalov, 1982).

Table 1 summarizes drug effects on aggression that is induced by environmental manipulations. The left column of Table 1 refers to the effects of several prototypic drugs on isolation-induced aggression. At rarely studied low doses, amphetamine, alcohol, diazepam, chlordiazepoxide, pargyline, and LSD may actually increase aggression in isolated mice under certain conditions. At higher doses, all of these drugs decrease aggression. This dose-dependent, biphasic pattern of effects appears to be characteristic of several different kinds of psychotropic drugs. A most significant issue concerns the specificity of drug effects on aggressive behavior vs nonaggressive motor activities (Miczek and Krsiak, 1979). Drugs differ from each other in the degree of specificity with which they suppress aggressive behavior in isolated mice (Malick, 1979). Anticholinergics, beta-blockers, opiate receptor blockers, and several recently developed drugs are considerably more specific than anxiolytics, antidepressants, or sedative hypnotics in decreasing isolation-induced aggression. Among the behaviorally least specific drugs with antiaggressive effects are the antipsychotics, whether of the phenothiazine, butyrophenone, or thioxanthine type.

The validity of isolation-induced aggression in mice to model some form of human aggression or other aspects of human behavior has been a matter of debate. When drug effects on aggressive behavior of isolated mice were first studied (Yen et al., 1959), this behavior was labeled "abnormal." This interpretation of aggressive, isolated mice as being abnormal and compulsive has been frequently reiterated and persists to date; it appears to be the basis for considering isolation-induced aggression as a model for affective disorders in humans (e.g., Valzelli, 1973; Garattini and Valzelli, 1981). Neither early nor present ethological analyses of aggressive behavior of mice have found it necessary or helpful to use psychiatric labels, such as "abnormal" or "compulsive," in describing or explaining this behavior (e.g., Ginsburg and Allee, 1942; Scott and Frederickson, 1951; Crowcroft, 1966; Brain, 1975).

Although there may be no direct analog in humans to the aggressive behavior of isolated mice, common neurochemical and physiological processes during species-specific patterns of aggression may provide similar targets for drug action in both species. Several impressive efforts have attempted to delineate a distinctive psychopharmacological

Table 1

Effects of Drugs on Aggression Induced by Environmental Manipulations[a]

Drug class prototype mg/kg	Isolation-induced aggression		Pain-induced aggression		Non-reinforcement induced aggression	
	Effect on aggression/motor	References	Effect on aggression/motor	References	Effect on aggression/motor	References
Stimulants						
d-Amphetamine						
<2.0	↑/?	Welch and Welch, 1969	↑/?	Kostowski, 1966		
	↑/?	Charpentier, 1969	↑/nc	Hoffmeister and Wuttke, 1969	↑/nc	Miczek, 1974
	↑/nc	Krsiak, 1979	↑/↑	Emley and Hutchinson, 1972	↓/↑↓	DeWeese, 1977
>2.0	↓/↑	Melander, 1960	↑/↑	Stille et al., 1963	↓/↑	Miczek, 1974
	↓/↑	DaVanzo et al., 1966	↓/?	Lal et al., 1968		
	nc/nc	Valzelli et al., 1967	↓/↑	Tedeschi et al., 1969		
	↓/?	Welch and Welch, 1969	nc/?	Carlini and Masur, 1970		
	↓/↑	LeDouarec and Broussy, 1969	nc/?	Eichelman and Thoa, 1973		
	↓/?	Scott et al., 1971	nc/?	Powell et al., 1973		
	↓↑/↑	Hodge and Butcher, 1975	↑/nc	Mukherjee and Pradhan, 1976		
	↓/↑	Miczek and O'Donnell, 1978	↑/?	Nath et al., 1982		
	↓/↑	Poshivalov, 1981				
	↓/↑	Sieber et al., 1982				

(*continued on next page*)

Table 1 (Continued)

Effects of Drugs on Aggression Induced by Environmental Manipulations[a]

Drug class prototype mg/kg	Isolation-induced aggression		Pain-induced aggression		Non-reinforcement induced aggression	
	Effect on aggression/motor	References	Effect on aggression/motor	References	Effect on aggression/motor	References
Caffeine						
<5.0					↓/↑	Cherek et al., 1983
					↓/↑	Cherek et al., 1984a
>5.0	↓/↓	Valzelli and Bernasconi, 1973	↑/↑	Hutchinson and Emley, 1973		
			↓/nc	Quenzer et al., 1974		
			↑/nc	Eichelman et al., 1978		
Opiates and Antagonists						
Morphine						
>0.5	↓/nc	Janssen et al., 1960	↓/↓	Emley and Hutchinson, 1972		
	↓/nc	DaVanzo et al., 1966				
	↓/↓	Poshivalov, 1974				
50 ng ICV	↓/↓	Puglisi-Allegra et al., 1984				
Morphine withdrawal						
			↑/?	Puri and Lal, 1974		
			↑/?	Stolerman et al., 1975		

(continued on next page)

Table 1 (Continued)
Effects of Drugs on Aggression Induced by Environmental Manipulations[a]

Drug class prototype mg/kg	Isolation-induced aggression		Pain-induced aggression		Non-reinforcement induced aggression	
	Effect on aggression/motor	References	Effect on aggression/motor	References	Effect on aggression/motor	References
Naloxone						
>1.0	↓/nc	Puglisi-Allegra et al., 1982	↑/?	Fanselow et al., 1980		
	↓/nc	Olivier and van Dalen, 1982	↑/?	Gorelick et al., 1981		
	↓/?	Lynch et al., 1983	↓/nc	McGivern et al., 1981		
	↓/?	Benton, 1984	↑/nc	Puglisi-Allegra., 1981		
			↑↓/?	Fanselow and Sigmundi, 1982		
			↓/nc	Rodgers, 1982		
Sedative-hypnotics						
Pentobarbital						
5–120	↓/↓	Janssen et al., 1960	↓/↓	Chen et al., 1963		
	↓/↓	Gray et al., 1961	↓/↓	Sofia, 1969		
	↓/↓	DaVanzo et al., 1966	↓/↓	Irwin et al., 1971		
	↓/↓	Cole and Wolf, 1966				
	(↓)/?	Valzelli et al., 1967				
	↓/nc	LeDouarec and Broussy, 1969				
	↓/↓	Sofia, 1969				
	nc/?	Krsiak, 1979				

(continued on next page)

Table 1 (Continued)
Effects of Drugs on Aggression Induced by Environmental Manipulations[a]

Drug class prototype mg/kg	Isolation-induced aggression		Pain-induced aggression		Non-reinforcement induced aggression	
	Effect on aggression/motor	References	Effect on aggression/motor	References	Effect on aggression/motor	References
Alcohol						
< 1000	↑/nc	Chance et al., 1973	nc/nc	Hutchinson et al., 1977	↑/nc	Miczek and Barry, 1977
	↑/nc	Krsiak, 1976	nc/nc	Bammer and Eichelman, 1983	↑/nc	Cherek et al., 1984b
> 1000	↓/nc	Krsiak, 1976	↓/↓	Irwin et al., 1971		
	nc/?	Lagerspetz and Ekqvist, 1978	↑/?	Weitz, 1974		
	↓/nc	Smoothy and Berry, 1983				
Axiolytics						
Diazepam						
< 1.0	↑/nc	Poshivalov, 1978	↓/nc	Sofia, 1969		
	(↑)/nc	Krsiak, 1979				
> 1.0	↓/nc	DaVanzo et al., 1966			↑/↑	Arnone and Dantzer, 1980
	↓/?	Valzelli et al., 1967				
	↓/?	Boissier et al., 1968				
	↓/↓	Sofia, 1969				
	↓/↓	Poshivalov, 1978				
	↓/↓	Delini-Stula and Vassout, 1979				
	↓/nc	Krsiak, 1979				
	↓/?	Poshivalov, 1981				
	↓/nc	Gardner and Guy, 1984				
chronic	↓/nc	Malick, 1978				

(continued on next page)

Table 1 (Continued)
Effects of Drugs on Aggression Induced by Environmental Manipulations[a]

Drug class prototype mg/kg	Isolation-induced aggression		Pain-induced aggression		Non-reinforcement induced aggression	
	Effect on aggression/motor	References	Effect on aggression/motor	References	Effect on aggression/motor	References
Chlordiazepoxide						
<5.0	↑/nc	Krsiak, 1979	↓/↓	Kostowski, 1966	↑/nc	Miczek, 1974
	↓/nc	Gardner and Guy, 1984	↓/↓	Sofia, 1969	↓/nc	Moore et al., 1976
>5.0	↓/↓	Scriabine and Blake, 1962	↓/nc	Hoffmeister and Wuttke, 1969		
	↓/nc	Cole and Wolf, 1966	↓/(↓)	Irwin et al., 1971		
	↓/?	Valzelli et al., 1967	↓/?	Manning and Elsmore, 1972		
	↓/↓	Sofia, 1969	(↓)/nc	Emley and Hutchinson, 1973		
	↓/nc	LeDouarec and Broussy, 1969	↓/nc	Goldberg et al., 1973		
	↓/↓	Hoffmeister and Wuttke, 1969	↓/↓	Quenzer et al., 1974		
	↓/?	Valzelli and Bernasconi, 1971	↓/?	Jarvix et al. (in press)		
	↓/?	Weischer and Opitz, 1972				
	↓/?	Poole, 1973				

(continued on next page)

Table 1 (Continued)
Effects of Drugs on Aggression Induced by Environmental Manipulations[a]

Drug class prototype mg/kg	Isolation-induced aggression		Pain-induced aggression		Non-reinforcement induced aggression	
	Effect on aggression/motor	References	Effect on aggression/motor	References	Effect on aggression/motor	References
Antidepressants						
Imipramine						
< 10 acute			nc/nc	Crowley, 1972		
acute						
> 10	(↓)/?	Valzelli et al., 1967, 1971	nc/nc	Lapin, 1967		
	↓/?	Boissier et al., 1968	nc/nc	Tedeschi et al., 1969		
	↓/nc	LeDouarec and Broussy, 1969	↓/↓	Sofia, 1969		
	↓/↓	Sophia, 1969	↓/↓	Irwin et al., 1971		
	↓/↓	Krsiak, 1976, 1979	↓/nc	Crowley, 1972		
	↓/nc	Delini-Stula and Vassout, 1979				
chronic						
10	↓/nc	Delini-Stula and Vassout, 1981	↑/?	Eichelman and Barchas, 1975		
	↑/?	Willner et al., 1981	↑/?	Mogilnicka and Przewlocka, 1981		
Pargyline						
< 50	↑/?	Welch and Welch, 1968				
> 50	↓/?	Welch and Welch, 1968				
Lithium						
acute						
1 mEq/kg	↓/?	Brain and Al-Maliki, 1979	↓/nc	Sheard, 1970		
			↓/nc	Mukherjee and Pradhan, 1976		
			(↓)/?	McGlone et al., 1980		

(continued on next page)

Table 1 (Continued)

Effects of Drugs on Aggression Induced by Environmental Manipulations[a]

Drug class prototype mg/kg	Isolation-induced aggression		Pain-induced aggression		Non-reinforcement induced aggression	
	Effect on aggression/motor	References	Effect on aggression/motor	References	Effect on aggression/motor	References
chronic						
>30.0	↓/?	Brain, 1972	↓/?	Eichelman and Thoa, 1973		
mEg/kg	↓/?	Eichelman et al., 1977	↓/?	Eichelman et al., 1973		
	↓/nc	Malick, 1978	↓/nc	Marini et al., 1979a		
			↓/?	Prasad and Sheard, 1982		
Hallucinogens						
LSD						
<0.2	↓/?	Uyeno and Benson, 1965	↑/?	Kostowski, 1966		
	nc/?	Valzelli et al., 1967	↑/?	Sheard et al., 1977		
	↓/?	Rewerski et al., 1971	↑/?	Marini et al., 1979a		
	↑/nc	Krsiak et al., 1971				
	↓/nc	Krsiak, 1979				
THC						
<1.0	↑/?	Carder and Olson, 1972				
>1.0	↓/?	Garattini, 1965	↑/?	Carlini and Masur, 1970	↓/(↓)	Cherek et al., 1972
	↓/nc	Santos et al., 1966	nc/↓	Manning and Ellsmore, 1972	↓/?	Cherek and Thompson, 1973
	↓/nc	Dubinsky et al., 1973b	↓/?	Carder and Olson, 1972	↓/nc	Miczek and Barry, 1974
	↓/?	ten Ham and van Noordwijk, 1973	↓/nc	Dubinsky et al., 1973b	↓/(↓)	Cherek et al., 1980
	↓/?	ten Ham and de Jong, 1974	↓↑/?	Pradhan et al., 1980		
	↓/nc	ten Ham and de Jong, 1975				

(continued on next page)

Table 1 (Continued)

Effects of Drugs on Aggression Induced by Environmental Manipulations[a]

Drug class prototype mg/kg	Isolation-induced aggression		Pain-induced aggression		Non-reinforcement induced aggression	
	Effect on aggression/motor	References	Effect on aggression/motor	References	Effect on aggression/motor	References
Antipsychotics Chlorpromazine >0.6	↓/?	Yen et al., 1959	↓/nc	Brunaud and Siou, 1959		
	↓/(↓)	Janssen et al., 1960	↓/↓	Chen et al., 1963		
	↓/↓	Gray et al., 1961	↓/↓	Kowstowski, 1966		
	↓/nc	Scriabine and Blake, 1962	↓/↓	Tedeschi et al., 1969		
	↓/↓	Cole and Wolf, 1966	↓/↓	Sofia, 1969		
	↓/nc	DaVanzo et al., 1966	↓/nc	Hoffmeister and Wuttke, 1969		
	↓/↓	Valzelli et al., 1967	↓/nc	Emley and Hutchinson, 1971		
	↓/?	Boissier et al., 1968	↓/↓	Barkov, 1973		
	↓/↓	Sofia, 1969	↓/?	Powell et al., 1973		
	↓/nc	LeDouarec and Broussy, 1969				
	↓/nc	Hoffmeister and Wuttke, 1969				
	↓/nc	Kletzkin, 1969				
	↓/?	Valzelli and Bernasconi, 1971				
	↓/↓	Dubinsky et al., 1973a				
	↓/↓	Poshivalov, 1974				
	↓/nc	Krsiak, 1979				
	↓/↓	Delini-Stula and Vassout, 1979				
	↓/?	Benton, 1984				
	↑/nc	Matte, 1975				
	↓/nc	Dorr and Steinberg, 1976				
	↓/↓	Miczek, 1978				

(continued on next page)

Table 1 (Continued)
Effects of Drugs on Aggression Induced by Environmental Manipulations[a]

Drug class prototype mg/kg	Isolation-induced aggression		Pain-induced aggression		Non-reinforcement induced aggression	
	Effect on aggression/motor	References	Effect on aggression/motor	References	Effect on aggression/motor	References
Drugs with specific antiagressive effects						
Scopolamine						
>0.05	↓/nc	Janssen et al., 1960	↓/↑	Lapin, 1967		
	↓/nc	DaVanzo et al., 1966	↓/?	Powell et al., 1973		
	↓/nc	Krsiak, 1979	↓/nc	Mukherjee and Pradhan, 1976		
	↓/nc	Krsiak, et al., 1981	↓/?	Pritchett et al., 1979		
	↓/nc	Donat and Krsiak, 1982	↓/?	Bell and Brown, 1980		
			↓/nc	Rolinski and Herbut, 1981		
			↓/nc	Rodgers and Brown, 1973		
Nicotine						
>0.1			↓/↓	Hutchinson and Emley, 1973	↓/nc	Cherek, 1981
			↓/nc	Rodgers, 1979		
			↓/?	Waldbillig, 1980		
			↓/nc	Driscoll and Baettig, 1981		
Sch 12679						
14.6	↓/nc	Barnett et al., 1974	↓/↓	Bean et al., 1978		
Fluprazine						
1.25–5.0	↓/nc	Olivier and van Dalen, 1982				
	↓/nc	Benton et al., 1983				
	↓/nc	Bradford et al., 1984	↓/nc	Bradford et al., 1984		

(continued on next page)

Table 1 (Continued)

Effects of Drugs on Aggression Induced by Environmental Manipulations[a]

Drug class prototype mg/kg	Isolation-induced aggression		Pain-induced aggression		Non-reinforcement induced aggression	
	Effect on aggression/motor	References	Effect on aggression/motor	References	Effect on aggression/motor	References
YG-19-256						
>2.5	↓/↓	Olivier and van Dalen, 1982	↓/nc	Bell and Brown, 1979		
cyclic CMP						
.25, 2.5	↓/nc	Benton and Newton, 1983				
Propranol						
acute						
>5.0	↓/nc	Delini-Stula and Vassout, 1979	↓/nc	Vassout and Delini-Stula, 1977		
	↓/nc	Weinstock and Weiss, 1980	↓/?	Hegstrand and Eichelman, 1983		
	(↓/↓)	Poshivalov, 1981	↓/nc	Mogilnicka et al., 1983		
chronic						
>5.0			↑/?	Hegstrand and Eichelman, 1983		
Clonidine						
0.05	↓/nc	Lassen, 1978				
62.5 ng ICV	↓/nc	Puglisi-Allegra et al., 1984				
GABA agonists						
Valproate						
≤300	↓/nc	Publisi-Allegra and Mandel, 1980				
	↓/nc	Puglisi-Allegra and Renzi, 1980				
	↓/nc	Sulcova et al., 1981				
	↓/?	Simler et al., 1983				

(continued on next page)

Table 1 (Continued)
Effects of Drugs on Aggression Induced by Environmental Manipulations[a]

Drug class prototype mg/kg	Isolation-induced aggression		Pain-induced aggression		Non-reinforcement induced aggression	
	Effect on aggression/motor	References	Effect on aggression/motor	References	Effect on aggression/motor	References
Aminooxyacetic acid						
≤40	↓/nc	DaVanzo and Sydow, 1979				
	↓/nc	Sulcova et al., 1981				

[a] Abbreviations ↓ = significant decrease; ↑ = significant increase; nc = no change; ? = not measured or not reported; (↓) = tends to decrease, not significant at $p < 0.05$; (↑) = tends to increase, not significant at $p < 0.05$.

profile for isolation-induced aggression during the past two decades (e.g., Janssen et al., 1960; DaVanzo et al., 1966; Valzelli et al., 1967; Sofia, 1969; Malick, 1979; Krsiak et al., 1981; Poshivalov, 1981). Drugs of many chemical and therapeutic classes exert similar effects on isolation-induced aggression, differing only in degree of behavioral specificity. Several investigators have probed whether or not isolation-induced aggression in mice could serve as a screen for drugs with antipsychotic properties (e.g., Janssen et al., 1960) or for anxiolytic (e.g., Garattini and Valzelli, 1981; Ross and Ogren, 1976) or antidepressant drugs (Delini-Stula and Vassout, 1981; Malick, 1979). Simple increases and decreases in aggressive behavior of isolated mice are insufficient measures to differentiate therapeutic agents. One of the most significant efforts has focused on those mice that do not become aggressive after isolated housing, but show escape and defensive reactions when paired with nonaggressive partners (Krsiak, 1975). A consistent pattern of drug effects identifies anxiolytics as most effectively and selectively reducing escape and defensive reactions that are referred to as "timid" (Krsiak et al., 1984).

2.1.2. Pain-Induced Aggression

Exposure to aversive stimuli, particularly painful electric shock pulses, may lead to distinct reactions that are called shock-induced fighting or pain-induced aggression. The major method consists of delivering electric shock pulses to pairs of rats or mice at an intensity that is sufficient to evoke postures, movements, and acts and vocalizations of a defensive nature. A further method requires the delivery of electric shock pulses to a restrained animal whose biting reactions can be automatically recorded.

The delivery of painful electric shock through the grid floor of a test cage to pairs of laboratory rats leads to a stereotyped pattern of defensive behavior (Fig. 1) (O'Kelly and Steckle, 1939; Ulrich and Azrin, 1962). In reaction to electric foot shock, pairs of rats eventually assume an upright posture, facing each other with mouth open and head angled upward, nipping each other's limbs or snout, and moving

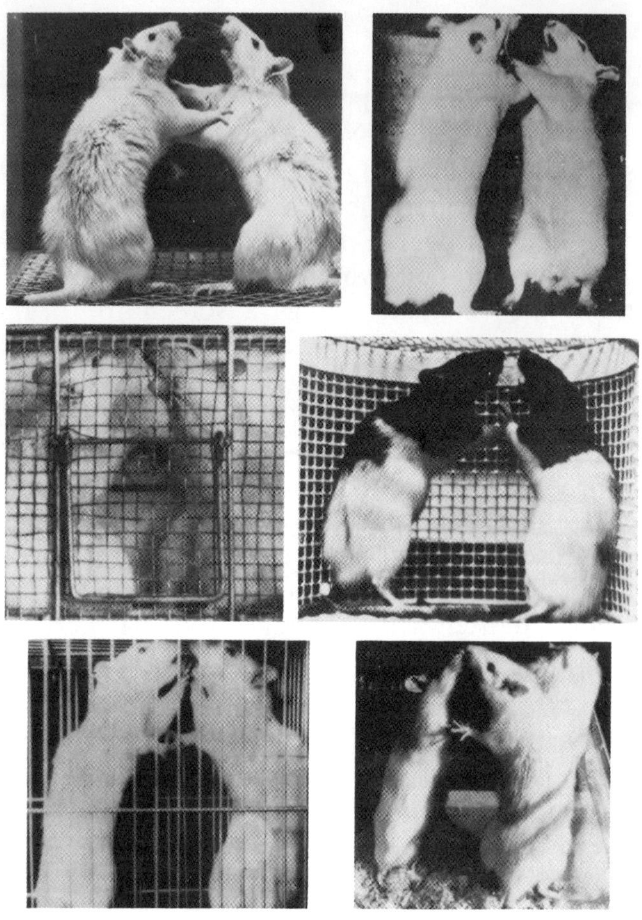

Fig. 1. Mutual upright postures, referred to in varying terminology during different kinds of experimental manipulations. (A)
top left: A dominant and a subordinate rat during an extinction-
induced aggression test (from Miczek, 1974). Top right: Two male
rats in "stereotyped fighting posture" while being exposed to pulses
of electric shock through the grid floor (Ulrich and Azrin, 1962).
Center left: Two male rats, 30 min after being injected iv with 1
mg/kg apomorphine, in fighting position (Senault, 1970). Center
right: Two male rats, 30 min after being injected sc with 20 mg/kg
apomorphine, in "aggressive attitude" (McKenzie, 1971). Bottom
left: Two rats, after being deprived of rapid-eye-movement sleep
for 4 d and then injected with 10 mg/kg of Δ^9-tetrahydro-

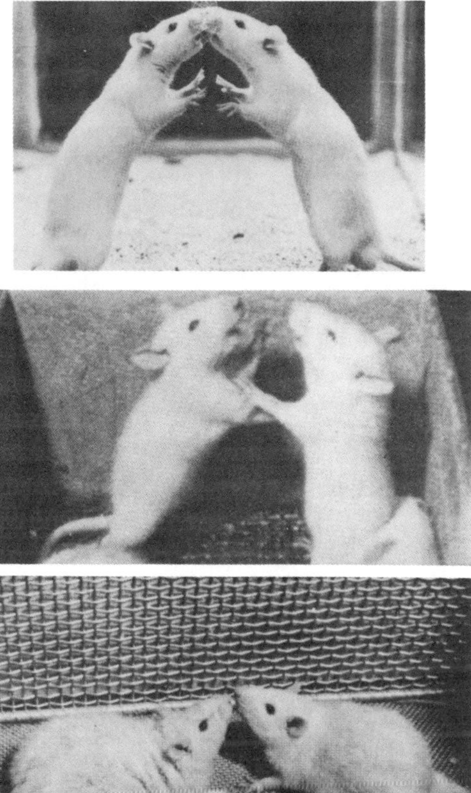

cannabinol, showing "mutual upright posture" (Carlini, 1977). Bottom right: Two male rats, about 30 min after ip injection of 8 mg/kg *p*-chloroamphetamine, showing "bizarre social behavior" (Korf and Kuiper, 1971). (B) top: Two rats, injected with the peripheral decarboxylase inhibitor Ro 4-4602 and L-DOPA (316 μmol/kg), showing "peculiar" and "bizarre" social behavior (Lammers and van Rossum, 1968). Center: Two male weanling Wistar rats, after being injected sc with 2.5 mg/kg apomorphine, showing "fighting" (Schneider, 1968). Bottom: Two rats, after sc injection of a monoamine oxidase inhibitor followed by 25 mg/kg L-DOPA, showing "mutual aggressiveness or rage" (Randrup and Munkvad, 1969).

forepaws up and down, all accompanied by loud vocalizations. Sometimes, anthropomorphic terms, such as "boxing posture," "sparring," and "exchanging blows" are used in reference to elements of pain-induced aggression in rats.

The behavior is simply tallied in terms of the percent of electroshocks that are followed by any of the elements of defensive behavior, or the frequency and duration of the defensive postures and movements (e.g., Halas et al., 1977). Ulrich and Azrin (1962) describe the optimal parameters for eliciting pain-induced aggression in pairs of rats as follows: 30–40 shocks/min, 2 mA intensity, 0.5 s duration, scrambled polarity between the bars of the grid floor, and a relatively small test cage (e.g., 15 × 15 cm). The strain, age, or sex of the rats have relatively little impact on pain-induced aggression.

A version of this test procedure for mice was introduced by Tedeschi et al. (1959). Pairs of mice were placed on a grid floor under an inverted 2-L beaker and exposed to five electric shock pulses/s (3 mA intensity, 0.2 s duration) for 3 min. After initial escape attempts, the mice assumed an upright posture facing their cage mate and moving their forepaws, similar to the rats' reactions. The proportion of mice displaying shock-induced aggression, the proportion of electric shock pulses that are followed by defensive acts and postures, and the duration of the interactions have been used as behavioral measures.

Further techniques were developed to improve the delivery method of the electric shock pulses and to automatically measure a given element of aggressive behavior in mice. Wagner et al. (1979) restrained mice in tubes, attached electrodes to their tails, and measured how often an inanimate object was bitten as the index of aggression. In another technique (Puglisi-Allegra and Renzi, 1977) pairs of mice were placed into a small enclosure, and their tails were connected to electrodes on the outside of the enclosure. Every 3 s a 2-mA electric shock of 0.5 s duration was delivered to both mice through the tail electrodes. The measure of aggression was the frequency of bites, as recorded by a contact sensor.

One of the earliest automated methods for eliciting and measuring pain-induced aggression was developed for squirrel monkeys (Hutchinson et al., 1966, 1968). Individual squirrel monkeys are restrained at the waist in a chair in front of a rubber hose. Electrodes are attached to shaved portions of the monkey's tail for the delivery of electric-shock pulses. In their pharmacological studies of pain-induced biting in squirrel monkeys, Emley and Hutchinson (1983) delivered electric shock pulses (400 V, 0.2 s in duration) every 4 min. The frequency of biting a rubber hose was measured automatically as the index of aggression.

The effects of prototypic drugs on pain-induced aggression are summarized in Table 1 (center). Additional neuropharmacological manipulations with drugs that lack direct therapeutic applications or abuse potential have recently been reviewed (Sheard, 1981). Psychomotor stimulants, such as amphetamines or caffeine, as well as hallucinogens, are most often found to enhance pain-induced defensive upright postures or biting, at low doses. This enhancement is usually based on the observation that the defensive reactions can be evoked at electric shock intensities that are lower than normal. In contrast to isolation-induced aggression, the group of sedative hypnotics and anxiolytics do not modulate pain-induced aggression in a dose-dependent, biphasic pattern; most reports indicate no significant changes in pain-induced aggression after administration of benzodiazepines or alcohol, and if suppression is seen, it appears to be associated with sedative doses. The effects of antidepressants and beta-blockers on pain-induced aggression depend on the treatment regimen; although acute doses of drugs, such as imipramine or propranolol, decrease pain-induced defensive upright reactions in rats, chronic treatment actually enhances these responses. Antipsychotic drugs decrease pain-induced defensive postures or biting in a nonspecific fashion, mainly as a result of their sedative properties. Lithium and the anticholinergics consistently decrease pain-induced aggression in a behaviorally specific manner, which appears independent of changes in motor and sensory functions.

Experimental protocols for pain-induced aggression have gained validity through the often-demonstrated systematic relationship between painful aversive stimuli and certain types of reactions that are subsumed under the label "aggression." This relationship appears to exist inside and outside of the laboratory across species ranging from invertebrates to primates (Ulrich, 1966). The topographic analysis of the reactions evoked by painful stimuli and their functional significance within the behavioral repertoire of a given species have been treated loosely, often giving rise to a great deal of acrimonious debate (e.g., Hutchinson, 1983; Blanchard and Blanchard, 1984). It seems that pharmacological research employs these protocols out of pragmatic considerations (i.e., ease of technique) and is less concerned with issues of functionally clearly defined behavior. Postures and bites that are evoked by painful aversive environmental stimuli, such as electric shock, resemble those by an animal in defense against an attacking opponent or a predator. This generalization has to remain tentative since measurements of pain-induced aggression rely on single behavioral indices without much information concerning behavioral context. For example, the exclusive focus on the bite response, particularly toward an inanimate object, does not permit an unambiguous functional analysis of this behavior. Bites are part of predatory behavior, attack behavior, and defensive reactions, and may also occur during copulatory behavior and in maternal retrieval. Measurement of a single criterion response is only informative after the face validity of the behavior is clearly established.

In distinction from isolation-induced aggression, a different profile of drug effects emerges with pain-induced aggression. Since the significance of pain-induced aggression in pathological human aggression and its treatment is not obvious, the predictive value of drug effects in this situation may be limited.

An intriguing experimental situation has been developed from the tradition of pain-induced aggression research that promises to be of value to psychopharmacology (Tadokoro, 1967). In this situation a monkey performs an operant response that is periodically reinforced by food pellets. During certain periods of the experimental session, the operant responses of this monkey deliver electric shock pulses to a second, larger monkey, who is restrained in close proximity. The shock-elicited behavior of the second monkey suppresses the food-reinforced responses of the first monkey. Anxiolytics, but neither chlorpromazine nor imipramine, attentuate the suppressive effects of the shock-elicited agonistic behavior of one monkey on the other's operant behavior (Kamioka et al., 1977). This pharmacological selectivity for anxiolytics and its underlying mechanism should be further explored since it may represent considerable predictive validity.

2.1.3. *Extinction-Induced Aggression and Aggression as Adjunct to Schedule-Controlled Behavior*

When a specific behavioral response is reinforced with clearly defined regularity, the omission of scheduled reinforcement (i.e., extinction) often induces aggressive behavior (Skinner, 1938; Azrin et al., 1966). For this type of aggression, earlier psychological theorists proposed the experience of frustration as the mediating event (Dollard et al., 1939). Surprisingly, in experimental psychopharmacological studies, extinction-induced aggression is considerably less frequently investigated than, for example, pain- or isolation-induced aggression.

When a behavioral response is not reinforced constantly, but intermittently, many responses are emitted that are actually not reinforced (Ferster and Skinner, 1957). Intermittent reinforcement, possibly as a result of the aversive properties of this intermittency, may induce aggressive behavior (Looney and Cohen, 1982). Several programs or "schedules" have been developed that specify which responses are followed by reinforcement and which are not. For example, when a specific response is reinforced only after a fixed period of time has elapsed (i.e., "fixed-interval schedule of reinforcement"), aggressive behavior may be seen during intervals between reinforcement (Cherek and Heistad, 1971). The term "adjunctive" has been applied to all those behaviors that are not directly controlled by the contingencies of the reinforcement schedule, but do occur in its context (Falk, 1971). Aggressive responses may be adjuncts to the conditions that provide intermittent access to positive reinforcement.

A major limitation of this approach derives from the focus on food-deprived pigeons as primary subjects for the study of schedule-induced aggression. Considerably fewer systematic demonstrations of schedule-induced aggression exist for rats, mice, pigs, and monkeys (Looney and Cohen, 1982), although recent studies in humans have produced systematic and consistent results (e.g., Cherek, 1981).

A sophisticated technology has been developed during the past 20 yr for accurate, objective, and automatic measurement of the aggressive responses induced by schedules of reinforcement. Usually, a single aspect of aggressive behavior, such as a pigeon's peck at a target or a monkey's bites of an object, is identified for unambiguous automated measurement (Fig. 2) (Looney and Cohen, 1982). For experimental work in humans, a comparable methodology has been developed (e.g., Cherek, 1981).

The effects of prototypic drugs on extinction- or schedule-induced aggression are summarized in Table 1 (right). These procedures have been used only rarely, and pharmacological information is rather limited. Alcohol and the benzodiazepines, at low doses, actually increase schedule-induced aggression in such different species as pigs (Arnone and Dantzer, 1980) and humans (Cherek et al., 1984b). Of course, these and other drugs decrease schedule-induced aggression at higher doses. A considerable degree of behavioral specificity in antiaggressive effects was seen with caffeine, THC, and nicotine.

The validity of extinction- or schedule-induced aggression inside and outside of the laboratory is more apparent than that of other forms of environmentally induced aggression. In terms of face validity, extinction-induced aggression ranks high; it is easily seen in humans, but more difficult to study in laboratory rodents. The pharmacological data, although sparse, show systematic dose–effect relationships and suggest differentiation among major drug classes. The limited database is insufficient to evaluate the predictive validity of this set of experimental procedures.

The conditioning procedures with carefully programmed periods of nonreinforcement engender a variety of excessive behaviors. The nature of the adjunctive behavior depends on the stimulus situation. In ethological terminology such

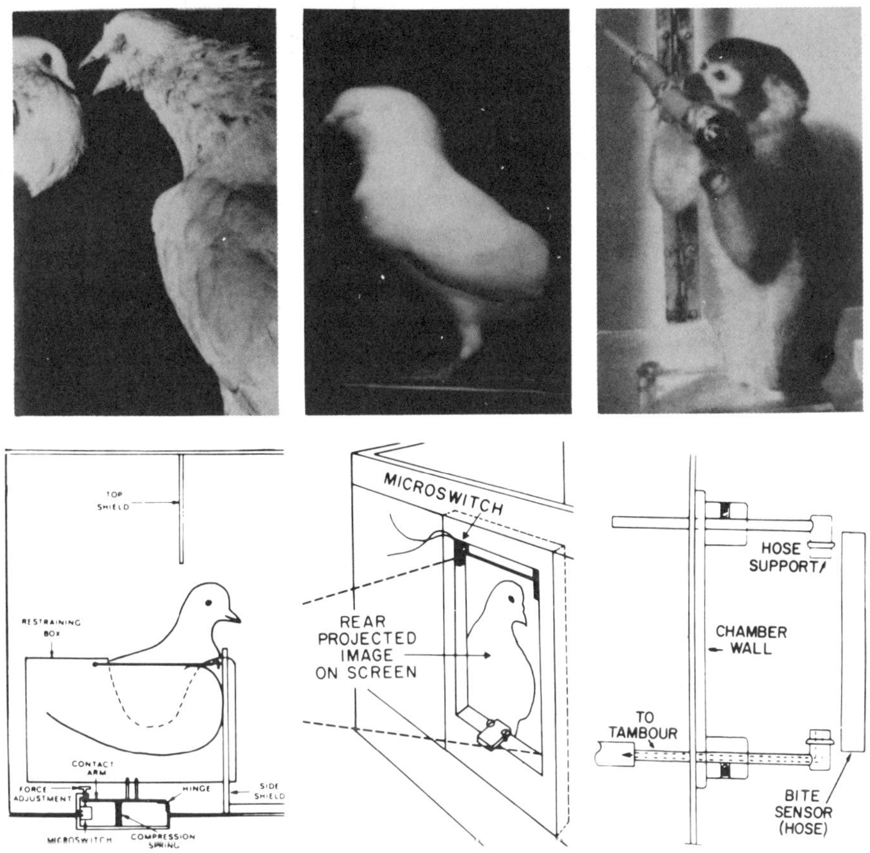

Fig. 2. With permission from Looney and Cohen, 1982.

adjunctive behaviors may be called displacement activities (Falk, 1977). For psychopharmacological research it may be significant that drugs that modulate schedule-induced aggression most likely act on processes that are common to a variety of adjunctive behaviors and are not specific to aggression.

2.2. Aggression Resulting From Neurological Manipulations

Integrated aggressive responses can be elicited by delivering microampere pulses of electric current to discrete subcortical brain structures. These behavioral phenomena and the prerequisite methodology were originally described by Hess (1928, 1948). Electrical stimulation of medial hypothalamic and brainstem structures in cats produces intense defensive responses, originally referred to as "affective defense" ("affektive Abwehr") (Hess and Brugger, 1943; de Molina and Hunsperger, 1962). In contrast to the affective defensive response pattern, electrical stimulation of more lateral hypothalamic sites in cats evokes a quiet biting attack toward a rat, including stalking and killing responses, but rarely eating (Flynn, 1967, 1969). The stimulation-evoked quiet biting attack resembles aspects of feline predatory behavior (Leyhausen, 1960). Psychopharmacological research has primarily used the stimulation protocol that leads to rage-like affective defensive behavior and, less often, the stimulation-evoked quiet biting attack. Damage to neural tissue resulting from ablations or electrolytic lesions has also served as an experimental preparation to induce aggression-like behavioral phenomena. For example, the "rage" and irritability after destruction of the septal forebrain area, medial hypothalamus, or olfactory bulbs of laboratory rats has been used occasionally in the evaluation of experimental drugs (e.g., Sofia, 1969).

2.2.1. Brain Stimulation-Induced Aggression and Defense

One of the early studies in experimental psychopharmacology was Masserman's (1937) investigation of the sedative effects of sodium amobarbital (20–50 mg/kg) on affective defensive responses that were elicited by electrical stimulation of the hypothalamus of cats. In the past two decades the most frequently used experimental protocol consists of implanting cats with intracranial electrodes. The tips of the electrodes are usually aimed at medial hypothalamic sites; the exact location is determined during initial exploratory experiments when the electrode is gradually lowered and permanently fixed as soon as a site is found that results in stimulation-bound behavior. Electrical stimulation is applied through the hypothalamic electrodes in trains of square wave pulses. Current intensity is gradually increased until one or several components of the defensive response pattern are seen. The method of limits, or similar psychophysical methods, are employed to establish the threshold current for the criterion response, which is often hissing, vocalization, or additional components of affective defense in the cat, such as dilated pupils, piloerection, retracted ears, arched back, growling, spitting, and strikes with unsheathed claws. This pattern of behavior resembles that of a cat defending itself. The experimenter measures changes in threshold current necessary to elicit this behavior as a result of drug action.

A more recent methodological development has applied the electrical brain stimulation technique to rats (Koolhaas, 1978; Kruk et al., 1979). In spite of early successes with brain stimulation-elicited aggressive responses in rats (e.g., Woodworth, 1971; Panksepp, 1971b), most experimental work, including psychopharmacological studies, is performed with cats. Although only limited data exist at present, the Dutch WE-zob strain of rats maybe useful in this context (van der Poel et al., 1982). The methods and techniques for electrical stimulation with rats are very similar to those used with cats. Behaviorally, however, the response pattern of the stimulated rat appears to resemble that of a resident attacking an intruder, including threat postures, attack jumps, and bites, whereas the behavior of cats is of a defensive nature.

Table 2 summarizes data concerning effects of drugs on brain stimulation-evoked aggression in cats. Prototypes of virtually all major drug classes increase the threshold current for eliciting affective defense or rage-like responses in cats; these drugs range from antidepressants, antipsychotics, and sedative-hypnotics to those drugs of various chemical classes that have been claimed to exert specific antiaggressive effects. If a larger amount of current is required to elicit the criterion response, the drug effect is considered to be decreasing the sensitivity of the neural substrate for affective defense. A low acute dose of ethanol appears to be the only exception to this general pattern of results, since it decreased the cats' latency to engage in defensive reactions in response to electrical hypothalamic stimulation (MacDonnell et al., 1971a,b).

Table 2
Effects of Drugs On Brain Stimulation—Evoked Affective Defense And Predatory Attack Behavior[a]

| Drug mg/kg | Affective defense | | Predatory attack | |
	Effect on aggression/motor	References	Effect on aggression/motor	References
Stimulants				
d-Amphetamine				
0.125–0.5			↑/↑	Sheard, 1967
			↑/↑	Marini et al., 1979b
1.0–1.5	nc/nc	Baxter, 1968	↓/↓	Marini et al., 1979b
methamphetamine				
2.0			↓/↓	Panksepp, 1971a
Antidepressants				
Imipramine				
8.0	nc/nc	Baxter, 1968	↓/nc	Dubinsky et al., 1973a
5.0	↓/?	Funderburk et al., 1970		
2.5, 5.0	↑/?	Penzola-Roja et al., 1961		
Antipsychotics				
Chlorpromazine				
2–8	nc/↓	Baxter, 1968	(↓)/↓	Dubinsky and Goldberg, 1971
5.0	↓/?	Funderburk et al., 1970		

(continued on next page)

Table 2 (*continued*)
Effects of Drugs On Brain Stimulation—Evoked Affective Defense
And Predatory Attack Behavior[a]

Drug mg/kg	Affective defense		Predatory attack	
	Effect on aggression/motor	References	Effect on aggression/motor	References
Anxiolytics				
Chlordiazepoxide				
5–20	nc/?	Baxter, 1968	nc/↓	Panksepp, 1971a
	↓/?	Funderburk et al., 1970		
	↓/nc	Delgado, 1973		
Diazepam				
0.5	↓/↓	Fukuda and Tsumagari, 1983		
Meprobamate				
100	↓/?	Apfelback, 1971		
	↓/↓	Delgado et al., 1971		
Sedative-Hypnotics				
Ethanol				
0.4–1.6 g/kg	↓/?	MacDonnell et al., 1971a	↓/nc	MacDonnell and Ehmer, 1969
0.37 g/kg	↑/?	MacDonnell et al., 1971a		
Phenobarbital				
40	↓/↓	Baxter, 1968		

(*continued on next page*)

Table 2 (*continued*)
Effects of Drugs On Brain Stimulation—Evoked Affective Defense
And Predatory Attack Behavior[a]

Drug mg/kg	Affective defense		Predatory attack	
	Effect on aggression/motor	References	Effect on aggression/motor	References
Amybarbital 20–50	↓/↓	Masserman, 1937		
Hallucinogens THC >1.0			nc/↓	Dubinsky et al., 1973b
Drugs with Specific Antiagressive Effects Atropine 4.0, 12.0	nc/↓	Baxter, 1968	nc/↑	Dubinsky and Goldberg, 1971
Scopolamine 0.6–2.0	(↓)/↓ ↓/?	Baxter, 1968 Katz, 1981	↓/?	Katz and Thomas, 1975
Sch 12679 10.0	↓/↓	Katz and Thomas, 1976	↓/↓	Katz and Thomas, 1976

[a] Abbreviations: ↓ = significant decrease; ↑ = significant increase; nc = no change; ? = not measured or not reported; (↓) = tends to decrease, not significant at $p < 0.05$; (↑) = tends to increase, not significant at $p < 0.05$.

2.2.2. Brain Stimulation-Induced Predatory Killing

In contrast to stimulation of medial hypothalamic sites that leads to defensive reactions, lateral hypothalamic stimulation elicits attack and kill responses directed toward prey (Wasman and Flynn, 1962; Flynn, 1969). The predatory-like behavior occurs even toward an anesthetized rat or mouse. The parameters of the electrical stimulation to elicit "quiet biting attack" are similar to those for "affective defense" (MacDonnell and Flynn, 1964; Bandler 1975). Behavioral measurements usually consist of determining the threshold current for eliciting attack on a prey; additionally, the threshold current for initiating motoric activity may also be assessed. Any drug effects are expressed as a change in threshold current for eliciting attack behavior as compared to nonaggressive motor activity or, alternatively, as change in latency to initiate movements after stimulation has been started.

Similar to the effects on "affective defense," the few known drug effects on predatory "quiet biting attack" elicited by hypothalamic stimulation are mostly inhibitory. Tricyclic antidepressants, anticholinergics, and ethanol increase the threshold current for eliciting predatory attack. Amphetamine appears to exert dose-dependent biphasic effects in this preparation, low doses facilitating attacks and higher doses decreasing them (Sheard, 1967; Marini et al., 1979b). As before, one of the chief concerns with drug effects on brain stimulation-elicited affective defense and quiet biting attack pertains to the behavioral specificity of the drug effects.

The validity of experimental preparations in which aggressive or defensive behavior is evoked by electrical stimulation of discrete brain structures is mainly derived from a sound theoretical rationale. Whether or not the neural processes for certain aggressive responses in cats and humans are homologous remains to be further explored. However, it is highly likely that drugs of various classes act on potentially similar neural mechanisms across species.

As with other experimental preparations, the prototypes of major drug classes alter behavior patterns that are evoked by electrical brain stimulation in a closely similar manner, differing only quantitatively in behavioral selectivity. Stimulation-evoked behaviors do not specifically predict the effectiveness or potency of a traditionally defined class of drugs. Of course, major affective disorders and brain stimulation-evoked aggression are neither directly related in symptomatology nor in underlying mechanisms. Instead, brain stimulation-evoked aggressive behavior patterns appear to constitute behavioral and neural systems with distinctive pharmacological characteristics.

2.3. Aggression Resulting From Pharmacological Manipulations

Some 40 years ago, Chance (1946) observed the emergence of "defensive encounters" among normally placid laboratory mice that were treated with large doses of amphetamine (i.e., in excess of 10 mg/kg, sc). Since then several distinct forms of drug-induced aggression have been studied: (1) groups of two or more animals of the same species are given a high drug dose and the resultant interactions are observed; (2) an individual animal receives a drug and its behavior toward a potential prey animal is examined; (3) an individual animal is treated with a high drug dose, mostly chronically, and the possibility of self-injurious behavior is investigated; and (4) chronic exposure to a psychotropic drug is terminated and the probability, intensity, and frequency of aggressive behavior during withdrawal are studied.

2.3.1. Drug-Induced Aggression in Groups of Animals

In the group test, animals of the same species, usually mice or rats, that do not exhibit aggressive behavior before drug treatment, are placed in a test cage in groups of 2–10. After a drug is administered, most commonly to all animals in a cage, a certain proportion of mice or rats will display an unusual constellation of behaviors, consisting of running and sudden rearing while facing each other, up and down movements of the forepaws, biting at the snout and limbs of the cagemate, and frequent vocalizations. Figure 1 portrays postures and movements that are produced by various treatments, all of which are referred to as drug-induced aggression or bizarre social behavior. These behaviors appear to be mainly of a defensive nature (e.g., Chance, 1946). Very high doses of catecholaminergic agonists (e.g., amphetamine, apomorphine, clonidine, L-Dopa, imipramine, and pargyline) or neurotoxins (e.g., 6-hydroxydopamine), or, alternatively, cholinergic agonists (e.g., carbachol, arecoline, and pilocarpine) or hallucinogens are able to induce bizarre social behavior in varying proportions of otherwise placid laboratory animals (Fig. 1) (Randrup and Munkvad, 1969; Senault, 1968; Ozawa et al., 1975; Maj et al., 1982; Van der Wende and Spoerlein, 1962; Fog, 1969; Scheel-Kruger and Randrup, 1968; Nakamura and Thoenen, 1972; Beleslin and Samardzic, 1977; Allikmets, 1974; Carlini, 1977; Schneider, 1968). This type of research will be illustrated with the example of apomorphine-induced aggression.

One of the most frequently studied forms of drug-induced aggression follows the injection of apomorphine. The highly unusual behavioral sequelae of apomorphine injections to grouped laboratory rats were initially observed in pharmacology laboratories (Senault, 1968, 1970, 1971; Schneider, 1968; Lammers and van Rossum, 1968; McKenzie, 1971). The most effective doses of apomorphine to induce these behavioral phenomena range from 1 to 20 mg/kg, suggesting action on postsynaptic dopamine receptors. Some of the prominent behavioral elements of apomorphine-induced aggression are portrayed in Fig. 1. The upright postures, leaps at the cagemate, and vocalizations that are induced by apomorphine resemble isolated elements of the defensive behavior pattern of rats. Often, the proportion of animals showing any of these behavioral elements is tallied or an aggression score is assigned, or the latency, duration, and frequency of individual elements are measured.

Apomorphine-induced aggression is effectively antagonized by drugs that interfere with catecholamine synthesis or release, or catecholamine receptors (Senault, 1968, 1970; Dlabac, 1973; Lal et al., 1975; Olpe, 1978). In addition to antipsychotic drugs, cholinergic agonists, such as pilocarpine, antiserotonergics, such as fenfluramine, and, to a lesser degree, antidepressants, anxiolytics, and morphine can also block apomorphine-induced aggression (Senault, 1968, 1974; Gianutsos and Lal, 1976, 1977; Rolinski and Herbut, 1979; McKenzie, 1981). However, many of the same drugs, when given chronically, actually increase apomorphine-induced aggression. Chronic treatment with antidepressants, phentolamine, haloperidol, clonidine, or morphine potentiate apomorphine aggression at lower doses or in larger proportions of animals (e.g., Lal and Puri, 1972; Puri and Lal, 1973; Gianutsos et al., 1974, 1976; Maj et al., 1979; Allikmets et al., 1979; Hahn et al., 1982). Similar enhancing effects have been seen after single doses of cyproheptadine, reserpine, or 6-hydroxydopamine (Rolinski and Herbut, 1979; Patni and Dandiya, 1974; Thoa et al., 1972).

Research on apomorphine-induced aggression seems to illustrate the increasing practice of searching for behavioral "markers" that identify a certain neurochemical process. In the case of apomorphine-induced aggression, this goal showed promise at first, since postsynaptic dopamine receptor activation seems to be the critical event for this phenomenon. Subsequent studies pointed to significant contributions by noradrenergic, serotonergic, and cholinergic systems to the constellation of behaviors induced by apomorphine. At present, increases and decreases in apomorphine aggression appear to be linked to several interacting neurochemical systems rather than to simple changes at a specific dopamine receptor. In addition to the pharmacological complexities, the behavioral significance of apomorphine-induced aggression remains obscure. The postures, movements, and vocalizations that are induced by apomorphine represent isolated elements of rat behavior of unusual appearance and out of functional context. Apomorphine-induced aggression is so far removed from the species-specific pattern of aggression in rats that it may be viewed as a pathological form of behavior. However, in order to use apomorphine aggression as a behavioral pathology, it is necessary to establish its behavioral validity.

2.3.2. Drug-Induced Killing

Drug-induced killing behavior is investigated by placing

drug-treated rats or cats with a likely prey, such as a mouse. Before drug treatment only those animals are selected that do not kill prey. However, it has been noted that prolonged cohabitation with a mouse retards the induction of mouse-killing behavior in nonkiller rats (e.g., Vergnes et al., 1977). Once administered a drug, the overall proportion of animals that are induced to kill is recorded, and the latency to attack, bite, kill, and consume the prey is measured. When the distribution of wounds on prey victims is analyzed, drug-induced killing appears less discriminate than predatory killing. Drug-induced killing may be more defensive in nature than predatory (Karli, 1981). Large acute doses or chronic treatments with cholinergic agonists (e.g., carbachol, physostigmine, and arecoline), serotonergic depletors, neurotoxins (e.g., *p*-chlorophenylalanine and 5,7-dihydroxytryptamine), or hallucinogens (e.g., cannabis) are among the most effective ways to induce killing behavior (e.g., Bandler, 1970; Vogel and Leaf, 1972; Berntson and Leibowitz, 1973; Sheard, 1969; Miczek et al., 1975; Miczek, 1976; Pucilowski and Kostowski, 1983; Vergnes et al., 1977). These studies are conducted for theoretical and pragmatic reasons; to learn about the neuropharmacological characteristics of the mechanisms that mediate killing (Karli, 1981) or, alternatively, to screen for antidepressant drugs.

2.3.3. Drug-Induced Self-Injurious Behavior

Drug-induced, self-injurious behavior may constitute a form of self-directed aggression. Large doses of pemoline, caffeine, or amphetamines, especially when given daily, induce self-directed biting in rats with injurious consequences (e.g., Genovese et al., 1969; Mueller and Nyhan, 1982, 1983; Mueller et al., 1982).

2.3.4. Aggression During Drug Withdrawal

Withdrawal from chronic exposure to opiates elicits complex physiological and behavioral reactions, including increased irritability and aggression (e.g., Gianutsos and Lal, 1978). The time course of the various symptoms of opiate withdrawal and of the enhanced aggression differs sufficiently in order to suggest a complex sequence of underlying processes (e.g., Blasig et al., 1973).

Chronic exposure to morphine is accomplished by varying methods; most often, animals are injected with increasing doses of morphine around the clock for 5–13 d. Alternatively, 75-mg morphine pellets are implanted subcutaneously. Duration of exposure to morphine and the quantity of morphine determine the intensity of withdrawal aggression (Gianutsos and Lal, 1978). Administration of an opiate antagonist, such as naloxone, after chronic exposure to morphine precipitates withdrawal symptoms, but does not always induce aggressive behavior (Gianutsos et al., 1975). Removal of the morphine pellet or termination of the injection schedule leads to the appearance of withdrawal aggression within 2–3 d. Most experimental studies on opiate withdrawal aggression are conducted in laboratory rats, but this phenomenon has also been seen in mice (Iorio et al., 1975), guinea pigs (Goldstein and Schulz, 1977), hamsters (Avis and Peeke, 1979), and rhesus monkeys (Seevers and Deneau, 1963). In laboratory rats, morphine withdrawal aggression consists of animals facing each other in upright postures, leaps at cagemates, forepaw movements, nips and bites directed at limbs and snout of opponent, and loud audible vocalizations. These behavioral elements are similar to those induced by apomorphine and are illustrated in Fig. 1.

Morphine withdrawal aggression is enhanced by several catecholaminergic agonists; L-dopa, amphetamine, methylphenidate, cocaine, and apomorphine increase the incidence of aggression during morphine withdrawal (Thor, 1971; Lal et al., 1971; Puri and Lal, 1973; Iorio et al., 1975; Ferrari and Baggio, 1982; Kantak and Miczek, 1982). Inversely, neuroleptics block morphine withdrawal aggression (Lal et al., 1975). Both increases and decreases in morphine withdrawal aggression have been found with the norepinephrine autoreceptor agonist clonidine (Gianutsos et al., 1976; Kantak and Miczek, 1982). Anticholinergics appear to increase, and cholinergic agonists appear to decrease, morphine withdrawal aggression (Hynes et al., 1976).

At present, the behavioral and pharmacological data on aggression during morphine withdrawal are incomplete. On the basis of the available data, it has been hypothesized that "reduced dopamine receptor activation after acute narcotic treatment and a compensatory receptor supersensitivity after chronic treatment comprehensively explain the behavioral effects of narcotics on aggression...." (Gianutsos and Lal, 1978; Lal, 1975b). Already, it appears that this hypothesis has to be expanded on behavioral and pharmacological grounds.

3. Ethopharmacological Analysis of Agonistic Behavior

The contributions of ethological aggression research to psychopharmacology have become apparent at several levels: Ethologists have focused on biologically significant situations in which aggression occurs in order to explore proximal causes for the behavior; and they have identified behavioral elements within the repertoire of a given species that are shown in situations of conflict, and quantitatively measured these elements of agonistic behavior (e.g., Eibl-Eibesfeldt, 1961; Scott, 1966).

It is possible to mimic the essential features of situations in which a certain species reliably exhibits agonistic behavior even under the constraints of the laboratory environment. For example, aggression by a solitary resident animal or a group of residents in encounters with an unfamiliar intruder can be seen under controlled laboratory conditions in many species ranging from invertebrates to primates. Most resident–intruder confrontations involve adult males. Female aggression is most readily studied during lactation ("maternal aggression"), but may also occur during pregnancy (Floody, 1983; Ogawa and Makino, 1984). In gregarious species, aggressive behavior is not only prominent during group formation, but is seen within established groups. These examples highlight the ethological emphasis on aggression with obvious biological functions. It has already proven feasible to study drug effects on aggression resulting from confrontations with an intruder, in association with certain reproductive activities, or within established groups (Miczek and DeBold, 1983).

The unambiguous, reliable recognition and identification of the behavioral elements that a given animal species displays during conflict constitute the basis for the representation of agonistic behavior in the form of an ethogram (Eibl-Eibesfeldt, 1970). Extensive catalogs of the behavioral elements that are shown before and during conflict have been prepared for the species most commonly studied in laboratory research, such as mice (Crowcroft, 1966; Grant and Mackintosh, 1963), rats (Barnett, 1975; Grant and Mackintosh, 1963), cats (Leyhausen, 1960), squirrel monkeys (Hopf et al., 1974), and rhesus monkeys (Sade, 1967; Altmann, 1962). Attack, threat, and pursuit are consistently characterized as offensive behaviors and differentiated from defensive and submissive responses as well as flight. In most species, such as those used in the laboratory, the distinction between offensive and defensive and, ultimately, submissive or flight behavior is readily accomplished; complex mixtures of offensive and defensive behavioral elements may occur (e.g., Leyhausen, 1960).

Ethological methods for the study of aggression, defense, flight, and submission attempt to capture the interactive, species-specific, sequential, and temporal patterned features of these behaviors (Miczek, 1983a). In situations of conflict, at least two individuals interact by exhibiting sequences of species-specific acts, postures, movements, displays, gestures, and vocalizations; these behavioral elements occur in distinctive temporal patterns, bursts of aggressive interactions alternating with periods of relative quiescence. Quantitative and reliable measurement over time of the salient behavioral elements that constitute attack, threat, defense, flight, and submission appears to be the prerequisite for an adequate assessment of drug effects on agonistic behavior (Miczek and Krsiak, 1979, 1981).

3.1. Agonistic Behavior During Resident–Intruder Confrontations

One of the most potent proximal causes for aggressive behavior is the approach by an unfamiliar conspecific, particularly the territorial intruder (e.g., Wilson, 1975). This phenomenon may be observed in most species ranging from insects to primates. The confrontation with an unfamiliar conspecific who intrudes into an established group or into a territory has been studied in psychopharmacological research on aggression since the 1950s, although in an unusual class—fish. Siamese fighting fish (*Betta splendens*) and Convict Cichlid fish (*Cichlasoma nigrofasciatum*) are the most frequently used species. After the initial studies on LSD, barbiturates, meprobamate, morphine, and reserpine (Abramson and Evans, 1954; Walaszek and Abood, 1956), subsequent research focused on alcohol and anxiolytics (e.g., Raynes et al., 1968; Raynes and Ryback, 1970; Peeke et al., 1973, 1975, 1981; Figler et al., 1973, 1975). The fish studies indicated behavioral specificity of drug action by comparing attack behavior to some measure of motor coordination. Alcohol, for example, modulated attack behavior in a dose-dependent biphasic fashion, low doses increasing, and higher doses decreasing, this behavior, in the absence of any detectable effects on nonaggressive motor activity. In format, the behavioral analysis of drug effects in these studies contrasted changes in two selected criterion measures, one aggressive, the other nonaggressive, comparable to those summarized in Table 1.

During the past decade, experimental protocols for resident–intruder confrontations in commonly used species have been developed, and the analysis of drug effects on aggression has included quantitative evaluation of the many constituent elements of agonistic behavior patterns. Agonistic behavior is embedded into the stream of many other on-going, nonagonistic behaviors. A comprehensive ethological analysis of drug effects on agonistic behavior attempts to assess concurrent changes in those segments of the behavioral repertoire that are not agonistic in function. This approach has begun to inform us of the true "behavioral costs" that are associated with the "benefit" of pharmacological control of aggression.

In addition to the cost-benefit aspect, the ethological analysis of drug effects on agonistic behavior attempts to represent drug-induced changes in a multicomponent, dynamic behavior pattern. From a practical viewpoint, a distinctive pharmacological profile of the various salient elements of agonistic behavior is beginning to emerge. Drugs may be grouped according to their characteristic profile of effects on (1) attack and threat; (2) defensive reactions; (3) flight or escape; (4) associative or nonagonistic social behavior; and (5) self-directed or nonsocial motor activities. These behaviors are illustrated in Fig. 3. Of course, it is possible to "split" the agonistic behavior patterns into finer elements instead of "lumping" elements together. In deciding on whether "to split or to lump" behavioral responses, it may be advisable to be guided by the data. Actually, drug-induced changes of the various behavioral elements often suggest the "lumping" of elements into functional categories, and it is this latter approach that will be illustrated.

Already, several independent studies on resident–intruder aggression have been conducted with sufficiently detailed behavioral measurements of drug effects to tentatively construct behavioral profiles for a few selected drugs; these are summarized in Table 3 and include amphetamines, chlordiazepoxide, diazepam, alcohol, chlorpromazine, Δ^9-tetrahydrocannabinol, scopolamine, and naloxone. Of course, not all studies report identical results because of significant variations in drug dose, animal species, and other methodological details.

Dose-dependent, biphasic effects on attack and threat behavior have been found with amphetamines, anxiolytics, and sedative-hypnotics. This confirms the data summarized earlier in Table 1. However, with more comprehensive ethological measurements, the enhancing and suppressing effects of amphetamine can be related to concurrent increases in defense and flight, disruption of social behavior, and activation of solitary motor activity. Effects in the opposite direction are obtained with alcohol and benzodiazepines. These latter drugs induce a similar pattern of effects not only on attack and threat, but also extending to other segments of the behavioral repertoire, the benzodiazepines showing slightly more specificity than alcohol at the aggression- and flight-decreasing doses.

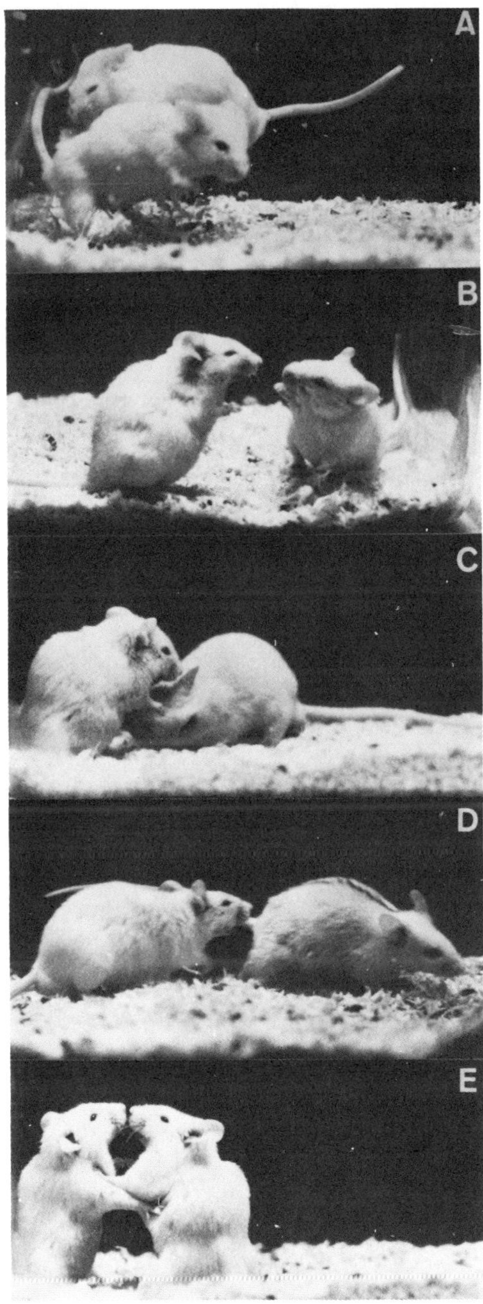

Fig. 3. Agonistic, nonagonistic, social, and individual motor behavior in mice during resident–intruder confrontations.

Table 3

Effects of Prototype Drugs on Components of Agonistic and Nonagonistic Behavior[a]

| Attack | | | | | Key | |
Drug dose	Threat	Defense	Flight	Social	motor	References
Amphetamines						
low	↑	nc	nc	nc	(↑)	Silverman, 1966
high	↓	↑	↑	↓	↑	Krsiak, 1975, 1979
						Miczek and O'Donnell, 1978
						Miczek, 1979
						Poshivalov, 1981
						Sieber et al., 1982
Chlordiazepoxide/						
Diazepam						
low	↑	(↓)	nc	↑	nc	Krsiak, 1975, 1979
high	↓	↓	(↓)	nc	nc	Poshivalov, 1981
						Olivier and van Dalen, 1982
						Miczek, 1984
Alcohol						
low	↑	nc	nc	(↑)	nc	Chance et al., 1973
high	↓	(↑)	nc	(↓)	(↓)	Cutler, 1976
						Krsiak, 1976
						Smoothy and Berry, 1983
						DeBold and Miczek, 1985

(Continued on next page)

Table 3 (continued)

Effects of Prototype Drugs on Components of Agonistic and Nonagonistic Behavior[a]

| Attack | | | | | Key | |
Drug dose	Threat	Defense	Flight	Social	motor	References
Chlorpromazine						
low	↓	nc	nc	↓	(↓)	Silverman, 1966
high	↓	(↓)	(↓)	↓	↓	Poshivalov, 1974
						Krsiak, 1975, 1979
						Olivier and van Dalen, 1982
THC	↓	?	↑	↓	(↑)	Cutler and Mackintosh, 1975
						Miczek, 1978
						Sieber et al., 1980, 1982
						Olivier et al., 1984
Naloxone	↓	nc	nc	nc	nc	Puglisi-Allegra et al., 1982
						Olivier and van Dalen, 1982
						Rodgers and Hendrie, 1983
						Benton et al., 1984
Scopolamine	↓	nc	nc	nc	nc	van der Poel and Remmelts, 1971
						Krsiak et al., 1981
						Donat and Krsiak, 1982

[a] Abbreviations: ↓ = significant decrease; ↑ = significant increase; nc = no change; ? = not measured or not reported; (↓) = tends to decrease, not significant at $p < 0.05$; (↑) = tends to increase, not significant at $p < 0.05$.

Among the drugs that consistently decrease attack and threat, only scopolamine and the opiate receptor antagonist naloxone reveal remarkable behavioral specificity, i.e., the antiaggressive effects in the resident–intruder situation occur in the absence of concurrent changes in other agonistic or nonagonistic behavioral responses. By contrast, chlorpromazine's antiaggressive effects are linked to a decrease in all behavior requiring the initiation of movement. Less extensive, but very promising, evidence for relatively selective antiaggressive effects in ethologically analyzed resident–intruder confrontations has also been obtained with lithium (Brain and Al-Maliki, 1979) and propranolol (Poshivalov, 1981; Miczek, 1981). the most significant "costs" associated with the antiaggressive effects of drugs, such as beta-blockers, anticholinergics, or lithium, appear to be their pronounced action on autonomic functions.

3.2. Maternal Aggression

Aggression by and toward females has mostly been studied for its hormonal basis, and even in this regard the evidence is sparse (Floody, 1983; Svare and Mann, 1983). One of the most significant recent developments in the psychopharmacology of aggression is the work on female aggression, during both pregnancy and lactation (Erskine et al., 1978; Gandelman, 1980; Ogawa and Makino, 1984). At present, only a handful of systematic pharmacological studies on aggression by females exists, but it appears that this neglected dimension of agonistic behavior, with obvious biological significance and validity, will receive increasing experimental attention.

Maternal aggression may be readily evoked in species that are common in laboratory research, such as mice, rats, and hamsters. The usual situation in which maternal aggression occurs is in confrontation with an intruder, particularly in the early lactation period (Erskine et al., 1978), and it may be viewed as defense of the nest. Suckling stimulation from the pups is necessary for maternal aggression in mice (Svare and Gandelman, 1976). Behavioral measurements of maternal aggression in mice and rats parallel those for inter-male, resident–intruder fighting; however, female mice and rats direct more frequent bites to the snout of the intruder than males do (DeBold and Miczek, 1981, 1984).

Pharmacological enhancement of maternal aggression in mice and rats has recently been found after administration of alcohol (DeBold and Miczek, 1985), chlordiazepoxide, and diazepam (Olivier et al., 1985; Yoshimura and Ogawa, personal communication). These results seem to parallel the effects of the same drugs on male aggression in resident–intruder confrontations (*see* Table 3). The aggression-enhancing effects of alcohol and anxiolytics in lactating mice and rats appear to be even larger in magnitude and more behaviorally specific than in males.

Pharmacological manipulations of catecholamines significantly alter maternal aggression, but the neurochemical, hormonal, and behavioral effects of these drugs appear to be related in a complex manner. Female rats given 6-hydroxydopamine, a catecholaminergic neurotoxin, icv, exhibit higher levels of maternal aggression (Sorenson and Gordon, 1975). However, this effect is not specific to maternal aggression, since such treatment also increases pain-elicited aggression and indices of "emotionality" in the open field. Ergot alkaloids that activate the D_2 subtype of dopamine receptors and inhibit prolactin secretion, appear to decrease aggression in lactating hamsters (Wise and Pryor, 1977), but leave this behavior unaltered in lactating mice (Mann et al., 1980). The involvement of prolactin in maternal aggression may be less significant than originally suspected, since the pituitary is not necessary for maternal aggression (Erskine et al., 1980). Amphetamine disrupts maternal aggression in mice only at higher doses, and it is unclear which of its neurochemical effects at these doses are the basis for this behavioral effect (DeBold and Miczek, in press). Additionally, lithium (0.2 mEq/d for 4 d) failed to alter maternal aggression in mice (Brain and Al-Maliki, 1979); a novel compound, fluprazine, with potentially specific antiaggressive effects decreased aggression in lactating rats in a behaviorally specific fashion (Olivier et al., 1985).

These initial experimental efforts suggest that aggression in postparturient females is a significant phenomenon, the neurochemical basis of which needs to be elucidated (Miczek and DeBold, 1983).

3.3. *Aggression Within Groups*

In species with higher forms of social organization, aggression occurs not only during group formation, but also after. This type of aggression, often related to social rank, status, and dominance, occupies only a small proportion of an individual's entire behavioral "budget," as is illustrated in "activity budgets" for dominant and subordinate squirrel monkeys (Fig. 4). Yet, it is this aspect of behavior that affects the individual's functioning at the neurochemical, physiological, and behavioral levels (e.g., Raleigh et al., 1984).

A first major rationale for these types of studies derives from the significant biological consequences of aggressive behavior in a social context. Success and failure in dyadic and higher-order interactions within a group lead to distinctive social stratification of the group members. In primate groups, social status and rank are not only based on an individual's

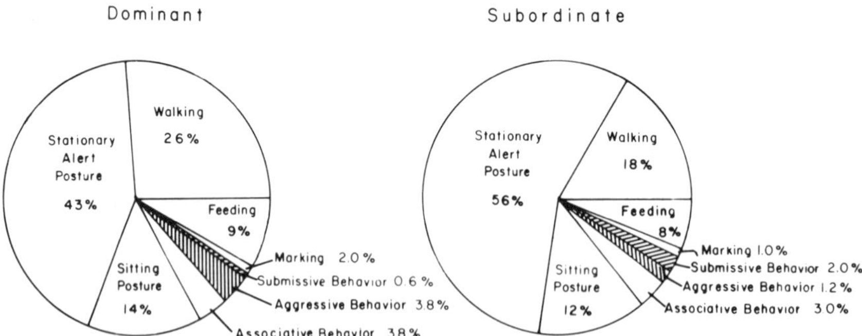

Fig. 4. Activity budgets for dominant and subordinate squirrel monkeys living in established groups. The proportion of time spent walking, sitting, in stationary alert posture, feeding, marking, aggressive, associative, and submissive behaviors (from Winslow and Miczek, 1985).

level of aggression and success in situations of conflict, but also on its genealogical position within the group (e.g., Hinde, 1983).

The significance of the active occupation of a social position that is based on the behavioral history of an individual was first illustrated by status-dependent endocrine profiles. Gonadal and adrenal hormone synthesis and secretion differ profoundly between high- and low-ranking animals (e.g., Sassenrath, 1971; Rose et al., 1971; Raab and Oswald, 1980; Sapolsky, 1982). Recently, the level of serotonin in the blood of vervet monkeys was not only found to be twice as high in dominant animals than in subordinates, but also depended on the active performance of the behavior pattern that is characteristic of dominant animals (Raleigh et al., 1984). This evidence has significant implications for drug effects on behavior in general and on aggressive behavior in particular. Pharmacological manipulations of an individual who is removed from its social context and exists in social isolation may result in unusual behavioral and physiological and neurochemical sequelae. In order to achieve a high degree of face validity, psychopharmacological studies of aggression must be pursued under conditions that preserve as closely as possible the natural social adaptations of a given species.

That the social status of an individual determines behavioral effects of drugs has been demonstrated experimentally for various psychoactive compounds. Especially social, competitive, aggressive, and submissive behaviors are the targets of status-dependent drug effects. For example, amphetamine may increase submissive postures and displays in subordinate rhesus monkeys (Haber et al., 1981) or, alternatively, in high-ranking stumptail macaques (Schlemmer and Davis, 1981); the same treatment may increase aggressive and threat behavior by dominant rhesus monkeys (Haber et al., 1981) or, conversely, disrupt this behavior by dominant squirrel monkeys (Miczek and Gold, 1983a) or pigtail macaques (Crowley et al., 1974). Even nonagonistic motor activity may be differentially altered by *d*-amphetamine, according to the social status of the drug recipient. Dominant squirrel monkeys differed from subordinate group members not only in the magnitude, but also in the direction, of amphetamine effects on time spent in locomotion (Fig. 5) (Miczek and Gold, 1983b). Amphetamine actually decreased locomotion in dominant monkeys, but increased the same behavior in subordinate animals.

Systematic shifts in the dose–effect curves for L-tryptophan's enhancement of approach and grooming in dominant vs nondominant vervet monkeys indicate higher drug sensitivity in dominant monkeys (Fig. 6) (Raleigh et al., 1983a,b). Chlordiazepoxide increased aggressive responses in a dominant rhesus monkey, but not in a low-ranking group member (Apfelbach and Delgado, 1974). Diazepam decreases motor activity of subordinate rhesus monkeys at lower doses than that of dominant group members (Delgado et al., 1976).

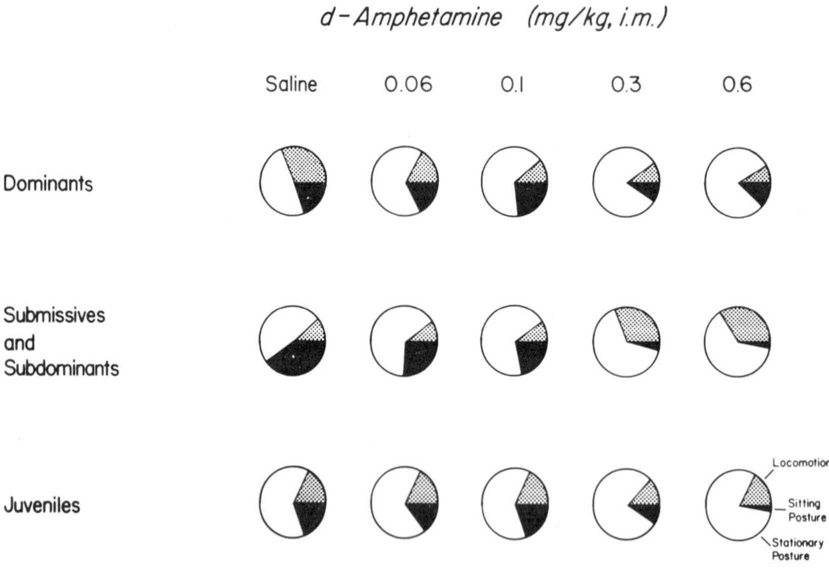

Fig. 5. Activity budget analysis for *d*-amphetamine effects on different kinds of motor activity in dominant, subdominant and submissive, and juvenile monkeys. Columns refer to different doses of *d*-amphetamine. The proportions of time spent in locomotion, sitting posture, and stationary alert posture are portrayed (from Miczek and Gold, 1983a).

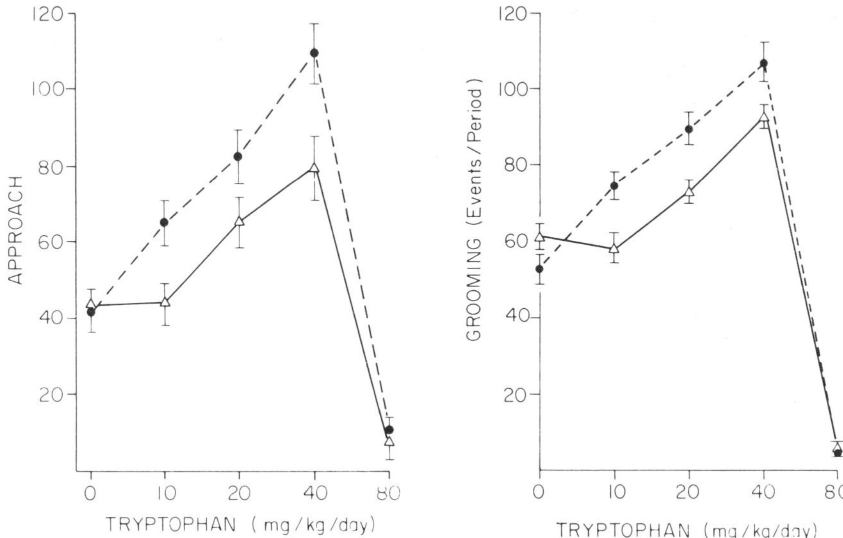

Fig. 6. The effects of L-tryptophan on approach and social grooming in dominant and nondominant male vervet monkeys (from Raleigh et al., 1983a,b).

Alcohol's enhancing effects on aggressive responses were evident only in the dominant members of four independent groups of squirrel monkeys, but the subordinates' low level of social and aggressive initiatives remained unaltered (Fig. 7) (Winslow and Miczek, 1985). These findings, although not always consistent across species, highlight the significance of an individual's social status as a powerful determinant of behavioral effects of drugs.

A further rationale for the study of drug effects on aggression as it occurs within established groups derives from this behavior's high sensitivity to drug effects. Different elements of agonistic behavior, including threat, attack, defense, submission, and flight, as well as associative responses, may be specifically modified by drug action. During the past decade, a substantial number of studies illustrates the unusual sensitivity of agonistic and social behavior to the effects of drugs of different pharmacological classes. Most of the work has focused on amphetamine because of its effects on aggres-

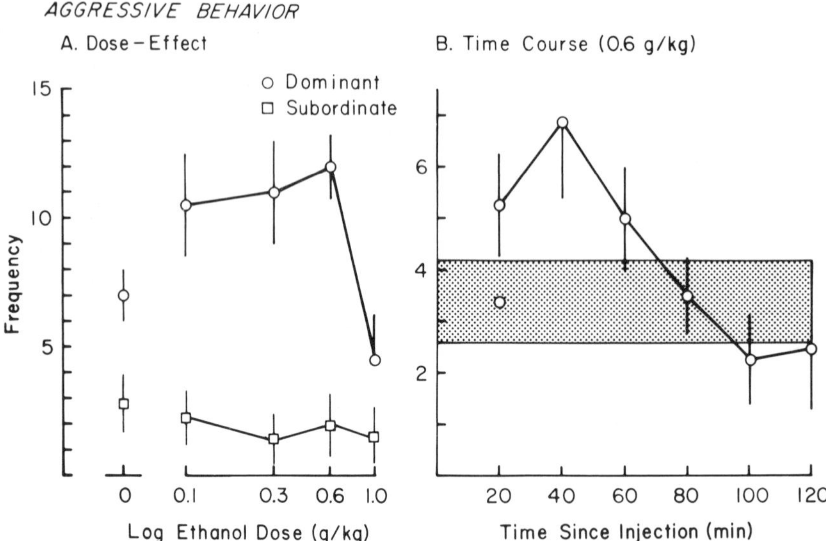

Fig. 7. The frequency of aggressive behavior toward group members in dominant and subordinate squirrel monkeys as a function of alcohol dose: (A) Dose–effect relationship; and (B) Time course of the effects of 0.6 g/kg alcohol in dominant monkeys. Vertical lines in each data point indicate ±1 SEM (from Winslow and Miczek, 1985).

sive and social behavior. Acute doses as low as 0.01 mg/kg, im may increase an individual stumptail macaque's aggressive behavior toward group members (Smith and Byrd, 1984), although, more often amphetamine in a range of 0.05–0.2 mg/kg starts to disrupt social grooming, sociosexual responses, and mother–infant contacts in vervet monkeys (Kjellberg and Randrup, 1973; Schiorring, 1979; Schiorring and Hecht, 1979) and decreases aggressive behavior in squirrel monkeys (Miczek and Gold, 1983a,b). As little as 1–3 ng/kg LSD was sufficient to alter social grooming and social spacing in stumptail macaques (Schlemmer and Davis, 1983). A major psychoactive ingredient in *Cannabis sativa*, Δ9-tetrahydrocannabinol, decreased aggressive responses in squirrel monkeys at doses as low as 0.25 mg/kg, po (Miczek, 1978); by contrast, alcohol increased aggressive displays and contacts at 0.3–0.6 g/kg in this species (Winslow and Miczek, 1985).

4. Limitations of the Observational Method

Studying drug effects on aggressive behavior by observation is limited in significant ways (Miczek and Gold, 1983b). Aggressive behavior within a group or during confrontations between a resident and an intruder occurs in an episodic manner; the triggering events are often obscured. No explicit experimental control over the behavioral measures is usually stipulated; a host of variables influence the intensity, frequency, and temporal pattern of their occurrence. On the other hand, social and agonistic interactions are often distorted by experimental manipulations as a result of their subtle nature. In order to study a behavioral process adequately and appropriately, the research method must not infringe on it (Altman, 1974). A great deal of experimental ingenuity is required to accommodate pharmacological objectives while maintaining aggressive behavior under field-like conditions.

Aggressive behavior within established groups or during resident–intruder confrontations is usually measured by direct observation, and these observations are encoded via keyboards into microprocessors (e.g., Miczek, 1979; Miczek and Yoshimura, 1982; Miczek and Gold, 1983a; Smith and Byrd, 1983). The observational method represents the strength and the weakness of ethopharmacological aggression research. Data collection based on direct observation may be biased by the observer's expectations, it may be inaccurate because of the speed of aggressive interactions, it may be selective because the observer records only those behavioral elements for which he or she is prepared, and it may be subjective because of the theoretical framework of the observer. Moreover, observation may be tedious and demands researchers who are dedicated to the task and are attuned to the fine details of behavior.

Many of these limitations are overcome by newly developed and constantly improving instruments, especially

economic, portable videosystems and microcomputers. Videorecords of the behavioral events allow the moment-to-
moment measurement of rapidly occurring aggressive interactions. The reliability of these measurements can be easily
established by repeated and independent reviews of the
videorecords (e.g., Miczek and Krsiak, 1979; Miczek, 1983a).
Error-free and automatic tabulation, transcription, and
analysis of the data are accomplished by microprocessor (e.g.,
Miczek, 1979; Winslow and Miczek, 1985). Recently, a very
promising methodological innovation was achieved by completely automating the process of recording social interactions
(Crawley et al., 1982). Individual animals are coded with
color spots and the color signals are recorded by a videocam-
era, digitized in the visual field, and analyzed in rapid succes-
sion with regard to changes in relative position. A host of
parameters of the animals' individual behavior and spatial
relationship in reference to each other may be measured.
Many of these parameters are sensitive to differential drug
action. For example, social interactions that are suppressed by
environmental manipulations can be selectively increased by
anxiolytic drugs (e.g., Crawley and Goodwin, 1980; File and
Hyde, 1978). Further development of automated techniques,
such as telemetry and digitized videosignals, promises to
enhance accuracy and objectivity of the recording of complex
social and aggressive behavior.

5. Microanalysis of Drug Effects on Aggressive Behavior Patterns

In order to determine with higher resolution the
"behavioral locus of action" for drug effects on aggressive
behavior, several quantitative ethological methods are
currently being explored for their usefulness. Assessing drug
action on temporal and sequential features will not only aid
in more adequately differentiating drugs from each other, but
will also pose relevant questions about the neurobiological
mechanisms that mediate aggressive behavior. As is evident
from a cursory inspection of Tables 1 and 2, and even the

more detailed behavioral profiles in Table 3, simple increases and decreases in a behavior are insufficient to convey distinct drug-induced changes in the patterning or sequencing of behavioral elements. The total frequency of a certain behavioral element over a fixed period of observation is often not a fully satisfactory and adequate representation of the complex pattern of aggressive behavior.

The starting point for most sequence analyses is a matrix in which the frequency of each behavioral element preceding and following other behavioral elements is summarized (van Hooff, 1982). Chi-square tests for goodness of fit may be applied when comparing the observed frequency of transitions from threats, for example, to attacks under certain drug conditions with those under vehicle conditions. In fact, amphetamine altered the probability of transitions between several elements of aggressive and flight behavior in mice at a dose (0.5 mg/kg) that was lower than that necessary for reliably changing the total incidence of these elements (Krsiak and Pribik, 1978). Discrete and continuous nonstationary models of transitions between elements of aggressive behavior have been illustrated in amphetamine-treated mice (Poshivalov and Khodko, 1984). However, it remains to be determined whether or not a sufficient number of transitions occur within the confines of a pharmacological experiment on aggressive behavior in order to fulfill the assumptions of a Markov-chain analysis. A single-link cluster analysis was performed on 37 elements of agonistic and nonagonistic behavior in drug-treated resident rats confronting an intruder (Olivier, 1981). The most apparent change in the patterning or structure of the resident's behavior was an increase in the variety of transitions between different behavioral elements when administered with a relatively specific antiaggressive drug. In order to visualize the shifts in the clusters of behavioral elements during the action of opiate antagonists, dendograms have been prepared (Brain et al., 1984).

An alternative to the sequence analyses of complex aggressive interactions appears to be the analysis of temporal aspects of these behaviors (Miczek, 1983b). Aggressive behavior during resident–intruder confrontations or within established groups follows a predictable time course. The episodic nature of aggressive behavior is already apparent when depicting the second-by-second occurrence of attack bites, sideways threats, and pursuits, as deflections from a time-line (Fig. 8A). The intervals between consecutive occurrences of aggressive acts may be tallied and conveniently portrayed in the form of a histogram (Fig. 8B). Frequency histograms of intervals between many different types of behavioral events often follow a negative exponential distribution. If one examines the intervals between aggressive acts as frequency histograms under several drug conditions, it is difficult to differentiate varying negative exponential curves. In order to ease this task, the distribution of intervals between aggressive acts may be portrayed in the form of a log survivor plot (Fig. 8C) (Fagen and Young, 1978; Van Hooff, 1982). Such a plot usually generates a straight line with a slope that is proportional to the probability of the aggressive act occurring a certain time after the last incidence of this event. A break in the straight line, such as in the example of the mouse's attack behavior, indicates that the probability of occurrence for this behavior has changed. Such a break point delimits, conveniently, a bout or epoch of aggressive behavior.

Figure 9 illustrates how log survivor plots represent the effects of acute low doses of alcohol on aggressive behavior by dominant monkeys toward group members. These data were shown earlier as dose–effect curves for session and group totals of aggressive behavior (Fig. 7) (Winslow and Miczek, 1985). The change in temporal pattern of aggressive behavior becomes apparent by the steep slope of the log survivor plot in comparison to the flat slope during control experiments.

The quantitative analysis of drug effects on patterns and sequences of aggressive behavior, in addition to those on frequency, emerges as an important topic of investigation for drug–behavior interactions. These analyses promise higher resolution and insight into the processes of aggressive interactions that are targets for drug action.

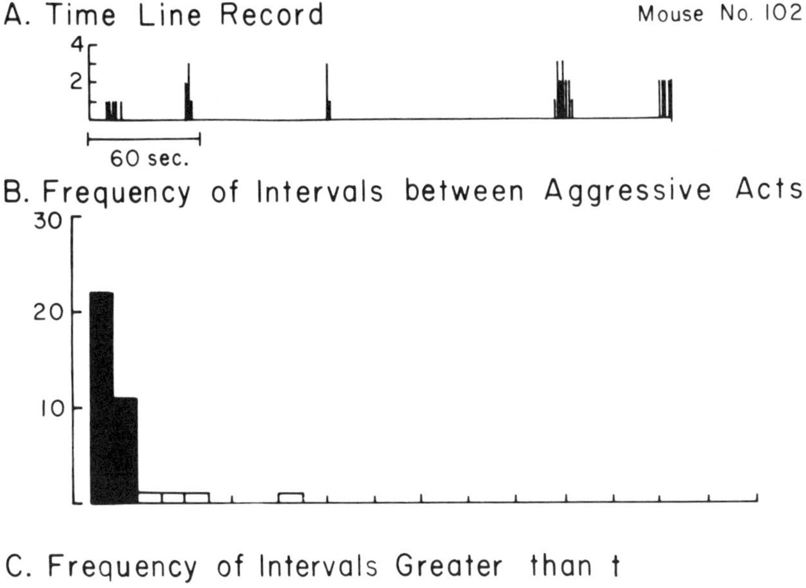

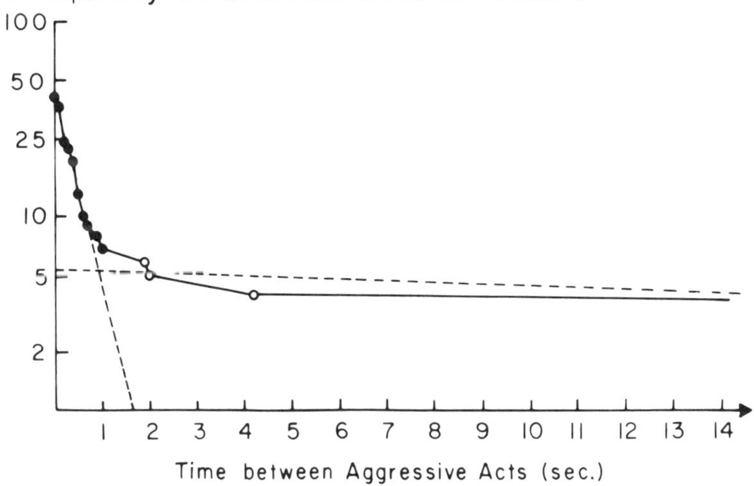

Fig. 8. Temporal pattern of attack behavior in a representative resident mouse confronting an intruder mouse: (A) Time-line record. The frequency of attack bites in each 300-s-long encounter is represented by an upward deflection from the time-line; (B) Frequency histogram of consecutive intervals between aggressive acts; and (C) Log survivor plot of the intervals between aggressive acts.

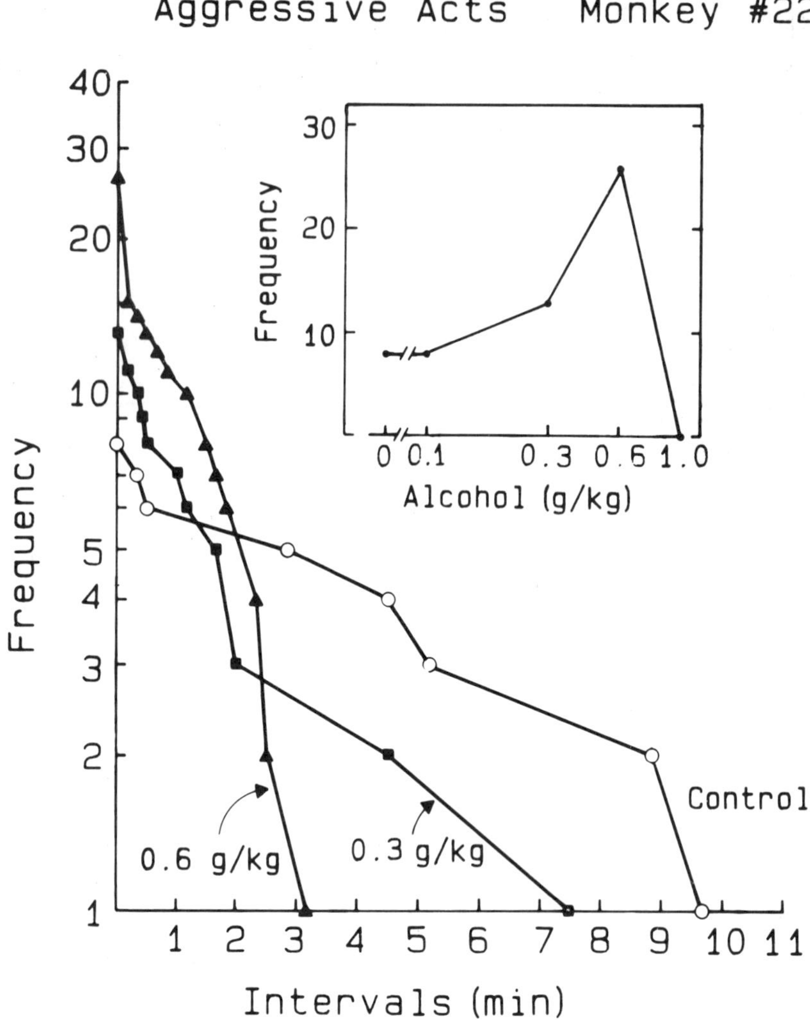

Fig. 9. Log survivor plots of the intervals between aggressive acts by the dominant squirrel monkey no. 22 after control treatment, 0.3 or 0.6 g/kg alcohol (po). The inset depicts the frequency of aggressive acts during the 40-min observation period as a function of alcohol dose.

6. Conclusions

Psychopharmacological research on aggression mirrors the significant advances in the neurobiological, as well as behavioral, methods and concepts during the past two decades. In view of the complexity of drug–behavior interactions, current psychopharmacological research on aggression has become more sophisticated at several levels: Reliance on a single drug at a single dose has given way to extensive dose–effect and time course determinations, comparing agents that share biochemical actions and exploring the mechanisms of action by antagonism, synergism, and other drug interaction protocols. At the behavioral level, the experimental imperative of accurate, objective, and reliable manipulations and measurements is beginning to be integrated with the ethological demand for biological validity. The clinical concern with abnormal or pathological forms of aggression and their treatment requires a thorough, detailed analysis of aggressive behavior patterns. Quantitative analysis of the behavioral elements that constitute aggressive interactions at the infrahuman level promises to enhance our understanding of adaptive, as well as maladaptive, patterns and sequences of behavior and how drugs modulate them. Here, as with the pharmacological and neurochemical aspects, more sophisticated approaches to the behavioral analysis of aggressive behaviors will become more widely accepted.

The agenda for future psychopharmacological research on aggression appears to be lengthy and challenging. The discoveries of neuropeptides and different types of receptors for endogenous substances, as well as for drugs, invite an assessment of their potential significance in the neurobiological mechanisms mediating aggressive behavior. Not only the causative neural processes for aggressive responses need to be delineated, but also the proximal and distal causes in the physical and social environment require further analysis. Pharmacological modulation of aggressive behavior may result from changes in the perception of aggression-triggering events (e.g., Dixon, 1982), in the motor capacities that are required for the performance of aggressive behavior, in the integrative mechanisms that are necessary for sequencing and patterning aggressive responses (e.g., Flynn, 1967), in the regulatory mechanisms for autonomic functions and arousal, or, alternatively, in neural processes specific to aggressive behavior. Interdisciplinary efforts will be required in order to accomplish such a comprehensive analysis of drug effects on aggressive behavior.

A new departure appears to be the use of drugs as probes for the functional state of neural processes that are altered by past and on-going aggressive behavior. An individual's interactions with environmental and social consequences alter neural, endocrinological, and sensory functions significantly. Not only a life history of aggressive or submissive behavior, but even a single experience of defeat profoundly changes neural processes (e.g., Miczek et al., 1982). These alterations become apparent when the individual is challenged pharmacologically. This research strategy employs drug effects as indices of functionally significant neurochemical alterations that result from engaging in aggressive behavior.

Acknowledgments

The preparation of this review and our own experimental work has been supported by research grants from the National Institute on Drug Abuse (DA02632) and the National Institute on Alcohol Abuse and Alcoholism (AA05122). We thank Drs. J. F. DeBold, K. Noda, and John Paul Scott for their constructive comments.

References

Abramson H. A., and Evans L. T. (1954) Lysergic acid diethylamide (LSD 25).II. Psychobiological effects on the Siamese fighting fish. *Science* **120,** 990–991.

Allikmets L. H. (1974) Cholinergic mechanisms in aggressive behaviour. *Med. Biol.* **52,** 19–30.

Allikmets L. H., Stanley M., and Gershon S. (1979) The effect of lithium on chronic haloperidol enhanced apomorphine aggression in rats. *Life Sci.* **25**, 165–170.

Altmann J. (1974) Observational study of behavior: Sampling methods. *Behaviour* **49**, 227–267.

Altmann S. A. (1962) A field study of the sociobiology of rhesus monkeys. *Ann. NY Acad. Sci.* **102**, 338–435.

Apfelbach R. (1971) Chemische unterdruckung elektrisch ausgeloster aggression. *Naturwissenschaften* **58**, 368.

Apfelbach R. and Delgado J. M. R. (1974) Social hierarchy in monkeys (*Macaca mulatta*) modified by chlordiazepoxide hydrochloride. *Neuropharmacology* **13**, 11–20.

Arnone M. and Dantzer R. (1980) Effects of diazepam on extinction induced aggression in pigs. *Pharmacol. Biochem. Behav.* **13**, 27–30.

Avis H. H. and Peeke H. V. S. (1979) Morphine withdrawal induced behavior in the syrian hamster (*Mesocricetus auratus*). *Pharmacol. Biochem. Behav.* **11**, 11–15.

Azrin N. H., Hutchinson R. R., and Hake D. F. (1966) Extinction-induced aggression. *J. Exp. Anal. Behav.* **9**, 191–204.

Bammer G. and Eichelman B. (1983) Ethanol effects on shock-induced fighting and muricide by rats. *Aggressive Beh.* **9**, 175–181.

Bandler R. (1975) Predatory aggression: Midbrain–pontine junction rather than hypothalamus as the critical structure?. *Aggressive Beh.* **1**, 261–266.

Bandler R. J. (1970) Cholinergic synapses in the lateral hypothalamus for the control of predatory aggression in the rat. *Brain Res.* **20**, 409–424.

Barkov N. K. (1973) Effect of neuroleptics on aggressive behavior. *Neurosci. Behav. Physiol.* **6**, 119–121.

Barnett S. A. (1975) *The Rat. A Study in Behavior.* University of Chicago, Chicago.

Barnett A., Taber R. I., and Steiner S. S. (1974) The behavioral pharmacology of Sch 12679. A new psychoactive agent. *Psychopharmacologia* **36**, 281–290.

Baxter B. L. (1968) The effect of selected drugs on the "emotional" behavior elicited via hypothalamic stimulation. *Int. J. Neuropharmacol.* **7**, 47–54.

Bean N. J., Loman K., and Conner R. (1978) Effects of benzazepine (Sch-12679) on shock-induced fighting and locomotor behavior in rats. *Psychopharmacology* **59**, 189–192.

Beleslin D. B. and Samardzic R. (1977) Muscarine- and carbachol-induced aggressions: Fear and irritable kinds of aggressions. *Psychopharmacology* **55**, 233–236.

Bell R. and Brown K. (1979) The effects of two "anti-aggressive" compounds, an indenopyridine and a benzothiazepin, on shock-induced defensive fighting in rats. *Prog. Neuropsychopharmacol.* **3**, 399–402.

Bell R. and Brown K. (1980) Shock-induced defensive fighting in the rat: Evidence for cholinergic mediation in the lateral hypothalamus. *Pharmacol. Biochem. Behav.* **12**, 487–491.

Benton D. (1984) The long-term effects of naloxone, dibutyryl cyclic CMP, and chlorpromazine on aggression in mice monitored by an automated device. *Aggressive Beh.* **10**, 79–89.

Benton D. and Newton R. P. (1983) The influence of dibutyryl cyclic CMP on aggression in the mouse. *Aggressive Beh.* **9**, 281–285.

Benton D., Brain P., Jones S., Colebrook E., and Grimm V. (1983) Behavioral examinations of the anti-aggressive drug fluprazine. *Behav. Brain Res.* **10**, 325–338.

Benton D., Brain S., and Brain P. F. (1984) Comparison of the opiate delta receptor antagonist ICI 154,129 and naloxone on social interaction and behaviour in an open field. *Neuropharmacology* **23**, 13–17.

Berntson G. G. and Leibowitz S. F. (1973) Biting attack in cats: Evidence for central muscarinic mediation. *Brain Res.* **51**, 366–370.

Blanchard D. C. and Blanchard R. J. (1984) Inadequacy of pain-aggression hypothesis revealed in naturalistic settings. *Aggressive Behav.* **10**, 33–46.

Bläsig J., Herz A., Reinhold K., and Zieglgänsberger S. (1973) Development of physical dependence on morphine in respect to time and dosage and quantification of the precipitated withdrawal syndrome in rats. *Psychopharmacologia* **33**, 19–38.

Boissier J. R., Grasset S., and Simon P. (1968) Effect of some psychotropic drugs on mice from a spontaneously aggressive strain. *J. Pharm. Pharmacol.* **20**, 972–973.

Bradford D. L., Olivier B., van Dalen D., and Schipper, J. (1984) Serenics: The Pharmacology of Fluprazine and DU 28412, in *Ethopharmacological Aggression Research* (Miczek K. A., Kruk M. R., and Olivier B., eds.), Alan R. Liss, New York.

Brain P. F. (1972) Oral lithium chloride, endocrine function and isolation-induced agonistic behaviour in male albino mice. *J. Endocrinol.* **55,** 1–2.

Brain P. F. (1975) What does individual housing mean to a mouse? *Life Sci.* **16,** 187–200.

Brain P. F. and Al-maliki S. (1979) Effects of lithium chloride injections on rank-related fighting, maternal aggression and locust-killing responses in naive and experienced "TO" strain mice. *Pharmacol. Biochem. Behav.* **10,** 663–669.

Brain P. and Poole A. (1974) Some studies on the use of "standard opponents" in intermale aggression testing in TT albino mice. *Behaviour* **50,** 100–110.

Brain P. F. and Nowell N. W. (1970) Some observations on intermale aggression testing in albino mice. *Commun. Behav. Biol.* **5,** 7–17.

Brain P. F., Jones S. E., Brain S., and Benton D. (1984) Sequence Analysis of Social Behavior Illustrating the Actions of Two Antagonists of Endogenous Opioids, in *Ethopharmacological Aggression Research* (Miczek K. A., Kruk M. R., and Olivier B., eds.), Alan R. Liss, New York.

Brunaud M. and Siou G. (1959) Action de Substances Psychotropes, Chez le Rat, sur un Etat d'Aggressivite Provoquee, in *Neuropsychopharmacology* (Bradley P. B., Deniker P., Radouco-Thomas C., eds.), Elsevier, Amsterdam.

Carder B. and Olson J. (1972) Marihuana and shock induced aggression in rats. *Physiol. Behav.* **8,** 599–602.

Carlini E. A. (1977) Further studies of the aggressive behavior induced delta-9-tetrahydrocannabinol in REM sleep-derived rats. *Psychopharmacology* **53,** 135–145.

Carlini E. A. and Masur J. (1970) Development of fighting behavior in starved rats by chronic administration of (–)delta-9-*trans*-tetrahydocannabinol and cannabis extracts. *Commun. Behav. Biol.* **5,** 57–61.

Chance M. R. A. (1946) A peculiar form of social behavior induced in mice by amphetamine. *Behaviour* **1,** 60–70.

Chance M. R. A., Mackintosh J. H., and Dixon A. K. (1973) The effects of ethyl alcohol on social encounters between mice. *J. Alcoholism* **8,** 90–93.

Charpentier J. (1969) Analysis and Measurement of Aggressive Behaviour in Mice, in *Aggressive Behaviour* (Garattini S. and Sigg E. G., eds.), Excerpta Medica Foundation, Amsterdam.

Chen G., Bohner B., and Bratton A. C. (1963) The influence of certain central depressants on fighting behavior of mice. *Arch. Int. Pharmacodyn. Ther.* **142,** 30–34.

Cherek D. R. (1981) Effects of smoking different doses of nicotine on human aggressive behavior. *Psychopharmacology* **75,** 339–345.

Cherek D. R. and Heistad G. T. (1971) Fixed-interval induced aggression. *Psychonomic Sci.* **25,** 7–8.

Cherek D. R. and Thompson T. (1973) Effects of Δ^9-tetrahydrocannabinol on schedule-induced aggression in pigeons. *Pharmacol. Biochem. Behav.* **1,** 493–500.

Cherek D. R., Steinberg J. L., and Brauchi J. T. (1983) Effects of caffeine on human aggressive behavior. *Psychiatry Res.* **8,** 137–145.

Cherek D. R., Steinberg J. L., and Brauchi J. T. (1984a) Regular or decaffeinated coffee and subsequent human aggressive behavior. *Psychiatry Res.* **11,** 251–258.

Cherek D. R., Steinberg J. L., and Vines R. V. (1984b) Low doses of alcohol affect human aggressive responses. *Biol. Psychiatry* **19,** 263–267.

Cherek D. R., Thompson T., and Heistad G. T. (1972) Effects of delta-9-tetrahydrocannabinol and food deprivation level on responding maintained by the opportunity to attack. *Physiol. Behav.* **9,** 795–800.

Cherek D. R., Thompson T., and Kelly T. (1980) Chronic delta-9-tetrahydrocannabinol administration and schedule-induced aggression. *Pharmacol. Biochem. Behav.* **12,** 305–309.

Cole H. G. and Wolf H. H. (1966) The effects of some psychotropic drugs on conditioned avoidance and aggressive behaviors. *Psychopharmacologia* **8,** 389–396.

Crawley J. N. and Goodwin F. K. (1980) Preliminary report of a simple animal behavior for the anxiolytic effects of benzodiazepines. *Pharmacol. Biochem. Behav.* **13,** 167–170.

Crawley J. N., Szara S., Pryor G. T., Creveling C. R., and Bernard B. K. (1982) Development and evaluation of a computer-automated color TV tracking system for automatic recording of the social and exploratory behavior of small animals. *J. Neurosci. Methods* **5**, 235–247.

Crowcroft P. (1966) *Mice All Over.* Foulis, London.

Crowley T. J. (1972) Dose-dependent facilitation or suppression of rat fighting by methamphetamine, phenobarbital, or imipramine. *Psychopharmacologia* **27**, 213–222.

Crowley T. J., Stynes A. J., Hydinger M., and Kaufman I. C. (1974) Ethanol, methamphetamine, pentobarbital, morphine, and monkey social behavior. *Arch. Gen. Psychiatry* **31**, 829–838.

Cutler M. G. (1976) Changes in the social behaviour of laboratory mice during administration and on withdrawal from non-ataxic doses of ethyl alcohol. *Neuropharmacology* **15**, 495–498.

Cutler M. G. and Mackintosh J. H. (1975) Effects of delta-9-tetrahydrocannabinol on social behaviour in the laboratory mouse and rat. *Psychopharmacologia* **44**, 287–289.

Dabac A. (1973) Apomorphine-induced aggressivity in rats and its alterations. *Act. Nerv. Super.* **15**, 133.

Daruna J. H. (1978) Patterns of brain monoamine activity and aggressive behavior. *Neurosci. Biobehav. Rev.* **2**, 101–113.

DaVanzo J. P., Daugherty M., Ruckart R., and Kang L. (1966) Pharmacological and biochemical studies in isolation-induced fighting mice. *Psychopharmacologia* **9**, 210–219.

DaVanzo J. P. and Sydow M. (1979) Inhibition of isolation-induced aggressive behavior with GABA transaminase inhibitors. *Psychopharmacology* **62**, 23–27.

DeBold J. F. and Miczek K. A. Effects of *d*-amphetamine on aggression in male or female mice: Changes in responsiveness with varying hormonal condition. *Pharmacol. Biochem. Behav.,* in press.

DeBold J. F. and Miczek K. A. (1981) Sexual dimorphisms in the hormonal control of aggressive behavior of rats. *Pharmacol. Biochem. Behav.* **14,S1,** 89–93.

DeBold J. F. and Miczek K. A. (1984) Aggression persists after ovariectomy in female rats. *Horm. Behav.* **18**, 177–190.

DeBold J. F. and Miczek K. A. (1985) Testosterone modulates the effects of ethanol on male mouse aggression. *Psychopharmacology* **86,** 286–290.

Delgado J. M. R. (1973) Antiaggressive Effects of Chlordiazepoxide, in *The Benzodiazepines* (Garattini S., Mussini E., and Randall L. O., eds.), Raven, New York.

Delgado J. M. R., Grau C., Delgado-Garcia J. M., and Rodero J. M. (1976) Effects of diazepam related to social hierarchy in rhesus monkeys. *Neuropharmacology* **15,** 409–414.

Delgado J. M. R., Lico M. C., Bracchitta H., and Snyder D. R. (1971) Brain excitability and behavioral reactivity in monkeys under meprobamate. *Arch. Int. Pharmacodyn. Ther.* **194,** 5–17.

Delini-Stula A. and Vassout A. (1979) Differential Effects of Psychoactive Drugs on Aggressive Responses in Mice and Rats, in *Psychopharmacology of Aggression* (Sandler M., ed.), Raven, New York.

Delini-Stula A. and Vassout A. (1981) The effects of antidepressants on aggressiveness induced by social deprivation in mice. *Pharmacol. Biochem. Behav.* **14,** 33–41.

De Molina A. F. and Hunsperger R. W. (1962) Organization of the subcortical system governing defense and flight reactions in the cat. *J. Physiol.* **160,** 200–213.

DeWeese J. (1977) Schedule-induced biting under fixed-interval schedules of food or electric-shock presentation. *J. Exp. Anal. Behav.* **27,** 419–431.

Dixon A. K. (1982) A possible olfactory component in the effects of diazepam on social behavior of mice. *Psychopharmacology* **77,** 246–252.

Dollard J., Doob L., Miller N., Mowrer O., and Sears R. (1939) *Frustration and Aggression,* Yale University, New Haven.

Donat P. and Krsiak M. (1982) Effects of scopolamine on agonistic behaviour of aggressive and non-aggressive mice. *Act. Nerv. Super.* **24,** 278–280.

Dorr M. and Steinberg H. (1976) Effects of delta-9-tetrahydrocannabinol on social behavior in mice. *Psychopharmacology* **47,** 87–91.

Driscoll P. and Baettig K. (1981) Selective inhibition by nicotine of shock-induced fighting in the rat. *Pharmacol. Biochem. Behav.* **14,** 175–179.

Dubinsky B. and Goldberg M. E. (1971) The effect of imipramine and selected drugs on attack elicited by hypothalamic stimulation in the cat. *Neuropharmacology* **10**, 537–545.

Dubinsky B., Karpowicz J. K., and Goldberg M. E. (1973a) Effects of tricyclic antidepressants on attack elicited by hypothalamic stimulation: Relation to brain biogenic amines. *J. Pharmacol. Exp. Ther.* **187**, 550–557.

Dubinsky B., Robichaud R. C., and Goldberg M. E. (1973b) Effects of Δ^9*trans*-tetrahydrocannabinol and its selectivity in several models of aggressive behavior. *Pharmacology* **9**, 204–216.

Eibl-Eibesfeldt I. (1961) The fighting behavior of animals. *Sci. Am.* **203**, 112–120.

Eibl-Eibesfeldt I. (1970) *Ethology. The Biology of Behavior.* Holt, Rinehart and Winston, New York.

Eichelman B. (1979) The Role of Biogenic Amines in Aggressive Behavior, in *Psychopharmacology of Aggression* (Sandler, M., ed.), Raven, New York.

Eichelman B. and Barchas J. (1975) Facilitated shock-induced aggression following anti-depressive medication in the rat. *Pharmacol. Biochem. Behav.* **3**, 601–604.

Eichelman B. S., Jr., and Thoa N. B. (1973) The aggressive monoamines. *Biol. Psychiatry* **6**, 143–164.

Eichelman B., Orenberg E., Hackley P., and Barchas J. (1978) Methylxanthine-facilitated shock-induced aggression in the rat. *Psychopharmacology* **56**, 305–308.

Eichelman B. Seagraves E., and Barchas J. (1977) Alkali metal cations: Effects on isolation-induced aggression in the mouse. *Pharmacol. Biochem. Behav.* **7**, 407–409.

Eichelman B., Thoa N. B., and Perez-Cruet J. (1973) Alkali metal cations: Effects on aggression and adrenal enzymes. *Pharmacol. Biochem. Beh.* **1**, 121–123.

Emley G. S. and Hutchinson R. R. (1972) Basis of behavioral influence of chlorpromazine. *Life Sci.* **11**, 43–47.

Emley G. S. and Hutchinson R. R. (1983) Unique influences of ten drugs upon post-shock biting attack and pre-shock manual responding. *Pharmacol. Biochem. Behav.* **19**, 5–12.

Erskine M. S., Barfield R. J., and Goldman B. D. (1978) Intraspecific fighting during late pregnancy and lactation in rats and effects of litter removal. *Behav. Biol.* **23**, 206–218.

Erskine M. S., Barfield R. J., and Goldman B. D. (1980) Postpartum aggression in rats: I. Effects of hypophysectomy. *J. Comp. Physiol. Psychol.* **94,** 484–494.

Everett G. M. (1975) Role of Biogenic Amines in the Modulation of Aggressive and Sexual Behavior in Animals and Man, in *Sexual Behavior: Pharmacology and Biochemistry* (Sandler M. and Gessa G. L., eds.), Raven, New York.

Fagen R. M. and Young D. Y. (1978) Temporal Patterns of Behavior: Durations, Intervals, Latencies and Sequences, in *Quantitative Ethology* (Colgan P. W., ed.), John Wiley, New York.

Falk J. L. (1971) The nature and determinants of adjunctive behavior. *Physiol. Behav.* **6,** 577–588.

Falk J. L. (1977) The origin and functions of adjunctive behavior. *Anim. Learning Behav.* **5,** 325–335.

Fanselow M. S. and Sigmundi R. A. (1982) The enhancement and reduction of defensive fighting by naloxone pretreatment. *Physiol. Psychol.* **10,** 313–316.

Fanselow M. S., Sigmundi R. A., and Bolles R. C. (1980) Naloxone pretreatment enhances shock-elicited aggression. *Physiol. Psychol.* **8,** 369–371.

Ferrari F. and Baggio G. (1982) Influence of lisuride on morphine withdrawal signs in the rat: A dopamine-mimetic effect. *Psychopharmacology* **78,** 326–330.

Ferster C. B. and Skinner B. F. (1957) *Schedules of Reinforcement.* Appleton-Century-Crofts, New York.

Figler M. H., Klein R. M., and Radford R. B. (1973) Effects of chlordiazepoxide (librium) on the attack behavior of male Siamese fighting fish, *Betta splendens. Psychopharmacologia* **33,** 277–292.

Figler M. H., Klein R. M., and Thompson C. S. (1975) Chlordiazepoxide (Librium)-induced changes in intraspecific attack and selected non-agonistic behaviors in male Siamese fighting fish. *Psychopharmacologia* **42,** 139–145.

File S. E. and Hyde J. R. G. (1978) Can social interaction be used to measure anxiety?. *Br. J. Pharmacol.* **62,** 19–24.

Floody O. R. (1983) Hormones and Aggression in Female Mammals, in *Hormones and Aggressive Behavior* (Svare B. B., ed.), *Plenum,* New York.

Flynn J. P. (1967) The Neural Basis of Aggression in Cats, in *Neurophysiology and Emotion* (Glass D. C., ed.), Rockefeller University, New York.

Flynn J. P. (1969) Neural aspects of attack behavior in cats. *Ann. NY Acad. Sci.* **159,** 1008–1012.

Fog R. (1969) Rage reactions produced in rats by a combination of thymoleptics and monoamine oxidase inhibitors. *Pharmacol. Res. Comm.* **1,** 79–83.

Fukuda T. and Tsumagari T. (1983) Effects of psychotropic drugs on the rage responses induced by electrical stimulation of the medial hypothalamus in cats. *Jpn. J. Pharmacol.* **33,** 885–890.

Funderburk W. H., Foxwell M. H., and Hakala M. W. (1970) Effects of psychotherapeutic drugs on hypothalamic-induced hissing in cats. *Neuropharmacology* **9,** 1–7.

Gandelman R. (1980) Gonadal hormones and the induction of intraspecific fighting in mice. *Neurosci. Biobehav. Rev.* **4,** 133–140.

Garattini S. (1965) Effects of a Cannabis Extract on Gross Behavior, in *Hashish: Its Chemistry and Pharmacology* (Wolstenholme G. E. W. and Knight J., eds.), J. & A. Churchill, London.

Garattini S. and Valzelli L. (1981) Is the isolated animal a possible model for phobia and anxiety? *Prog. Neuropsychopharmacol.* **5,** 159–165.

Garattini S., Giacalone E., and Valzelli L. (1967) Isolation, aggressiveness and brain 5-hydroxytryptamine turnover. *J. Pharm. Pharmacol.* **19,** 338–339.

Gardner C. R. and Guy A. P. (1984) A social interaction model of anxiety sensitive to acutely administered benzodiazepines. *Drug Dev. Res.* **4,** 207–216.

Genovese E., Napoli P. A., and Bolego-Zonta N. (1969) Self-aggressiveness: A new type of behavioral change induced by pemoline. *Life Sci.* **8,** 513–515.

Gianutsos G. and Lal H. (1976) Blockade of apomorphine-induced aggression by morphine or neuroleptics: Differential alteration by antimuscarinics and naloxone. *Pharmacol. Biochem. Behav.* **4,** 639–642.

Gianutsos G. and Lal H. (1977) Modification of apomorphine induced aggression by changing central cholinergic activity in rats.*Neuropharmacology* **16,** 7–10.

Gianutsos G. and Lal H. (1978) Narcotic Analgesics and Aggression, in *Psychopharmacology of Aggression* (Valzelli L., ed.). S. Karger, New York.

Gianutsos G., Hynes M. D., Drawbaugh R. B., and Lal H. (1975) Paradoxical absence of aggression during naloxone-precipitated morphine withdrawal. *Psychopharmacologia* **43,** 43–46.

Gianutsos G., Hynes M. D., and Lal H. (1976) Enhancement of morphine-withdrawal and apomorphine-induced aggression by clonidine. *Psychopharmacol. Commun.* **2,** 165–171.

Gianutsos G., Hynes M. D., Puri S. K., Drawbaugh R. B., and Lal H. (1974) Effect of apomorphine and nigrostriatal lesions on aggression and striatal dopamine turnover during morphine withdrawal: Evidence for dopaminergic supersensitivity in protracted abstinence. *Psychopharmacologia* **34,** 37–44.

Ginsburg B. and Allee W. C. (1942) Some effects of conditioning on social dominance and subordination in inbred strains of mice. *Physiol. Zool.* **15,** 485–506.

Goldberg M. E., Insalaco J. R., Hefner M. A., and Salama A. I. (1973) Effect of prolonged isolation on learning, biogenic amine turnover and aggressive behaviour in three strains of mice. *Neuropharmacology* **12,** 1049–1058.

Goldstein A. and Schulz R. (1977) Morphine tolerant longitudinal muscle strip from guinea-pig ileum. *Br. J. Pharmacol.* **42,** 655–666.

Gorelick D. A., Elliott M. L., and Sbordone R. J. (1981) Naloxone increases shock-elicited aggression in rats. *Res. Commun. Subst. Abuse* **2,** 419–422.

Grant E. C. and MacKintosh J. H. (1963) A comparison of the social postures of some common laboratory rodents. *Behaviour* **21,** 246–259.

Gray W. D., Osterberg A. C., and Rauth C. E. (1961) Neuropharmacological actions of mephenoxalone. *Arch. Int. Pharmacodyn. Ther.* **134,** 198–215.

Haber S., Barchas P. R., and Barchas J. D. (1981) A primate analogue of amphetamine-induced behaviors in humans. *Biol. Psychiatry* **16,** 181–195.

Hahn R. A., Hynes M. D., and Fuller R. W. (1982) Apomorphine-induced aggression in rat chronically treated with oral clonidine: Modulation by central noradrenergic mechanisms. *J. Pharmacol. Exp. Ther.* **220,** 389–393.

Halas E., Reynolds G., Rowe M., Heinrich M., and Pirc M. (1977) Comparison of frequency, intensity, and duration of aggressive responses in rats. *Physiol. Behav.* **18,** 975–977.

Hegstrand L. R. and Eichelman B. (1983) Increased shock-induced fighting with supersensitive beta-adrenergic receptors. *Pharmacol. Biochem. Behav.* **19,** 313–320.

Hess W. R. (1928) Stammganglien-Reizversuche. *Berichte uber die gesamte. Physiol. Exp. Pharmakol.* **42,** 554–555.

Hess W. R. (1948) *Das Zwischenhirn.* Benno Schwabe, Basel.

Hess W. R. and Brugger M. (1943) Das subkortikale Zentrum der affektiven Abwehrreaktion. *Helv. Physiol. Acta* **1,** 33–52.

Hinde R. A. (Ed.) (1983) *Primate Social Relationships.* Blackwell, Oxford.

Hodge G. K. and Butcher L. L. (1975) Catecholamine correlates of isolation-induced aggression in mice. *Eur. J. Pharmacol.* **31,** 81–93.

Hoffmeister F. and Wuttke W. (1969) On the Actions of Psychotropic Drugs on the Attack- and Aggressive-Defensive Behaviour of Mice and Cats, in *Aggressive Behaviour* (Garattini S. and Sigg E. B., ed.) *Excerpta Medica Foundation*, Amsterdam.

Hopf S., Hartmann-Weisner E., Kuhlmorgen B., and Mayer S. (1974) The behavioral repertoire of the squirrel monkey. *Folia Primatol.* **21,** 225–249.

Hutchinson R. R. (1983) The pain–aggression relationship and its expression in naturalistic settings. *Aggressive Behav.* **9,** 229–242.

Hutchinson R. R. and Emley G. S. (1973) Effects of Nicotine on Avoidance, Conditioned Suppression and Aggression Response Measures in Animals and Man, in *Smoking Behavior: Motives and Incentives* (Dunn W. L., ed.), V. H. Winston, Washington.

Hutchinson R. R., Azrin N. H., and Hake D. F. (1966) An automatic method for the study of aggression in squirrel monkeys. *J. Exp. Anal. Behav.* **9,** 233–237.

Hutchinson R. R., Azrin N. H., and Renefrew J. W. (1968) Effects of shock intensity and duration on the frequency of biting attack by squirrel monkeys. *J. Exp. Anal. Behav.* **11,** 83–88.

Hutchinson R. R., Emly G. S., and Krasnegor N. A. (1977) The Effect of Cocaine on the Aggressive Behavior of Mice, Pigeons, and Squirrel Monkeys, in *Cocaine and Other Stimulants* (Ellinwood E. H., Jr. and Kilbey M. M., eds.), Plenum, New York.

Hynes M. D., Gianutsos G., and Lal H. (1976) Effects of cholinergic agonists and antagonists on morphine-withdrawal syndrome. *Psychopharmacology* **49,** 191–195.

Iorio L. C., Deacon M. A., and Ryan E. A. (1975) Blockade by narcotic drugs of naloxone precipitated jumping in morphine-dependent mice. *J. Pharmacol. Exp. Ther.* **192,** 58–63.

Irwin S., Kinohi R., Van Sloten M., and Workman M. P. (1971) Drug effects on distress-evoked behavior in mice: Methodology and drug class comparisons. *Psychopharmacologia* **20,** 172–185.

Janssen P. A. J., Jageneau A. H., and Niemegeers J. E. (1960) Effects of various drugs on isolation-induced fighting behavior of male mice. *J. Pharmacol. Exp. Ther.* **129,** 471–475.

Jarvis M. F., Kreiger M., Cohen G., and Wagner G. C. (1985) The effects of phencyclidine and chlordiazepoxide on target-biting of confined male mice. *Aggressive Behav.* **11,** 201–205.

Kamioka T., Nakayama I., Akiyama S., and Takagi H. (1977) Effects of oxazolam, cloxazolam, and CS-386, new anti-anxiety drugs, on socially induced suppression and aggression in pairs of monkeys. *Psychopharmacology* **52,** 17–23.

Kantak K. and Miczek K. A. (1982) Pharmacological separation of aggression from other symptoms of morphine withdrawal. *Neurosci. Abst.* **8,** (2), 592.

Karczmar A. G., Richardson D. C., and Kindel G. (1978) Neuropharmacological and related aspects of animal aggression. *Prog. Neuropsychopharmacol.* **2,** 611–631.

Karli P. (1981) Conceptual and Methodological Problems Associated With the Study of Brain Mechanisms Underlying Aggressive Behavior, in *The Biology of Aggression* (Brain P. F. and Benton D., eds.), Sijthoff and Noordhoff, Rockville, Maryland.

Katz R. J. (1981) Possible muscarinic-cholinergic mediation of patterned aggressive reflexes in the cat. *Prog. Neuropsychopharmacol.* **5,** 49–56.

Katz R. J. and Thomas E. (1975) Effects of scopolamine and alpha-methyl-para-tyrosine upon predatory attack in cats. *Psychopharmacologia* **42,** 153–157.

Katz R. J. and Thomas E. (1976) Effects of a novel antiaggressive agent upon two types of brain stimulated emotional behavior. *Psychopharmacology* **48,** 79–82.

Kjellberg B. and Randrup A. (1973) Disruption of social behavior of vervet monkeys (*Cercopithecus*) by low doses of amphetamines. *Pharmakopsychiatrie* **6**, 287–293.

Kletzkin M. (1969) An Experimental Analysis of Aggressive-Defensive Behaviour in Mice, in *Aggressive Behavior* (Garattini S. and Sigg E. B., eds.), Excerpta Medica Foundation, Amsterdam.

Koolhaas J. M. (1978) Hypothalamically induced intraspecific aggressive behavior in the rat. *Exp. Brain Res.* **32**, 365–375.

Korf J. and Kuiper H. E. (1971) Induction of bizarre behaviour in rats by *p*-chloroamphetamine, a serotonin depletor, after repeated drug administration. *Psychopharmacologia* **21**, 328–337.

Kostowski W. (1966) A note on the effects of some psychotropic drugs on the aggressive behaviour in the ant, *Formica Rufa. J. Pharm. Pharmacol.* **18**, 747–749.

Krsiak M. (1974) Behavioral changes and aggressivity evoked by drugs in mice. *Res. Commun. Chem. Pathol. Pharmacol.* **7**, 237–257.

Krsiak M. (1975) Timid singly-housed mice: Their value in prediction of psychotropic activity of drugs. *Br. J. Pharmacol.* **55**, 141–150.

Krsiak M. (1976) Effect of ethanol on aggression and timidity in mice. *Psychopharmacology* **51**, 75–80.

Krsiak M. (1979) Effects of drugs on behaviour of aggressive mice. *Br. J. Pharmacol.* **65**, 525–533.

Krsiak M. and Pribik V. (1978) Effect of amphetamine on sequences of behavioral activities in mice. *Act. Nerv. Super.* **20**, 9–11.

Krsiak M., Borgesova M., and Kadlecova O. (1971) LSD-accentuated individual type of social behavior in mice. *Act. Nerv. Super.* **13**, 211–212.

Krsiak M., Sulcova A., Donat P., Tomasikova Z., Dlohozkova N., Kosar E., and Masek K. (1984) Can Social and Agonistic Interactions be Used to Detect Anxiolytic Activity of Drugs, in *Ethopharmacological Aggression Research* (Miczek K. A., Kruk M. R., and Olivier B., eds.), Alan R. Liss, New York.

Krsiak M., Sulcova A., Tomasikova Z., Dlohozkova N., Kosar E., and Masek K. (1981) Drug effects on attack, defense and escape in mice. *Pharmacol. Biochem. Behav.* **14**, 47–52.

Kruk M. R., Van Der Poel A. M., and De Vos-Frerichs T. P. (1979) Induction of aggressive behaviour by electrical stimulation in the hypothalamus of male rats. *Behaviour* **70**, 292–322.

Lagerspetz K. M. J. and Ekqvist K. (1978) Failure to induce aggression in inhibited and in genetically non-aggressive mice through injections of ethyl alcohol. *Aggressive Behav.* **4**, 105–113.

Lal H. (1975a) Narcotic dependence, narcotic action and dopamine receptors. *Life Sci.* **17**, 483–496.

Lal H. (1975b) Morphine-Withdrawal Aggression, in *Methods in Narcotic Research* (Ehrenpreis S., and Neidel E. A., eds.), Marcel Dekker, New York.

Lal H. and Puri S. K. (1972) Morphine-Withdrawal Aggression: Role of Dopaminergic Stimulation, in *Drug Addiction: Experimental Pharmacology* (Singh J. M., Miller L., and Lal H., eds.), Futura, New York.

Lal H., Defeo J. J., and Thut P. (1968) Effect of amphetamine on pain-induced aggression. *Commun. Behav. Biol.* **1**, 333–336.

Lal H., Gianutsos G., and Puri S. K. (1975) A comparison of narcotic analgesics with neuroleptics on behavioral measures of dopaminergic activity. *Life Sci.* **17**, 29–34.

Lal H., O'Brien J., and Puri S. K. (1971) Morphine-withdrawal aggression: Sensitization by amphetamines. *Psychopharmacologia* **22**, 217–223.

Lammers A. J. J. C. and van Rossum J. M. (1968) Bizzare social behavior in rats induced by a combination of a peripheral decarboxylase inhibitor and DOPA. *Eur. J. Pharmacol.* **5**, 103–106.

Lapin I. P. (1967) Simple pharmacological procedures to differentiate antidepressants and cholinolytics in mice and rats. *Psychopharmacologia* **11**, 79–87.

Lassen J. B. (1978) Piperoxane reduces the effects of clonidine on aggression in mice and noradrenaline dependent hypermotility in rats. *Eur. J. Pharmacol.* **47**, 45–49.

LeDouarec J. C. and Broussy L. (1969) Dissociation of the Aggressive Behavior of Mice Produced by Certain Drugs, in *Aggressive Behavior* (Garattini S. and Sigg E. B., eds.), Excerpta Medica Foundation, Amsterdam.

Leyhausen P. (1960) *Verhaltensstudien an Katzen.* Paul Parey Verlag, Berlin.

Looney T. A. and Cohen P. S. (1982) Aggression induced by intermittent positive reinforcement. *Biobehav. Rev.* **6**, 15–37.

Lynch W. C., Libby L., and Johnson H. F. (1983) Naloxone inhibits intermale aggression in isolated mice. *Psychopharmacology* **79**, 370–371.

MacDonnell M. F. and Ehmer M. (1969) Some effects of ethanol on aggressive behavior in cats. *Quart. J. Stud. Alcohol* **30**, 312–319.

MacDonnell M. and Flynn J. P. (1964) Attack elicited by stimulation of the thalamus of cats. *Science* **5**, 1249–1250.

MacDonnell M. F., Fessock L., and Brown S. H. (1971a) Ethanol and the neural substrate for affective defense in the cat. *Q. J. Stud. Alcohol* **32**, 406–419.

MacDonnell M. F., Fessock L., and Brown S. H. (1971b) Aggression and associated neural events in cats. Effects of *p*-chlorophenylalanine compared with alcohol. *Q. J. Stud. Alcohol* **32**, 748–763.

Maj J., Molgilnika E., and Kordecka A. (1979) Chronic treatment with antidepressant drugs: Potentiation of apomorphine-induced aggressive behavior in rats. *Neurosci. Lett.* **13**, 337–341.

Maj J., Rogoz Z., Skuza G., and Sowinska H. (1982) Effects of chronic treatment with antidepressants on aggressiveness induced by clonidine. *J. Neural Transm.* **55**, 19–25.

Malick J. B. (1978) Selective antagonism of isolation-induced aggression in mice by diazepam following chronic administration. *Pharmacol. Biochem. Behav.* **8**, 497–499.

Malick J. B. (1979) The Pharmacology of Isolation-Induced Aggressive Behavior in Mice, in *Current Developments in Psychopharmacology* (Essman W. B. and Valzelli L., eds.), SP Medical & Scientific Books, New York.

Mann M., Michael S. D., and Svare B. (1980) Ergot drugs suppress plasma prolactin and lactation but not aggression in parturient mice. *Horm. Behav.* **14**, 319–328.

Manning F. J. and Elsmore T. F. (1972) Shock-elicited fighting and delta-9-tetrahydrocannabinol. *Psychopharmacologia* **25**, 218–228.

Marini J. L., Sheard M. H., and Kosten T. (1979a) Study of the role of serotonin in lithium action using shock-elicited fighting. *Commun. Psychopharmacol.* **3**, 225–233.

Marini J. L., Walters J. K., and Sheard M. H. (1979b) Effects of *d*- and *l*-amphetamine on hypothalamically-elicited movement and attack in the cat. *Agressolgie* **20**, 155–160.

Masserman J. H. (1937) Effects of sodium amytal and other drugs on the reactivity of the hypothalamus of the cat. *Arch. Neurol. Psychiatry* **37**, 617–628.

Matte A. C. (1975) Effects of hashish on isolation induced aggression in wild mice. *Psychopharmacologia* **45**, 125–128.

McGivern R. F., Lobaugh N. J., and Collier A. C. (1981) Effect of naloxone and housing conditions on shock-elicited reflexive fighting: Influence of immediate prior stress. *Physiol. Psychol.* **9**, 251–256.

McGlone J. J., Ritter S., and Kelley K. W. (1980) The antiaggressive effect of lithium is abolished by area postrema lesion. *Physiol. Behav.* **24**, 1095–1100.

McKenzie G. M. (1971) Apomorphine-induced aggression in the rat. *Brain Res.* **34**, 323–330.

McKenzie G. M. (1981) Dissociation of the antiaggression and serotonin-depleting effects of fenfluramine. *Can. J. Physiol. Pharmacol.* **59**, 830.

Melander B. (1960) Psychopharmacodynamic effects of diethylpropion. *Acta Pharmacol. Toxicol.* **17**, 182–190.

Miczek K. A. (1974) Intraspecies aggression in rats: Effects of *d*-amphetamine and chlordiazepoxide. *Psychopharmacologia* **39**, 275–301.

Miczek K. A. (1976) Does THC Induce Aggression? Suppression and Induction of Aggressive Reactions by Chronic and Acute delta-9-Tetrahydrocannabinol Treatment in Laboratory Rats, in *Pharmacology of Marihuana* (Braude M., and Szara S., eds.), Raven, New York.

Miczek K. A. (1978) delta-9-Tetrahydrocannabinol: Antiaggressive effects in mice, rats, and squirrel monkeys. *Science* **199**, 1459–1461.

Miczek K. A. (1979) A new test for aggression in rats without aversive stimulation: Differential effects of *d*-amphetamine and cocaine. *Psychopharmacology* **60**, 253–259.

Miczek K. A. (1981) Differential antagonism of *d*-amphetamine effects on motor activity and agonistic behavior in mice. *Neurosci. Abs.* **7**, 343.

Miczek K. A. (1983a) Ethological Analysis of Drug Action on Aggression, Defense and Defeat, in *Behavioral Models and the Analysis of Drug Action* (Spiegelstein M. Y. and Levy A., eds.), Elsevier, Amsterdam.

Miczek K. A. (1983b) Ethological analysis of drug action on aggression and defense. *Prog. Neuropsychopharmacol. Biol. Psychiatry* **7**, 519–524.

Miczek K. A. (1984) Separate mechanisms for diazepam's effects on aggression and punished drinking. *Neurosci. Abs.* **10**, 17.

Miczek K. A. (1986) Diazepam increases aggressive behavior and punishment-suppressed drinking: Antagonism by Ro15–1788. *Psychopharmacology* (in press).

Miczek K. A. and Barry H., III (1974) delta-9-Tetrahydrocannabinol and aggressive behavior in rats. *Behav. Biol.* **11**, 261–267.

Miczek K. A. and Barry H., III (1977) Effects of alcohol on attack and defensive–submissive reactions in rats. *Psychopharmacology* **52**, 231–237.

Miczek K. A. and DeBold J. F. (1983) Hormone-Drug Interactions and Their Influence on Aggressive Behavior, in *Hormones and Aggressive Behavior* (Svare, B. B., ed.), Plenum, New York.

Miczek K. A. and Gold L. H. (1983a) Ethological Analysis of Amphetamine Action on Social Behavior in Squirrel Monkeys (*Saimiri sciureus*), in *Ethopharmacology: Primate Models of Neuropsychiatric Disorders* (Miczek K. A., ed.), Alan R. Liss, New York.

Miczek K. A. and Gold L. H. (1983b) *d*-Amphetamine in squirrel monkeys of different social status: Effects on social and agonistic behavior, locomotion, and stereotypies. *Psychopharmacology* **81**, 183–190.

Miczek K. A. and Krsiak M. (1979) Drug Effects on Agonistic Behavior, in *Advances in Behavioral Pharmacology* (Thompson T. and Dews P. B., eds.), Academic, New York.

Miczek K. A. and Krsiak M. (1981) Pharmacological Analysis of Attack and Flight, in *A Multidisciplinary Approach to Aggression Research* (Brain P. F. and Benton D., eds.), Elsevier, Amsterdam.

Miczek K. A. and O'Donnell J. M. (1978) Intruder-evoked aggression in isolated and nonisolated mice: Effects of psychomotor stimulants and L-dopa. *Psychopharmacology* **57**, 47–55.

Miczek K. A. and Yoshimura H. (1982) Disruption of primate social behavior by *d*-amphetamine and cocaine: Differential antagonism by antipsychotics. *Psychopharmacology* **76,** 163– 171.

Miczek K. A., Thompson M. L., and Shuster L. (1982) Opioid-like analgesia in defeated mice. *Science* **215,** 1520–1522.

Miczek K. A., Altman J. L., Appel J. B., and Boggan W. O. (1975) Para-chlorophenylalanine, serotonin and killing behavior. *Pharmacol. Biochem. Behav.* **3,** 355–361.

Miller N. (1965) Chemical coding of behavior in the brain. *Science* **148,** 328–338.

Mogilnicka E. and Przewlocka B. (1981) Facilitated shock-induced aggression after chronic treatment with antidepressant drugs in the rat. *Pharmacol. Biochem. Behav.* **14,** 129–132.

Mogilnicka E., Boissard C. G., Waldmeier P. C., and Delini-Stula A. (1983) The effects of single and repeated doses of maprotiline, oxaprotiline and its enantiomers on foot-shock induced fighting in rats. *Pharmacol. Biochem. Behav.* **19,** 719–723.

Moore M. S., Tychson R. L., and Thompson D. M. (1976) Extinction-induced mirror responding as a baseline for studying drug effects on aggression. *Pharmacol. Biochem. Behav.* **4,** 99–102.

Mueller K. and Nyhan W. L. (1982) Pharmacologic control of pemoline induced self-injurious behavior in rats. *Pharmacol. Biochem. Behav.* **16,** 957–963.

Mueller K. and Nyhan W. L. (1983) Clonidine potentiates drug induced self-injurious behavior in rats. *Pharmacol. Biochem. Behav.* **18,** 891–894.

Mueller K., Saboda S., Palmour R., and Nyhan W. L. (1982) Self-injurious behavior produced in rats by daily caffeine and continuous amphetamine. *Pharmacol. Biochem. Behav.* **17,** 613–617.

Mukherjee B. P. and Pradhan S. N. (1976) Effects of lithium on foot shock-induced aggressive behavior in rats. *Arch. Int. Pharmacodyn. Ther.* **222,** 125–131.

Nakamura K. and Thoenen H. (1972) Increased irritability: A permanent behavior change induced in the rat by intraventricular administration of 6-hydroxydopamine. *Psychopharmacologia* **24,** 359–372.

Nath C., Gulati A., Dhawan K. N., Gupta G. P., and Bhargava K. P. (1982) Evidence for central histaminergic mechanism in foot shock aggression. *Psychopharmacology* **76,** 228–231.

Ogawa S. and Makino J. (1984) Aggressive behavior in inbred strains of mice during pregnancy. *Behav. Neural Biol.* **40,** 195–204.

O'Kelly L. I. and Steckle L. C. (1939) A note on long enduring emotional responses in the rat. *J. Psychol.* **8,** 125–131.

Olivier B. (1981) Selective anti-aggressive properties of DU 27725: Ethological analyses of intermale and territorial aggression in the male rat. *Pharmacol. Biochem. Behav.* **14,S1,** 61–77.

Olivier B. and van Dalen D. (1982) Social behavior in rats and mice: An ethologically based model for differentiating psychoactive drugs. *Aggressive Behav.* **8,** 163–168.

Olivier B., Mos J., and van Oorschot R. (1985) Maternal aggression in rats: Effects of chlordiazepoxide and fluprazine. *Psychopharmacology* **86,** 68–76.

Olivier B., van Aken H., Jaarsma I., van Oorschot R., Zethof T., and Bradford D. (1984) Behavioral Effects of Psychoactive Drugs on Agonistic Behavior of Male Territorial Rats (Resident–Intruder Model), in *Ethopharmacological Aggression Research* (Miczek K. A., Kruk M. R., and Olivier B., eds.), Alan R. Liss, New York.

Olpe H. R. (1978) Pharmacological manipulations of the automatically recorded biting behavior evoked in rats by apomorphine. *Eur. J. Pharmacol.* **51,** 441–448.

Ozawa H., Michauchi T., and Sugawara K. (1975) Potentiating effect of lithium chloride on aggressive behaviour induced in mice by nialamide plus *L*-DOPA and by clonidine. *Eur. J. Pharmacol.* **34,** 169–179.

Panksepp J. (1971a) Drugs and stimulus-bound attack. *Physiol. Behav.* **6,** 317–320.

Panksepp J. (1971b) Aggression elicited by electrical stimulation of the hypothalamus in albino rats. *Physiol. Behav.* **6,** 321–329.

Patni S. K. and Dandiya P. C. (1974) Apomorphine induced biting and fighting behaviour in reserpinized rats and an approach to the mechanism of action. *Life Sci.* **14,** 737–745.

Peeke H. V. S., Cutler L., Ellman G., Figler, M., Gordon, D., and Peeke, S. C. (1981) Effects of alcohol, congeners, and acetaldehyde on aggressive behavior of the Convict Cichlid. *Psychopharmacology* **75,** 245–247.

Peeke H. V. S., Ellman G. E., and Herz M. J. (1973) Dose dependent alcohol effects on the aggressive behavior of the Convict Cichlid (*Cichlasoma nigrofaciatum*). *Behav. Biol.* **8,** 115–122.

Peeke H. V. S., Peeke S. C., Avis H. H., and Ellman G. (1975) Alcohol, habituation and the patterning of aggressive responses in a cichlid fish. *Pharmacol. Biochem. Behav.* **3,** 1031–1036.

Penaloza-Rojas J. H., Bach-y-Rita G., Rubio-Chevannier H. F., and Hernandez-Peon R. (1961) Effects of imipramine on hypothalamic and amygdaloid excitability. *Exp. Neurol.* **4,** 205–213.

Poole T. B. (1973) Some studies on the influence of chlordiazepoxide on the social interaction of golden hamsters (*Mesocricetus auratus*). *Br. J. Pharmacol.* **48,** 538–545.

Poshivalov V. P. (1974) Pharmacological analysis of aggressive behaviour of mice induced by isolation. *J. Higher Nerv. Activity* **24,** 1079–1081.

Poshivalov V. P. (1978) Ethological analysis of the action exerted by medazepam and diazepam on the zoosocial behavior of isolated mice. *Farmacol. Toksikol.* **41,** 263–266.

Poshivalov V. P. (1981) Pharmaco-ethological analysis of social behaviour of isolated mice. *Pharmacol. Biochem. Behav.* **14,S1,** 53–59.

Poshivalov V. P. (1982) Ethological analysis of neuropeptides and psychotropic drugs: Effects on intraspecies aggression and sociability of isolated mice. *Aggressive Behav.* **8,** 355–369.

Poshivalov V. P. and Khodko S. T. (1984) Mathematical Description and Experimental Pharmaco-Ethological Analysis of Animal Intraspecific Agonistic Behavior, in *Ethopharmacological Aggression Research* (Miczek K. A., ed.), Alan R. Liss, New York.

Powell D. A., Walters K., Duncan S., and Holley J. R. (1973) The effects of chlorpromazine and *d*-amphetamine upon shock-elicited aggression. *Psychopharmacologia* **30,** 303–314.

Pradhan S. N. (1975) Aggression and Central Neurotransmitters, in *International Review of Neurobiology* (Pfeiffer C. C. and Smythies J. M., eds.), Academic, New York.

Pradhan S. N., Ghosh B., Aulakh C. S., and Bhattacharyya A. K. (1980) Effects of delta-9-tetrahydrocannabinol on foot shock-induced aggression in rats. *Commun. Psychopharmacol.* **4,** 27–34.

Prasad V. and Sheard M. H. (1982) Effect of lithium upon desipramine enhanced shock-elicited fighting in rats. *Pharmacol. Biochem. Behav.* **17,** 337–378.

Pritchett J., Cole B. T., and Powell D. A. (1979) Effects of prior shock and scopolamine on aggressive behavior and blood glucose levels in the rat. *Behav. Neural Biol.* **25,** 176–189.

Pucilowski O. and Kostowski W. (1983) Aggressive behaviour and the central serotonergic systems. *Behav. Brain Res.* **9,** 33–48.

Puglisi-Allegra S. and Mandel P. (1980) Effects of sodium n-dipropyl-acetate, muscimol hydrobromide and (R,S) nipecotic acid amide on isolation-induced aggressive behavior in mice. *Psychopharmacology* **70,** 287–290.

Puglisi-Allegra S. and Renzi P. (1977) A technique for the measurement of aggressive behavior in mice. *Behav. Res. Meth. Inst.* **9,** 503–504.

Puglisi-Allegra S. and Renzi P. (1980) An automated device for screening the effects of psychotropic drugs on aggression and motor activity in mice. *Pharmacol. Biochem. Behav.* **13,** 287–290.

Pulgisi-Allegra S. and Oliverio A. (1981) Naloxone potentiates shock-induced aggressive behavior in mice. *Pharmacol. Biochem. Behav.* **15,** 513–514.

Puglisi-Allegra S., Mele A., and Cabib S. (1984) Involvement of Endogenous Opioid Systems in Social Behavior of Individually Housed Mice, in *Ethopharmacological Aggression Research* (Miczek K. A., Kruk M. R., and Olivier B., eds.), Alan R. Liss, New York.

Puglisi-Allegra S., Olivierio A., and Mandel P. (1982) Effects of opiate antagonists on social and aggressive behavior of isolated mice. *Pharmacol. Biochem. Behav.* **17,** 691–694.

Puri S. K. and Lal H. (1973) Effect of dopaminergic stimulation or blockade on morphine-withdrawal aggression. *Psychopharmacology* **32,** 113–120.

Puri S. K. and Lal H. (1974) Reduced threshold to pain induced aggression specifically related to morphine dependence. *Psychopharmacology* **35,** 237–241.

Quenzer L. F., Feldman R. S., and Moore, J. W. (1974) Toward a mechanism of the anti-aggression effects of chlordiazepoxide in rats. *Psychopharmacologia* **34,** 81–94.

Raab A. and Oswald R. (1980) Coping with social conflict: Impact on the activity of tyrosine hydroxylase in the limbic system and in the adrenals. *Physiol. Behav.* **24,** 387–394.

Raleigh M. J., Brammer G. L., and McGuire M. T. (1983a) Male Dominance, Serotonergic Systems, and the Behavioral and

Physiological Effects of Drugs in Vervet Monkeys (*Cercopithecus aethiops sabaeus*), in *Ethopharmacology: Primate Models of Neuropsychiatric Disorders* (Miczek K. A., ed.), Alan R. Liss, New York.

Raleigh M. J., Brammer G. L., McGuire M. T., Yuwiler A., Geller E., and Johnson C. K. (1983b) Social Status Related Differences in the Behavioral Effects of Drugs in Vervet Monkeys (*Cercopithecus aethiops sabaeus*), in *Hormones, Drugs and Social Behavior in Primates* (Stecklis H. D. and Kling A. S., eds.), Spectrum, New York.

Raleigh M. J., McGuire M. T., Brammer G. L., and Yuwiler A. (1984) Social and environmental influences on blood serotonin concentrations in monkeys. *Arch. Gen. Psychiatry* **41,** 405–410.

Randrup A. and Munkvad I. (1969) Relation of Brain Catecholamines to Aggressiveness and Other Forms of Behavioral Excitation, in *Aggressive Behavior* (Garattini S. and Sigg E. B., eds.), Excerpta Medica Foundation, Amsterdam.

Raynes A., Ryback R. S. (1970) Effect of alcohol and congeners on aggressive response in *Betta splendens. Q. J. Studies on Alcohol* **5,** 130–135.

Raynes A., Ryback R., and Ingle D. (1968) The effect of alcohol on aggression in *Betta splendens. Commun. Behav. Biol.* **2,** 141–146.

Reis D. J. (1974) The Chemical Coding of Aggression in Brain, in *Neurohumoral Coding of Brain Function* (Myers R. D. and Drucker-Colin R. R., eds.), Plenum, New York.

Rewerski W. J., Piechocki T., and Rylski M. (1973) Effects of Hallucinogens on Aggressiveness and Thermoregulation in Mice, in *The Pharmacology of Thermoregulation* (Schonbaum E. and Lomax P., eds.), Karger, New York.

Rodgers R. J. (1979) Effects of nicotine, mecamylamine, and hexamethonium on shock-induced fighting, pain reactivity, and locomotor behaviour in rats. *Psychopharmacology* **66,** 93–98.

Rodgers R. J. (1982) Differential effects of naloxone and diprenorphine on defensive behavior in rats. *Neuropharmacology* **21,** 1291–1294.

Rodgers R. J. and Brown K. (1973) The inhibition of shock-induced attack in rats by scopolamine. *IRCS Med. Sci.* **1,** 36.

Rodgers R. J. and Hendrie C. A. (1983) Social conflict activates status-dependent endogenous analgesic or hyperalgesic mechanisms in male mice: Effects of naloxone on nociception and behaviour. *Physiol. Behav.* **30**, 775–780.

Rolinski Z. and Herbut M. (1979) Determination of the role of serotonergic and cholinergic systems in apomorphine–induced aggressiveness in rats. *Pol. J. Pharmacol. Pharm.* **31**, 97–106.

Rolinski Z. and Herbut M. (1981) The role of the cholinergic system in footshock-induced mouse aggression. *Pol. J. Pharmacol. Pharm.* **33**, 177–183.

Rose R. M., Holaday J. W., and Bernstein I. S. (1971) Plasma testosterone, dominance rank and aggressive behavior in a group of male rhesus monkeys. *Nature* **231**, 366–368.

Ross S. B. and Ogren S. -O. (1976) Anti-aggressive action of dopamine-beta-hydroxylase inhibitors in mice. *J. Pharm. Pharmacol.* **28**, 590–592.

Sade D. S. (1967) Determinants of Dominance in a Group of Free-ranging Rhesus Monkeys, in *Social Communication among Primates* (Altmann S. A., ed.), University of Chicago, Chicago.

Santos M., Sampaio M. R. P., Fernandez N. S., and Carlini E. A. (1966) Effects of *Cannabis sativa* (marihuana) on fighting behavior of mice. *Psychopharmacologia* **8**, 437–444.

Sapolsky R. M. (1982) The endocrine stress-response and social status in the wild baboon. *Horm. Behav.* **16**, 279–292.

Sassenrath E. N. (1971) Increased adrenal responsiveness related to social stress in rhesus monkeys. *Horm. Behav.* **1**, 283–298.

Scheel-Kruger J. and Randrup A. (1968) Aggressive behavior provoked by pargyline in rats pretreated with diethyldithiocarbamate. *J. Pharm. Pharmacol.* **20**, 948–949.

Schiorring E. (1979) Social isolation and other behavioral changes in groups of adult vervet monkeys (*Cercopithecus aethiops*) produced by low, nonchronic doses of *d*-amphetamine. *Psychopharmacology* **64**, 297–302.

Schiorring E. and Hecht A. (1979) Behavioral effects of low, acute doses of *d*-amphetamine on the dyadic interaction between mother and infant vervet monkeys (*Cercopithecus aethiops*) during the first six postnatal months. *Psychopharmacology* **64**, 219–224.

Schlemmer R. F. and Davis J. M. (1981) Evidence for dopamine mediation of submissive gestures in the stumptail macaque monkey. *Pharmacol. Biochem. Behav.* **14,S1**, 95–102.

Schlemmer R. F. and Davis J. M. (1983) A Comparison of Three Psychomimetic-Induced Models of Psychosis in Non-Human Primate Social Colonies, in *Ethopharmacology: Primate Models of Neuropsychiatric Disorders* (Miczek K. A., ed.), Alan R. Liss, New York.

Schneider C. (1968) Behavioral effects of some morphine antagonists and hallucinogens in the rat. *Nature* **220,** 586–587.

Scott J. P. (1966) Agonistic behavior of mice and rats: A review. *Am. Zool.* **6,** 683–701.

Scott J. P. and Fredericson E. (1951) The causes of fighting in mice and rats. *Physiol. Zool.* **24,** 273–309.

Scott J. P., Lee C., and Ho J. E. (1971) Effects of fighting, genotype, and amphetamine sulfate on body temperature of mice. *J. Comp. Physiol. Psychol.* **76,** 349–352.

Scriabine A. and Blake M. (1962) Evaluation of centrally acting drugs in mice with fighting behavior induced by isolation. *Psychopharmacologia* **2,** 224–226.

Seevers M. H. and Deneau G. A. (1963) Physiological Aspects of Tolerance and Physical Dependence, in *Physiological Pharmacology* (Root W. S. and Hoffmann F. G., eds.), Academic, New York.

Senault B. (1968) Syndrome agressif induit par l'apomorphine chez le rat. *J. Physiol.* **60,** 543–544.

Senault B. (1970) Comportement d'aggressivité intraspecifique induit par l'apomorphine chez la rat. *Psychopharmacologia* **18,** 271–287.

Senault B. (1971) Influence de l'isolement sur le comportement d'agressivité intraspecifique induit par l'apomorphine chez le rat. *Psychopharmacoogia* **20,** 389–394.

Senault B. (1974) Amines cerebrales et comportement d'agressivité intraspecifique induit par l'apomorphine chez le rat. *Psychopharmacologia* **34,** 143–154.

Sheard M. H. (1967) The effects of amphetamine on attack behavior in the cat. *Brain Res.* **5,** 330–338.

Sheard M. H. (1969) The effect of *p*-chlorophenylalanine on behavior in rats: Relation to 5-hydroxytryptamine and 5-hydroxyindole acetic acid. *Brain Res.* **15,** 303–307.

Sheard M. H. (1970) Effect of lithium on foot shock aggression in rats. *Nature* **228,** 284–285.

Sheard M. H. (1981) Shock-induced fighting (SIF): Psychopharmacology studies. *Aggressive Behav.* **7**, 41–49.

Sheard M. H., Astrachan D. I., and Davis M. (1977) The effect of *d*-lysergic acid diethylamide (LSD) upon shock-elicited fighting in rats. *Life Sci.* **20**, 427–430.

Sieber B., Frischknecht H., and Waser P. G. (1980) Behavioral effect of hashish in mice III. Social interactions between two residents and an intruder male. *Psychopharmacology* **70**, 273–278.

Sieber B., Frishknecht H., and Waser P. (1982) Behavioral effects of hashish in mice in comparison with psychoactive drugs. *Gen. Pharmacol.* **13**, 315–320.

Silverman A. P. (1966) The social behaviour of laboratory rats and the action of chlorpromazine and other drugs. *Behaviour* **27**, 1–38.

Simler S., Puglisi-Allegra S., and Mandel P. (1983) Effects of n-dipropylacetate on aggressive behavior and brain GABA level in isolated mice. *Pharmacol. Biochem. Behav.* **18**, 717–720.

Skinner B. F. (1938) *The Behavior of Organisms.* MacMillan, New York.

Smith E. O. and Byrd L. D. (1983) Studying the Behavioral Effects of Drugs in Group-Living Nonhuman Primates, in *Ethopharmacology: Primate Models of Neuropsychiatric Disorders* (Miczek K. A., ed.), Alan R. Liss, New York.

Smith E. O. and Byrd L. D. (1984) Contrasting effects of *d*-amphetamine on affiliation and aggression in monkeys. *Pharmacol. Biochem. Behav.* **20**, 255–260.

Smith D. E., King M. B., and Hoebel B. G. (1970) Lateral hypothalamic control of killing: Evidence for a cholinoceptive mechanism. *Science* **167**, 900–901.

Smoothy R. and Berry M. S. (1983) Effects of ethanol on behavior of aggressive mice from two different strains: A comparison of simple and complex behavioral assessments. *Pharmacol. Biochem. Behav.* **19**, 645–653.

Sofia R. D. (1969) Effects of centrally active drugs on four models of experimentally-induced aggression in rodents. *Life Sci.* **8**, 705–716.

Sorenson C. A. and Gordon M. (1975) Effects of 6-hydroxydopamine on shock-elicited aggression, emotionality and maternal behavior in female rats. *Pharmacol. Biochem. Behav.* **3**, 331–335.

Stille G., Ackermann H., Eichenberger E., and Lauener H. (1963) Vergleichende pharmakologische Untersuchung eines neuen zentralen Stimulans, 1-*p*-tolyl-1-oxo-2-pyrro-lidino-*n*-pentan-HCL. *Arzneimittelforsch.* **13,** 871–877.

Stolerman I. P., Johnson C. A., Bunker P., and Jarvik M. P. (1975) Weight loss and shock-elicited aggression as indices of morphine abstinence in rats. *Psychopharmacologia* **45,** 157–161.

Sulcova A., Krsiak M., and Masek K. (1981) Effects of calcium valproate and aminooxyacetic acid on agonistic behaviour in mice. *Act. Nerv. Super.* **23,** 287–289.

Svare B. and Gandelman R. (1976) Postpartum aggression in mice: the influence of suckling stimulation. *Horm. and Behav.* **7,** 407–416.

Svare B. B. and Mann M. A. (1983) Hormonal Influences on Maternal Aggression, in *Hormones and Aggressive Behavior* (Svare B. B., ed.), Plenum, New York.

Tadokoro S. (1967) Effects of psychotropic drugs on socially induced suppression and aggression in rhesus monkeys. *Nipon Ishikai Zasshi* **58,** 21–27.

Tedeschi D. H., Fowler P. J., Miller E. B., and Macko E. (1969) Pharmacological Analysis of Footshock-Induced Fighting Behaviour, in *Aggressive Behavior* (Garattini S. and Sigg E. B., eds.), Excerpta Medica Foundation, Amsterdam.

Tedeschi R. E., Tedeschi D. H., Mucha A., Cook L., Mattis P. A., and Fellow E. J. (1959) Effects of various centrally acting drugs on fighting behavior. *J. Pharmacol. Exp. Ther.* **125,** 28–34.

ten Ham M. and de Jong Y. (1974) Tolerance to the hypothermic and aggression-attenuating effect of delta-8- and delta-9-tetrahydrocannabinol in mice. *Eur. J. Pharmacol.* **28,** 144–148.

ten Ham M. and de Jong Y. (1975) Absence of interaction between delta-9-tetrahydrocannabinol and cannabidiol (CBD) in aggression, muscle control and body temperature experiments in mice. *Psychopharmacologia* **41,** 169–174.

ten Ham M. and van Noordwijk J. (1973) Lack of tolerance to the effect of two terahydrocannabinols on aggressiveness. *Psychopharmacologia* **29,** 171–176.

Thoa N. B., Eichelman B., and Ng K. Y. (1972) Aggression in rats treated with dopa and 6-hydroxydopamine. *J. Pharm. Pharmacol.* **24,** 337–338.

Thor D. H. (1971) Amphetamine induced fighting during morphine withdrawal. *J. Gen. Psychol.* **84,** 245–250.

Thurmond J. B. (1975) Technique for producing and measuring territorial aggression using laboratory mice. *Physiol. Behav.* **14,** 879–881.

Ulrich R. (1966) Pain as a cause of aggression. *Am. Zool.* **6,** 643–662.

Ulrich R. E. and Azrin N. H. (1962) Reflexive fighting in response to aversive stimulation. *J. Exp. Anal. Behav.* **5,** 511–520.

Uyeno E. T. and Benson W. M. (1965) Effects of lysergic acid diethylamide on attack behaviour of male albino mice. *Psychopharmacologia* **7,** 20–26.

Valzelli L. (1969) Aggressive Behavior Induced by Isolation, in *Aggressive Behavior* (Garattini S. and Sigg E. B., eds.), John Wiley, New York.

Valzelli L. (1973) The "Isolation syndrome" in mice. *Psychopharmacologia* **31,** 305–320.

Valzelli L. and Bernasconi S. (1971) Differential activity of some psychotropic drugs as a function of emotional levels in animals. *Psychopharmacologia* **20,** 91–96.

Valzelli L. and Bernasconi S. (1973) Behavioral and neurochemical effects of caffeine in normal and aggressive mice. *Pharmacol. Biochem. Behav.* **1,** 251–254.

Valzelli L., Giacalone E., and Garattini S. (1967) Pharmacological control of aggressive behavior in mice. *Eur. J. Pharmacol.* **2,** 144–146.

Van der Poel A. M. and Remmelts M. (1971) The effects of anticholinergics on the behavior of the rats in a solitary and a social situation. *Arch. Int. Pharmacodyn. Ther.* **189,** 394–396.

Van der Poel A. M., Mos J., Kruk M. R., and Olivier B. (1984) A Motivational Analysis of Ambivalent Actions in the Agonistic Behaviour of Rats in Tests Used to Study the Effects of Drugs on Aggression, in *Ethopharmacological Aggression Research* (Miczek K. A., Kruk M. R., and Olivier B., eds.), Alan R. Liss, New York.

Van der Poel A. M., Olivier B., Mos J., Kruk M. R., Meelis W., and van Aken J. H. M. (1982) Antiaggressive effects of a new phenylpiperazine compound (DU 27716). *Pharmacol. Biochem. Behav.* **17,** 147–153.

Van der Wende C. and Spoerlein M. T. (1962) Psychotic symptoms induced in mice by the intravenous administration of solutions of 3,4 dihydroxyphenylalanine (DOPA). *Arch. Int. Pharmacodyn. Ther.* **137**, 145–154.

van Hooff J. A. R. A. M. (1982) Categories and Sequences of Behavior: Methods of Description and Analysis, in *Handbook of Methods in Nonverbal Behavior Research* (Scherer K. R. and Ekman P., eds.), Cambridge University, Cambridge.

Vassout A. and Delini-Stula A. (1977) Effets de β-bloqueurs (propranolol et oxprenolol) et du diazepam sur differents modeles d'agressivité chez le rat. *J. Pharmacol.* **8**, 5–14.

Vergnes M., Penot C., Kempf E., and Mack G. (1977) Lesion selective des neurones serotonergiques du raphe par 5,7 dihydroxytryptamine: Effets sur le comportment d'aggression interspecifique du rat. *Brain Res.* **133**, 167–171.

Vogel J. R. and Leaf R. C. (1972) Initiation of mouse killing in non-killer rats by repeated pilocarpine treatment. *Physiol. Behav.* **8**, 421–424.

Wagner G. C., Beuving L. J., and Hutchinson R. R. (1979) Androgen-dependency of aggressive target-biting and paired fighting in mice. *Physiol. Behav.* **22**, 43–46.

Walaszek E. and Abood L. (1956) Effect of tranquilizing drugs on fighting response of Siamese fighting fish. *Science* **124**, 440–441.

Waldbillig E. J. (1980) Suppressive effects of intraperitoneal and intraventricular injections of nicotine on muricide and shock-induced attack on conspecifics. *Pharmacol. Biochem. Behav.* **12**, 619–623.

Wasman M. and Flynn J. P. (1962) Directed attack elicited from hypothalamus. *Arch. Neurol.* **6**, 220–227.

Weinstock M. and Weiss C. (1980) Antagonism by propranolol of isolation-induced aggression in mice: Correlation with 5-hydroxytryptamine receptor blockade. *Neuropharmacology* **19**, 653–656.

Weischer M.-L. and Opitz K. (1972) Einfluss von Fenfluramin, Chlorphentermine und verwandten Verbindungen auf das Verhalten von aggressiven Mausen. *Arch. Int. Pharmacodyn. Ther.* **195**, 252–259.

Weitz M. K. (1974) Effects of ethanol on shock-elicited fighting behavior in rats. *Q. J. Studies on Alcohol* **35**, 953–958.

Welch B. L. and Welch A. S. (1968) Rapid modification of isolation-induced aggressive behavior and elevation of brain catecholamines and serotonin by the quick-acting monoamine-oxidase inhibitor pargyline. *Commun. Behav. Biol.* **1,** 347–351.

Welch B. L. and Welch A. S. (1969) Aggression and the Biogenic Amine Neurohumors, in *Aggressive Behaviour* (Garattini, S. and Sigg, E. B., eds.), Excerpta Medica Foundation, Amsterdam.

Willner P., Theodorou A., and Montgomery A. (1981) Subchronic treatment with the tricyclic antidepressant DMI increases isolation-induced fighting in rats. *Pharmacol. Biochem. Behav.* **14,** 475–479.

Wilson E. O. (1975) *Sociobiology.* Harvard University, Cambridge, Massachusetts.

Winslow J. T. and Miczek K. A. (1985) Social status as determinant of alcohol effects on aggressive behavior in squirrel monkeys (*Saimiri sciureus*). *Psychopharmacology* **85,** 167–172.

Wise D. and Pryor T. L. (1977) Effects of ergocornine and prolactin on aggression in the postpartum golden hamster. *Horm. Behav.* **8,** 30–39.

Woodworth C. H. (1971) Attack elicited in rats by electrical stimulation of the lateral hypothalamus. *Physiol. Behav.* **6,** 345–353.

Yen C. I., Stanger R. L., and Millman N. (1959) Ataractic suppression of isolation-induced aggressive behavior. *Arch. Int. Pharmacodyn. Ther.* **1234,** 179–185.

Psychopharmacology of Food and Water Intake

Steven J. Cooper and Suzanne Turkish

1. Introduction

This chapter provides a brief introduction to the psychopharmacology of food and water intake. Particular topics are not dealt with in depth, and neither is it possible to offer a satisfactory integrated view of the field. Instead, representative experimental examples have been chosen to illustrate general trends in research, methodological issues, and important findings.

A considerable advantage in the study of food and water intake is that the dependent variables are unambiguously defined and reliably quantified on ratio scales of measurement. Food intake, expressed in grams or milliliters, is a measure of the food the subject consumes over a chosen time period. Water intake can be similarly measured.

Unless food or water intake is being used merely to quantify the effects of drugs, there is often a wish to go beyond the observed intake measures to infer something of the organizational principles that underlie the subject's behavior. When a subject has experienced a period without food, and then responds to the presentation of food with vigorous feeding, we may think in terms of the motivation to eat, of hunger, or of appetite. The subject is aroused, and its behavior may be fairly described in terms of organization to obtain and ingest food. Our confidence in this interpretation is strengthened when the subject ceases to feed, and we find that the amount of food that has been consumed is related to the duration of the preceding period without food. These considerations prompt questions about the factors that influence the initiation, maintenance, and termination of feeding and drinking responses. Measurements of food and water intake alone are insufficient to address questions concerning motivational variables, unless they are set in an experimental context designed to assess motivation and steps are taken to control for nonspecific changes in ingestive responses.

1.1. Behavioral Considerations
1.1.1. Initiation and Maintenance of Feeding and Drinking

A straightforward experiment is to maintain the subject on free access to food and water and to monitor spontaneous food and water intake. In the rat, drinking usually occurs in association with eating the dry diet that is normally provided. Thus, any manipulation that tends to decrease food intake will also tend to affect drinking commensurately. Similarly, enhanced food intake will tend to elevate drinking. If excessive drinking occurs following drug treatment, a check has to be made that the polydipsia is not secondary to polyuria. Some drugs are potent diuretics, and excess drinking may occur to compensate for the loss of water and electrolytes.

Feeding and drinking can be elicited reliably by well-defined stimuli or experimental manipulations. One of the more obvious maneuvers is to precede a test of feeding or drinking with a period of deprivation. For example, an animal maintained on a 23-h food-deprivation schedule would have a 1-h/d access to food, with free access to water. Alternatively, deprivation can be arranged to maintain a lowered body weight. Adaptation to a deprivation schedule is also an important consideration, since animals show adaptive behavioral, physiological, and biochemical changes. Usually, the ingestive pattern becomes more regular and efficient, and animals develop strong forms of anticipatory behavior.

There are other procedures to choose from. Depletions of body fluid from intracellular- and extracellular-fluid compartments can be achieved by hemorrhage, injections of hypertonic saline, administration of polyethylene glycol, and injection of a variety of hormones and drugs (Fitzsimons, 1979). Manipulations of this sort are usually undertaken when some attempt is being made to assess mechanisms by which drug treatments affect drinking. A parallel set of experiments can be used in feeding studies, for example, eliciting feeding responses by injections of insulin, or 2-deoxyglucose.

Variations in environmental temperature will affect feeding and drinking responses. In high ambient temperatures, animals may drink more to compensate for increased fluid loss, whereas in low ambient temperatures, animals may eat more to maintain body temperature at a constant level (Kraly and Blass, 1976).

Increased feeding and drinking can be achieved by manipulating palatability as a factor. Thus, rats will consume more fluid if sweet or salty solutions are available for drinking (Ernits and Corbit, 1973; Rolls et al., 1978). Access to palatable foods can induce excess feeding, and these can be provided in the form of sweetened liquids, semisolid mashes, or supermarket foods. High levels of feeding and drinking can be achieved in nondeprived animals by the appropriate selection of highly palatable foods and fluids, respectively. The level of ingestion can be conveniently manipulated by varying the composition of the ingredients.

A mild pinch to a rat's tail can induce feeding (Antelman and Szechtman, 1975). The feeding response has been attributed to stress (Antelman and Caggiula, 1977), or can be seen as example of a response to nonspecific arousal (Robbins and Fray, 1980).

Electrical stimulation of certain sites within the brain (in particular at sites within the hypothalamus) can elicit stimulation-bound eating and drinking (Coons and Cruce, 1968; Mogenson and Stevenson, 1967). The responses may reflect the excitation of specific neural pathways that normally subserve the responses (Wise, 1974), or the relationship between the brain stimulation and the observed response may be considerably more plastic (Valenstein et al., 1969).

An interesting example of excessive drinking is a phenomenon described as schedule-induced drinking, which was first described by Falk (1961). If food-deprived rats are given small pellets of food to eat on a periodic basis (for example, a 45-mg food pellet every 60 s), and a bottle of water is available with a drinking spout, frequent drinking develops in the intervals between the deliveries of food. The cumulative intake of water over a typical test session can reach high levels. Recent evidence suggests that it may be quite different in character from the regulatory drinking that occurs in response to water loss (Cooper and Holtzman, 1983; Porter et al., 1984).

1.1.2. Satiation and Reduction in Feeding and Drinking

The termination of eating or drinking is often described in terms of satiety, on the assumption that learned and unlearned factors arising as a consequence of consumption actively terminate the ingestional response. One method of demonstrating the phenomenon is to use the sham-feeding or -drinking preparation. For example, rats can be surgically equipped with a gastric fistula, which when open allows drainage of ingested liquid diet from the stomach. Antin et al. (1975) have shown that rats that were deprived of food for 17 h before the sham-feeding test eat continuously when the liquid diet is made available and fail to show behavioral signs of satiety. When the fistula was closed, and the food was retained, cessation of feeding ensued and behavioral signs of satiety were evident.

Feeding or drinking may cease for reasons other than satiety. Adulterating the food or water with an unpleasant taste can reduce or completely inhibit ingestion. Feeding can be inhibited by novelty; a novel environment, a novel food container, or the presence of novel food, for example (Corey 1978). Previous experience of a distinctive flavor paired with sickness can result in a conditioned taste aversion (Garcia et al., 1955), so that a food or fluid identified with the flavor is avoided. The experimental subject may be distracted, sleepy, or ill. A range of factors, therefore, can inhibit feeding responses or bring about the termination of feeding, yet have nothing specifically to do with satiety. The same can be said for drinking responses. In order to interpret drug effects on feeding and drinking responses sensibly, an attempt must be made to identify the causes of increases or decreases.

1.1.3. Analysis of Meal Patterns

Rats, like people, eat and drink in discrete episodes that are referred to as meals. Within a meal, eating may not be continuous; instead, it is likely to be interrupted by pauses of varying duration. The question arises, therefore, as to how long an interval between consecutive bouts of eating must last to be considered an intermeal interval, and how short, to be considered a within meal pause?

A typical experimental situation in which the question arises is the automatic monitoring of feeding using a food-pellet dispenser and some means to detect the delivery or removal of the pellet (Kissileff, 1970). An on-line computer can be used to log the time of occurrence of each pellet delivery. For purposes of data reduction and analysis, it is useful to discriminate between meals, particularly when the monitoring is maintained over an appreciable period of time. There is insufficient space available here to consider in what ways the problem of defining meals, and intermeal intervals can or should be resolved. It is worth noting, however, that once criteria have been established, a set of parameters can be established based simply on the temporal distribution of discrete feeding events, such as the removal of small food pellets. These derived measures include meal size (amount), meal duration, bout size within meals, rate of eating within bouts, intermeal intervals, and more. This microstructural analysis of feeding can be applied to the description of the effects of drug treatments on food intake (Blundell and McArthur, 1981).

2. Food Intake

2.1. Drug-Induced Increments

Relatively little attention has been paid in the past to drug treatments that increase food intake. More interest has been shown in drugs that can be used to decrease feeding because of their potential use as aids to dieting. Yet, the psychopharmacology of food intake would be deficient if it did not pursue the question of drug-induced stimulation of feeding. Several drugs, members of various classes, have been reported to enhance food consumption (Hoebel, 1977; Silverstone and Kyriakides, 1982). Cyproheptadine, methysergide, chlorpromazine, and amitriptyline are examples. For present purposes, further examples will be drawn from drugs that are the subject of considerable current interest.

2.1.1. *Norepinephrine*

Of the central neurotransmitters involved in the control of feeding responses, most effort has been devoted to understanding the functions of norepinephrine (NE) in discrete hypothalamic nuclei. The starting point for this research was Grossman's (1962a,b) important and original observation that the direct injection of *l*-NE into the hypothalamus elicited a vigorous eating response in nondeprived rats. The most sensitive hypothalamic site has been localized to a small medial region. Leibowitz (1973a, 1978a) undertook a systematic search in over 800 rats, each with a cannula implant in one of 30 forebrain structures. All injections sites outside the hypothalamus were relatively or completely unresponsive to adrenergic stimulation. Leibowitz's search revealed that, within the hypothalamus, the most effective site for increasing feeding was the medial paraventricular nucleus (PVN). NE injected into the PVN elicited eating frequently within 2 min (Leibowitz, 1978a), and the threshold dose was between 1.0 and 4.2 ng (Leibowitz, 1978b).

A thorough pharmacological analysis has shown that the receptors in the PVN that mediate the NE effect are α-adrenergic receptors (Leibowitz, 1980). Bilateral electrolytic lesions of the PVN produce a major attenuation of the feeding response to NE injected unilaterally into the left lateral ventricle (Leibowitz et al., 1983). Furthermore, NE receptors in the PVN may be involved in the modulation or control of spontaneous eating in the normal rat. Perhaps NE acts to enhance food consumption by inhibiting the effects of a satiety system controlled from the PVN. In support of this view, it has been shown that PVN lesions cause hyperphagia and obesity (Leibowitz et al., 1981).

2.1.2. Neuropeptide Y

Neuropeptide Y (NPY) is a member of the pancreatic polypeptide family, which has recently been isolated from the brain (Tatemoto, 1982). When injected in very small amounts into the PVN, NPY produced a large, dose-dependent increase in food intake (Allen et al., 1985; Stanley and Leibowitz, 1985). It is currently thought that hypothalamic NPY may have an important role in feeding behavior.

2.1.3. Benzodiazepines

The benzodiazepines (BZ) include familiar compounds like chlordiazepoxide, diazepam, lorazepam, oxazepam, and many others. They are used extensively in the management of anxiety symptoms and for their anticonvulsant, muscle-relaxing, and sleep-inducing properties. The prototype 1,4-benzodiazepine is chlordiazepoxide (CDP). In the first full account of its pharmacology, it was noted that acute administration of the drug increased food intake in rats and approximately doubled the food consumption of dogs when given over a 5-d period (Randall et al., 1960). Since this initial observation, hyperphagia induced by several BZ treatments has been described in many mammalian species (Cooper, 1980a). Benzodiazepines also enhance the readiness to seek and ingest food. Thus, the latency to initiate feeding is reduced (Cooper and Francis, 1979) and "food-anticipatory" responses are selectively enhanced (Neito and Posadas-Andrews, 1984) following CDP administration.

Interestingly, the hyperphagia induced by BZ does not appear to interact with the animal's level of food deprivation (Cole, 1983). The two stimuli to feed appear to act independently. Furthermore, BZ treatments strongly enhance food ingestion in nondeprived animals given access to a highly palatable diet (Cooper and Estall, 1985; Cooper and Gilbert, 1985). Even in animals that have been partially satiated on the palatable diet before drug administration, BZ treatments continue to enhance food intake (Cooper and Estall, 1985).

2.1.4. Kappa Opiate Agonists

There is considerable evidence to suggest that endogenous opioid peptides are involved in the control of feeding responses (Morley et al., 1983; Sanger, 1981, 1983). Several types of receptor for opiate compounds have been distinguished, and Martin et al. (1976) proposed three distinct receptors based on the patterns of physiological changes induced in the chronic spinal dog preparation. They suggested that opiate-like effects are mediated by three classes of receptors called mu, kappa, and sigma after the prototype morphine, ketocyclazocine, and SKF10,047 (*n*-allylnormetazocine), respectively. To these have been added an enkephalin receptor, delta. Using selectively acting agonists, therefore, it becomes possible to ask if any or all of these distinguishable receptor types are involved in the mediation of feeding responses.

There has been a convergence of interest on the kappa-receptor, and on the actions of drugs and neuropeptides that act at these receptors (Morley and Levine, 1983; Morley et al., 1984). Sanger and McCarthy (1981) administered ethylketocyclazocine (EKC, a kappa-agonist) to nondeprived rats with free access to food and water. Food intake was increased within 1 h following injections of 0.1 and 0.3 mg/kg EKC. Morley et al. (1982a) also noted that food intake was stimulated in nondeprived rats 4 h after the administration of ketocyclazocine (10 mg/kg) or EKC (10 mg/kg). Locke et al. (1982) familiarized nondeprived rats and squirrel monkeys with a highly palatable sweetened condensed milk diet. Both EKC (0.03 mg/kg) and ketocyclazocine (0.01–10 mg/kg), administered subcutaneously, significantly enhanced milk consumption in rats. In contrast, the only effect of the two drugs in the squirrel monkey was to depress milk consumption. U-50,488H is a highly selective kappa-agonist (von Voigtlander et al., 1983). Recent studies have confirmed that this compound is effective in stimulating food consumption (Cooper et al., 1984; Morley and Levine, 1983).

The endogenous opioid peptide—dynorphin—is considered to be an endogenous ligand for the kappa-receptor

(Chavkin et al., 1982; Huidobro-Toro et al., 1981). This suggests that dynoorphin, acting at kappa-receptors, may be involved in the control of feeding responses. In support of this view, intracerebroventricular (icv) administration of dynorphin-(1-13) or dynorphin-(1-17) induces feeding in nondeprived rats (Morley and Levine, 1981, 1982; Morley et al., 1982b). It seems probable, therefore, that dynorphin and the kappa-agonists (EKC, ketazocine, U-50,488H) may act at the same receptor sites to produce an overconsumption of food.

2.2. Drug-Induced Decrements

For many years, the possibility of losing weight through the use of drugs has held considerable attraction. Considerable research energy has been expended in trying to understand mechanisms by which drugs reduce food consumption.

2.2.1. Amphetamine and Fenfluramine

In the past, amphetamine was used extensively as a dietary aid in the treatment of obesity. Imaginative laboratory studies led to the conclusion that the reduction in food intake after amphetamine administration stems from a reduction in the motivation for food (Miller 1956). Amphetamine has its disadvantages, however. It produces potent peripheral sympathomimetic effects and central stimulant effects. Consequently, treatment with amphetamine results in heightened arousal, hyperactivity, and insomnia. It was deemed particularly unacceptable for clinical use once it was realized that many individuals could become dependent on amphetamine. Other drugs, e.g., phenmetrazine, diethylpropion, mazindol, and phentermine have been introduced as anorectics, but show a similar profile of anorectic action coupled with stimulant activity (Hoebel, 1977; Silverstone and Kyriakides, 1982). Fenfluramine represented a new departure, although in chemical structure it is a phenylethylamine derivative, which relates it to amphetamine and other anorectics (*see* Maickel and Zabik, 1977, for structures). Food intake is reduced by fenfluramine, but it has a sedating action, which distinguishes it from amphetamine and similar drugs.

Experimental comparisons between amphetamine and fenfluramine became common in attempts to determine similarities and differences in their modes of action. It emerged that amphetamine-induced anorexia could be linked with increased release of catecholamines in the central nervous system (CNS), but fenfluramine's effects were thought to depend on serotonin (5-hydroxytryptamine; 5-HT) mechanisms (Blundell, 1977; Hoebel, 1977; Samanin and Garattini, 1982). An early attempt to characterize their distinctive behavioral effects suggested that amphetamine reduces hunger, but fenfluramine enhances satiety (Blundell et al., 1976).

Thus, there were attempts to analyze the anorectic effects of the two drugs at behavioral and neurochemical levels and subsequently, of course, to interrelate changes at the two levels (Blundell, 1981). However, more detail is required in the specification of their effects. Catecholamines and 5-HT are widely distributed throughout the CNS and in peripheral tissues. "Hunger" and "satiety" are short-hand terms that are used to cover many processes that can be described in motivational, physiological, or biochemical terms.

If we consider the case of amphetamine, one way to approach the question of neuroanatomical specificity is to destroy catecholamine pathways in the brain, in a selective fashion, and thus determine if the anorectic effect is retained. Ahlskog (1974) attempted selective lesions of either the dorsal or ventral noradrenergic bundles in the rat brain, and reported hyperphagia in animals that had sustained lesions to the ventral pathway. In the same animals, amphetamine-induced anorexia was antagonized. Ahlskog's suggestion that the ventral noradrenergic system may serve as a neural substrate for amphetamine-induced anorexia, however, has been challenged by more recent findings. Sahakian et al. (1983) reported that lesions of the ventral noradrenergic projection failed to disturb amphetamine-induced anorexia. These authors suggest that the procedure they used resulted in more restricted damage to the ventral bundle and less damage to other structures.

An alternative approach, to localize sites of action of amphetamine within the brain, is to microinject small quantities of amphetamine into specific sites within the brain. This approach has been used to great effect by Leibowitz (1975a). When amphetamine was injected into the perifornical region of the lateral hypothalamus (LH), food intake was markedly suppressed. Virtually all sites outside the hypothalamus and preoptic area were unresponsive to a moderately large dose of amphetamine. Within the hypothalamus, medial sites were also unresponsive. These data provide a strong argument for the location of mechanisms within the LH that mediate amphetamine's effect. Leibowitz (1975b) went on to show that in the LH, amphetamine-induced anorexia can be blocked by β-adrenergic and dopamine receptor antagonists, but not by α-adrenergic, serotonergic, or cholinergic receptor antagonists. Hence, amphetamine may cause the release of NE and dopamine within this region of the brain, and thereby produce the anorectic effect. Liebowitz has also assessed the role of 5-HT, the neurotransmitter that has been most implicated in fenfluramine's anorectic effect. When 5-HT was injected into the medial PVN, an inhibition of feeding was obtained in the absence of effects on general arousal (Leibowitz, 1980; Leibowitz and Papadakos, 1978).

Tordoff et al. (1982) provided evidence that, at least in part, anorexia induced by amphetamine may depend on peripheral sympathetic innervation. They performed celiac ganglionectomy in rats and found that the animals were protected from the anorectic effects of low doses of amphetamine (0.2 and 0.4 mg/kg, ip). Although the celiac ganglion innervates most of the abdominal viscera, they favor the liver as the most likely site for amphetamine's peripheral anorectic action. The anorexia may arise because of increased hepatic glycogenolysis, with a subsequent stimulation of hepatic receptors involved in metabolic control. A peripheral locus of action has also been proposed for fenfluramine. Davies et al. (1983) found that fenfluramine slowed gastric emptying rate and prolonged the postmeal interval when it was administered immediately after a meal. They proposed that part of fenfluramine's anorectic effect may be a result of the reduced gastric emptying rate and so the animals remain satiated longer.

The effects of fenfluramine and *d*-amphetamine on human feeding responses have been studied (Blundell and Rogers, 1980; Rogers and Blundell, 1979). Twelve volunteers (six male, six female) each underwent four treatment conditions: 10 mg *d*-amphetamine; 30 and 60 mg fenfluramine; and placebo. After drug administration, they were offered a test meal, and feeding performance was observed through a one-way screen and recorded for later analysis on videotape. Before and after the meal, each subject was asked to complete bodily sensation and food preference questionnaires. Fenfluramine (60 mg) and *d*-amphetamine (10 mg) significantly reduced total food intake. However, amphetamine reduced protein intake, but not carbohydrate intake, whereas fenfluramine had the opposite effect (Blundell and Rogers, 1980). This dichotomy was consistent with the results of animal experiments (Blundell and McArthur 1979). Both drug treatments affected subjective reports of hunger, but neither affected reports of satiety feelings. As in animal studies, the human subjects showed a slow rate of eating throughout the meal following fenfluramine treatment, which could account for its anorectic effect (Rogers and Blundell, 1979). During the postmeal period, 60 mg fenfluramine caused subjects to experience feelings of sedation. This effect may be the result of an intensification of the sedating consequences of having consumed a meal (Blundell and Rogers, 1980).

2.2.2. *Naloxone and Other Opiate Receptor Antagonists*

The first report that the opiate receptor antagonist—naloxone—reduces food intake in food-deprived rats, came from Holtzman (1974). Subsequently, this finding was confirmed in many other studies and extended to several other opiate receptor antagonists (including naltrexone, diprenorphine, Mr 2266) and to many additional species, including mice (Brown and Holtzman, 1979), cats (Foster et al., 1981), guinea pigs (Schulz et al., 1980), squirrel monkeys (Locke et al., 1982), and pigeons (Cooper and Turkish 1981). Naloxone has also been reported to reduce food intake in human subjects (Atkinson, 1982; Trenchard and Silverstone, 1983; Thompson et al., 1982).

There are numerous important factors that modulate the anorectic effect of naloxone. First, obese animals may be more sensitive, in some cases, to the effects of naloxone than lean animals (Apfelbaum and Mandenoff, 1981; Cooper et al., 1985; Margules et al., 1978). Second, rats that have been adapted to a schedule of reported daily food deprivation were less sensitive to naloxone's effects than animals that had been deprived of food for the first time, immediately prior to the feeding test (Sanger and McCarthy, 1982). Nevertheless, opiate receptor antagonists have been shown to retain their anorectic potency over chronic treatments in monkeys (Herman and Holtzman, 1984) and rats (Jalowiec et al., 1981; Brands et al., 1979).

2.2.3. *Cholecystokinin*

It has been suggested that the gut peptide— cholecystokinin (CCK)—plays a part in the control of feeding responses. Specifically, the entry of food into the gut stimulates the release of endogenous CCK, which then produces a satiety effect. Evidence for this hypothesis first came in a report that CCK significantly reduced food intake in rats (Gibbs et al., 1973). Water consumption in 12-h water-deprived rats was unaffected. There are several reports concerning the effects of CCK on food consumption and appetite in human subjects. For example, intravenous infusion of CCK significantly reduced the intake of a liquified blend of several foods in nonobese men (Kissileff et al., 1981). In obese subjects, similar infusions of CCK reduced food intake in a majority of cases (Pi-Sunyer et al., 1982). Several authors suggest that CCK acts as a short-term satiety signal. It does not affect the initial rate of eating within a meal, but terminates feeding sooner and so reduces the meal size (Gibbs et al., 1973, Hsiao et al., 1979). The intermeal interval, that is the time until the next meal, may be extended (Hsiao et al., 1979).

A major controversy has arisen over the physiological vs the pharmacological nature of CCK's effects. The proponents of the physiological view suggest that food-related release of endogenous CCK is a significant factor in short-term satiety that brings feeding to an end (Smith and Gibbs, 1979). Their opponents, however, maintain that the effects of CCK are pharmacological and that it causes malaise and, therefore, nonspecifically upsets feeding (Deutsch, 1978). Aversive consequences of administration have been detected using the conditioned-taste aversion paradigm (Deutsch and Hardy, 1977) and the conditioned-place preference paradigm (Swerdlow et al., 1983).

Trying to resolve this problem, Billington et al. (1983) suggested that a satiety factor should be less effective in inhibiting feeding in a hungrier animal, whereas an aversive treatment would affect feeding regardless of hunger. Applying this criterion, they confirmed that CCK had more pronounced effects in less-hungry animals. In contrast, lithium chloride, which has aversive effects, produced decreases in food consumption that were unrelated to food deprivation levels. Billington et al. (1983) concluded that CCK probably acts as a short-term satiety signal. West et al. (1984) also present data that argues against the effects of CCK on feeding being a result of temporary malaise. In their study, CCK was infused in the rat via indwelling intraperitoneal catheter at the onset of each meal, over several days. CCK continued to reduce the average meal size over the period of testing, but the animals showed no signs of illness since they maintained normal growth rate after an initial loss of body weight.

3. Water Intake

3.1. Drug-Induced Increments

3.1.1. Angiotensin II

Angiotensin II occupies a central position in the study of thirst mechanisms. Fitzsimons (1966, 1969) first proposed that the kidney renin-angiotensin system has an important part to play in the control of drinking. Juxtaglomerular (JG) cells of the kidneys secrete the proteolytic enzyme renin, which acts on its substrate angiotensinogen to produce an inactive decapeptide angiotensin I. This product is converted to the physiologically active octapeptide—angiotensin II—by the action of a converting enzyme. Some of the factors that bring about renin release are the actions of vasodilators (e.g., bradykinin and prostaglandins), α-adrenergic stimulation (e.g., isoproterenol), arousal of the sympathetic nervous system, and renal vasodilatation following a fall in blood pressure.

Fitzsimons (1969) found that saline extracts of rat renal cortex caused increased drinking by nephrectomized rats, and that iv injection of partly purified pig renin stimulated drinking in normal and nephrectomized rats. Since all known physiological actions of renin are mediated through angiotensin II, the next step was to determine if angiotensin II, itself, had dipsogenic activity. Fitzsimons and Simons (1969) then showed that iv infusion of angiotensin II caused rats in normal water balance to drink water. The effect of angiotensin II was greater in nephrectomized animals. Epstein and Hsiao (1975), using rats that had already experienced the effects of iv angiotensin, found that drinking could be elicited after infusion of doses of 300–400 ng/kg, at a rate of 32 ng/min for 4–5 min. The question of how angiotensin elicits drinking was examined by Epstein et al., (1970), who found that it acts in the CNS.

Considerable attention has been directed toward identifying the site or sites of action of angiotensin. In the first experiments in rats and cats, the preoptic area was found to be particularly sensitive to the dipsogenic action of angiotensin II (Epstein et al., 1970). However, these results were difficult to interpret, since circulating angiotensin should not reach the preoptic area, which lies beyond the blood–brain barrier. Interest was diverted, instead, to a group of small structures that are present in the vicinity of the third ventricle (circumventricular organs), which are not beyond the barrier. Circulating substances can gain access to these structures from either their blood supply or the cerebrospinal fluid that occupies the ventricles.

One of these structures is the subfornical organ (SFO). Angiotensin II, in doses as small as 0.1–1.0 pg injected directly into the SFO of rats, causes drinking to occur (Simpson and Routtenberg, 1973; Simpson et al., 1978). Ablation of the SFO attenuates or abolishes the drinking that occurs in response to intracranial or iv angiotensin II (Simpson et al., 1978; Hoffman and Phillips, 1976). The drinking induced by iv angiotensin II can be blocked by injection of saralasin, an angiotensin II antagonist, into the SFO (Simpson et al., 1978). A further site of action for angiotensin II is the organum vasculosum lamina terminalis (OVLT). A dose of 0.05 pg angiotensin II elicits drinking when injected into the anteroventral third ventricle (AV3V), where the OVLT is located (Phillips et al., 1978). Lesions of AV3V attentuate drinking in response to intraventricular and iv angiotensin (Buggy et al., 1977).

Angiotensin II stands as an important example of a single substance that can organize and integrate the combined activities of several organs to produce adaptive responses. In the periphery, angiotensin II is involved in the regulation of circulating blood volume and arterial blood pressure and brings about vasoconstriction and renal sodium retention. Acting centrally, angiotensin promotes thirst and sodium appetite, causes a rise in arterial blood pressure via an activation of the sympathetic-adrenal axis, and stimulates vasopressin release. Simultaneous activation of behavioral, endocrine and physiological responses combine, therefore, to compensate for the loss of plasma volume; blood pressure is prevented from falling, sodium and water are retained, and ingestion of water and salt are vigorously promoted.

Together, the effects of angiotensin suggest that as far as drinking is concerned, it may operate in cases of emergency to prevent the deleterious effects of the loss of plasma. But does it have a role in normal drinking? Ledingham et al. (1983) infused angiotensin II iv into fluid-replete male human subjects. For plasma levels of angiotensin II within the physiological range, thirst and drinking were not stimulated. In humans, and possibly in other species too, angiotensin II may not be essential to the arousal of drinking, and other factors need to be considered, particularly in the case of normal drinking.

3.1.2. Isoproterenol

Subcutaneous injections of the β-adrenergic agonist— isoproterenol—cause substantial drinking in rats in water-balance, together with antidiuresis (Lehr et al., 1967). In contrast, the α-adrenergic agonist—metaraminol—caused an increase in urine flow, which was not accompanied by any increased drinking. The isoproterenol-induced drinking was prevented by the β-adrenergic antagonist—propranolol—but was not affected by tolazoline—an α-adrenergic antagonist.

Isoproterenol may induce drinking by the activation of the renal renin-angiotensin system. Houpt and Epstein (1971) found that the drinking response to isoproterenol, nylidrine, and isoxsuprine (all β-adrenergic agonists) was abolished in the rat by bilateral nephrectomy. Controlling for the hypotensive effects of isoproterenol, Rettig et al. (1981) confirmed that a renal-related factor (probably angiotensin II) has a major responsibility in the mediation of the induced drinking. Lesions of the periventricular tissue surrounding the AV3V attentuated the drinking response to isoproterenol (Lind and Johnson, 1981), presumably by removing sites of action for increased circulating angiotensin II.

3.1.3. 5-Hydroxytryptamine

5-hydroxytryptophan (5-HTP), which is the immediate precursor of 5-HT, causes an increase in drinking when administered to rats (Fregly et al., 1980). The dipsogenic response to 5-HTP is inhibited by the peripheral decarboxylase inhibitor—carbidopa—and by the peripheral 5-HT receptor antagonist—methysergide (Kikta et al., 1981)—suggesting that it depends on the peripheral conversion of 5-HTP to 5-HT. In confirmation, subcutaneous administration of 5-HT itself proves to be a potent stimulus to drink (Lehr and Goldman, 1973; Kikta et al., 1983).

There is evidence that suggests that the dipsogenic effect of peripherally-acting 5-HT depends on the renal renin-angiotensin system. Administration of captopril, an angiotensin converting enzyme inhibitor, blocked the drinking response to 5-HTP (Threatte et al., 1981), and to 5-HT (Kikta et al., 1983). Suppression of renin release from the kidneys by clonidine, an α_2-adrenergic agonist, attenuated 5-HT-induced drinking (Kikta et al., 1983).

Serotonin may induce drinking in rats by acting at a point before the activation of β-adrenergic receptors, leading to the release of renin from the kidneys. Whereas propanolol, a β-adrenergic antagonist, blocked the drinking response to 5-HTP and 5-HT, methysergide, a 5-HT receptor antagonist, failed to reduce isoproterenol-induced drinking (Kikta et al., 1983; Threatte et al., 1981). The site of action of 5-HT leading to the stimulation of drinking has not been established. However, 5-HT increases the release of catecholamines from the adrenal medulla, and this may result in an enhanced effect mediated by renal β-adrenergic receptors.

3.1.4. Histamine

Subcutaneous administration of histamine in rats causes increased water intake and elevates plasma renin activity (Gutman and Krausz, 1973). The effect was only partly reduced by nephrectomy or following treatment with propranolol.

Kraly has proposed that histamine release plays a major role in spontaneous drinking, which occurs in association with eating in the rat. Pharmacological blockade of peripheral histamine receptors inhibits drinking that is elicited by eating (Kraly, 1983; Kraly and Specht, 1984). Antagonists of histamine receptors did not affect spontaneous eating or drinking after water deprivation (Kraly and Specht, 1984) when given in doses that were effective in blocking feeding-related drinking. In sham-feeding rats equipped with a gastric fistula, the drinking that was associated with feeding was attenuated by complete bilateral subdiaphragmatic vagotomy and was abolished by histamine receptor antagonists (Kraly, 1984). Kraly proposes that preabsorptive stimulation by food elicits a vagally-mediated release of histamine from the gastric mucosa, and that the histamine contributes to drinking by acting at peripheral histamine receptors.

It has also been shown that histamine elicits drinking in rats when injected into LH, anterior hypothalamus, and preoptic area (Leibowitz, 1973b). Subsequent studies revealed that the medial PVN was the most sensitive to the dipsogenic effect of directly administered histamine (Liebowitz, 1979).

3.1.5. Benzodiazepines

Benzodiazepines similarly enhance water consumption in water-deprived rats, in animals challenged with an osmotic thirst stimulus, and in nondeprived animals (Cooper, 1982b, 1983a; Leander, 1983; Maickel and Maloney, 1973). Treatment with the BZ receptor antagonist—RO 15-1788—blocked BZ-induced hyperdipsia (Cooper, 1982a; Turkish and Cooper, 1984a). Hence, their effects on drinking are mediated by specific receptors, although the location of the receptors needs to be established.

3.2. Drug-Induced Decrements

3.2.1. Amphetamine, Fenfluramine, and β-Phenylethylamine

Administration of amphetamine, in its racemic form (*d,l-*) or as the separate isomers (*d-, l-*), reduces water consumption when it is given acutely (Epstein, 1959; Soulairac and Soulairac, 1970). This hypodipsic effect is also induced by structurally related compounds such as fenfluramine (Soulairac and Soulairac, 1970; Stolerman and D'Mello, 1978).

There are numerous possible explanations for the hypodipsic effect of amphetamine. One possibility is that it is secondary to the anorectic effect of amphetamine; some drinking is closely associated with eating (prandial drinking), and therefore, any reduction in feeding will also lower water consumption. Neill and Grossman (1971), using rats, reported that the hypodipsic effect of amphetamine was enhanced when food was present. Nielsen and Lyon (1973), in contrast, reported that the presence or absence of food did not affect drinking results. Furthermore, there are examples in which amphetamine reduced water drinking in thirsty rats when food was not available (e.g., Maickel and Webb, 1972).

Possibly, the reduction in water intake may be explained in terms of aversive consequences of amphetamine administration. Indeed, conditioned taste aversions have been induced using amphetamine (Booth et al., 1977; Cappell and Le Blanc, 1973). However, in a study of seven compounds, Stolerman and D'Mello (1978) compared their potency for producing suppression of water intake with that for inducing a conditioned taste aversion (Booth et al. 1977) and found a dissociation between the two effects. Hence, the hypodipsia may not simply be a consequence of aversive effects of the drug treatments.

β-Phenylethylamine (PEA) is a structural analog of amphetamine that occurs endogenously in human, rat, and other mammalian tissue (Boulton and Juorio, 1982). PEA, in contrast to amphetamine, is rapidly metabolized by type B monoamine oxidase, and therefore has a considerably shorter duration of action. Cooper and Dourish (1984) found that PEA induced a transient hypodipsia in water-deprived rats. Water intake recovered as a result of a compensatory hyperdipsia, which occurred during a period 15–60 min after injection of the drug. Similar observations have been made with amphetamine, although changes take place over a more extended period (Soulairac and Soulairac, 1970; Stolerman and D'Mello, 1978). PEA in moderate doses induces locomotor stimulation and in larger doses induces a behavioral stereotypy syndrome. Cooper and Dourish (1984) suggest that the induced hyperactivity and stereotypy may have interfered with drinking responses. Hence, the hypodipsic effect of PEA may not reflect a direct inhibitory action on drinking responses. Since amphetamine also produces potent behavioral stimulation, it seems possible that it too reduces drinking by producing competing behavioral responses.

Central administration of amphetamine to hypothalamic sites attenuates water consumption (Leibowitz, 1980). Such experiments provide good evidence for a dissociation between amphetamine-induced anorexia and its hypodipsic effect. When amphetamine is injected directly into the perifornical region of LH, it induces a suppression of feeding that can be blocked by the β-adrenergic antagonists—propranolol and sotalol (Leibowitz, 1975a,b; Leibowitz and Rossakis, 1978). Antagonists of α-adrenergic, serotonergic, or cholinergic receptors were ineffective. Hence, amphetamine may release NE in LH and thereby activate β-adrenergic receptors and cause a reduction in feeding.

Norepinepherine, when injected into the PVN of the thirsty rat, inhibits water consumption. The receptors that mediate the drinking suppression appear to be α-adrenergic. Intrahypothalamic injection of amphetamine can also inhibit drinking in thirsty rats, and this effect can be reversed with hypothalamic injection of an α-adrenergic receptor antagonist (Leibowitz, 1980). Hence, amphetamine may suppress drinking, in part at least, by increasing the release of hypothalamic NE acting at α-receptors.

3.2.2. Ethylketocyclazocine

The kappa-opiate receptor agonist—EKC—enhances fluid intake in nondeprived rats (Sanger and McCarthy, 1981; Turkish and Cooper, 1984b). This hyperdipsia is most likely also a secondary effect, following polyuria. Kappa-agonists are potent diuretic compounds (Leander, 1984; Slizgi and Ludens, 1982). In water-deprived rats, EKC (0.01–3.0 mg/kg) induced a dose-related suppression of drinking (Turkish and Cooper, 1984b). Its effect on drinking aroused by other forms of thirst stimuli have not been investigated.

3.2.3. Naloxone and Other Opiate Antagonists

Naloxone—an opiate receptor antagonist—has been shown to produce dose-dependent suppression of drinking in water-deprived rats, mice, and monkeys (Brown and Holtzman, 1979, 1981b). Other opiate receptor antagonists, including naltrexone, diprenorphine, and Mr2266, have been shown to exert the same effect (Leander and Hynes, 1983; Turkish and Cooper, 1984b).

Naloxone reduces drinking aroused by a variety of stimuli: angiotensin II, isoproterenol, or osmotic thirst challenge with hypertonic saline (Brown and Holtzman, 1980; Cooper, 1980b; Czech and Stein, 1980; Rowland, 1982). Naloxone also reduces spontaneous drinking in nondeprived rats (Cooper, 1980b).

Naloxone and other opiate antagonists do not affect drinking responses *per se,* since schedule-induced drinking remains unaffected following naloxone, naltrexone, or diprenorphine administration (Brown and Holtzman, 1981a; Cooper and Holtzman, 1983). Furthermore, the initiation of drinking remains unaffected. Naloxone-induced reductions in water intake in rehydrating animals occurs some minutes following the start of drinking (Cooper and Holtzman, 1983; Siviy et al., 1982). It appears possible that opiate receptor antagonists in some way contribute to signals of drinking satiety and so bring drinking to a premature termination.

The sites of action for the antidipsogenic effects of opiate antagonists appear to be centrally located (Brown and Holtzman, 1981c). Czech et al. (1983) reported that naloxone was effective in reducing drinking in water-deprived rats when injected into LH, preoptic area, and zona incerta, but was ineffective at several other diencephalic sites.

3.2.4. Substance P and Tachykinins

When the peptides substance P and related tachykinins are injected icv into rats, they exert a profound antidipsogenic effect. For example, substance P inhibits the drinking elicited by angiotensin II, carbachol, water deprivation, and hypertonic sodium chloride (de Caro et al., 1978). In contrast, iv administration of tachykinins did not affect feeding responses in rats. It appears that neuropeptides belonging to this family may feature prominently in mechanisms that inhibit drinking in rats (Cooper, 1985).

4. Preference and Acceptance

All foods or fluids are not treated equally by either humans or other animals; some are preferred to others. Familiar foods may be preferred to novel ones; cold drinks to hot ones in a hot climate; salty or sweet foods to bland. Some flavors are rejected, being too bitter or too salty, or because in the past they had been uniquely associated with illness or dietary deficiency. The investigation of factors that determine the acceptance or rejection of particular types of food or fluid is fascinating, but the psychopharmacological approach is still in its infancy. Falk (1971) recommends that a distinction be drawn between a measure of acceptance on the one hand and a measure of preference on the other. The "single-stimulus method" has been used in drinking studies in which a single fluid at a time is presented to the subject (Weiner and Stellar,

1951). Rats will drink more sweet-tasting solutions than water, when tested by the single-stimulus method (e.g., Ernits and Corbit, 1973). Falk suggests that this method yields an acceptance measure, and is not, strictly speaking, a preference test. The amount of fluid consumed will vary according to the concentration of the solution, and Falk recommends Young's term "acceptance–rejection function" to refer to the relationship. The term "preference test" can be used when two or more fluids (or two or more foods) are simultaneously available, and the animal has a choice.

In the function that relates concentration of the solution to the measure of preference, several features can usually be described. First, there is the threshold for preference, i.e., the concentration at which animals begin to prefer the solution to water. Second, there is a region of preference (often rising to a peak value) at which the animal consumes more of the solution than the water. Third, there is a point of indifference, at which concentration the animal consumes as much water as it does the solution. Finally, there may be a region of aversion, at which the animal chooses water in preference to the solution. The behavior of the animal, then, is markedly affected both by the type of fluid it has available to consume and the concentration of the solution. Measures of acceptance or preference will also depend on the duration of the period over which the behavior is sampled.

In the sections that follow, examples will be limited for illustrative purposes to studies of drinking. There are, nevertheless, some recent investigations in the psychopharmacology of food preference and dietary selection (e.g., Blundell and McArthur, 1981; Cooper, 1981).

4.1. Increased Acceptance

In a single-stimulus test, water-deprived rats drink considerably more sodium chloride solution than if they are offered water. The level of consumption first rises as the salt concentration increases, peaking around an isotonic value (0.9% or 0.15M solution), and than falls. Animals in sodium balance will reject strongly hypertonic salt solutions.

In an early study, it was shown that CDP increased the intake of a 1.5% NaCl solution in rats that had been adapted to a 23-h water-deprivation schedule (Falk and Burnidge, 1970). The authors interpreted their data, at that stage, in terms of an attenuation by CDP of the aversive quality of a concentrated salt solution. However, it has since been shown that CDP also produces drinking of a maximally acceptable 0.9% NaCl solution in rehydrating rats (Turkish and Cooper 1984a). Hence, the hypothesis that the attenuation of aversion is responsible is not tenable. The most complete data on the effects of CDP on salt solutions come from a study by Falk and Tang, (1984). Using a single-stimulus method, they offered rehydrating rats salt concentrations ranging from 0.1 to 3.0%. Peak acceptance was reached with a 0.9% NaCl solution, then acceptance declined markedly with solutions of greater concentration. Chlordiazepoxide treatments increased the intake of all salt concentrations to produce an upward shift in the entire acceptance curve, without altering the peak acceptance concentration.

4.2. *Decreased Preference*

Rats, whether thirsty or not, will ingest large quantities of sweet-tasting solutions (Ernits and Corbit, 1973; Rolls et al., 1978). Presumably, the reward value of the sweet taste plays an important part in maintaining the high levels of consumption. If the preference for sweet solutions can be blocked, some correlate of the sweet reward can perhaps be inhibited by the drug treatments.

Several laboratories have now reported that naloxone attenuates the preference for sweet solutions in water-deprived rats (LeMagnen et al., 1980; Cooper, 1983b; Siviy and Reid, 1983; Lynch and Libby, 1983). Together, these results suggest that naloxone suppresses the palatability of sweet taste and implies that endogenous opioid peptides are involved in the reward processes associated with gustatory stimulation.

5. Summary

There has been a growth in the number of drugs shown to affect feeding and drinking responses. In addition, the discovery of active peptides in the gut, brain, and elsewhere adds considerably to the number of possible candidate endogenous substances that play some part in the control of food and water intake. It is a task for physiologists and psychologists to assess the functional significance of the effects of these substances. An ultimate aim is to describe the events that lead to the initiation of ingestional responses—their maintenance and their satiation—and to comprehend their organization. A pharmacological approach emphasizes the interaction of chemical entities (hormones, neurotransmitters, neurosecretory products, and metabolites) with potentially identifiable receptors and offers a powerful methodology for understanding the nature and outcome of the interactions. Harnessing the skills and knowledge of these disciplines into a working team, promises, in the long run at least, an increased understanding of the complexities that lie behind the deceptively simple acts of feeding and drinking.

Acknowledgment

We wish to thank Dr. Colin T. Dourish for his comments on an earlier version of this chapter.

References

Ahlskog J. E. (1974) Food intake and amphetamine anorexia after selective norepinephrine loss. *Brain Res.* **82,** 211–240.

Allen L. G., Kalra P.S., Crowley W. R., and Kalra S. P. (1985) Comparison of the effects of neuropeptide Y and adrenergic transmitters on LH release and food intake in male rats. *Life Sci.* **37,** 617–623.

Antelman S. M. and Caggiula A. R. (1977) Tails of Stress-Related Behavior: A Neuropharmacological Approach, in *Animal*

Models in Psychiatry and Neurology (Hanin I. and Usdin E., eds.) Pergamon, Oxford.

Antelman S. M. and Szechtman H. (1975) Tail-pinch induces eating in sated rats which appears to depend on nigrostriatal dopamine. *Science* **189**, 731–733.

Antin J., Gibbs J., Holt J., Young R. C., and Smith G. P. (1975) Cholecystokinin elicits the complete behavioral sequence of satiety in rats. *J. Comp. Physiol. Psychol.* **89**, 784–790.

Apfelbaum M. and Mandenoff A. (1981) Naltrexone suppresses hyperphagia induced in the rat by a highly palatable diet. *Pharmacol. Biochem. Behav.* **15**, 89–91.

Atkinson R. L. (1982) Naloxone decreases food intake in obese humans. *J. Clin. Endocrinol. Metab.* **56**, 196–198.

Billington C. J., Levine A. S., and Morley J. E. (1983) Are peptides truly satiety agents? A method of testing for neurohumoral satiety effects. *Am. J. Physiol.* **245**, R920–926.

Blundell J. E. (1977) Is there a role for serotonin (5-hydroxytryptamine) in feeding? *Int. J. Obes.* **1**, 15–42.

Blundell J. E. (1981) Bio-Grammar of Feeding: Pharmacological Manipulations and Their Interpretation, in *Theory in Psychopharmacology* vol. 1 (Cooper S. J., ed.), Academic, London.

Blundell J. E. and McArthur R. A. (1979) Investigation of food consumption using a dietary self-selection procedure: Effects of pharmacological manipulation and feeding schedules. *Br. J. Pharmacol.* **67**, 436–438P.

Blundell J. E. and McArthur R. A. (1981) Behavioural Flux and Feeding: Continuous Monitoring of Food Intake and Food Selection, and the Video-recording of Appetitive and Satiety Sequences for the Analysis of Drug Action, in *Anorectic Agents: Mechanisms of Action and Tolerance* (Garattini S. and Samanin R., eds), Raven, New York.

Blundell J. E. and Rogers P. J. (1980) Effects of anorexic drugs on food intake, food selection and preferences and hunger motivation and subjective experiences. *Appetite* **1**, 151–165.

Blundell J. E., Latham C. J., and Leshem M. B. (1976) Differences between the anorexic actions of amphetamine and fenfluramine—possible effects on hunger and satiety. *J. Pharm. Pharmacol.* **28**, 471–477.

Booth D. A., D'Mello G. D., Pilcher C. W. T., and Stolerman I. P. (1977) Comparative potencies of amphetamine, fenfluramine and related compounds in taste aversion experiments in rats. *Br. J. Pharmacol.* **61,** 669–677.

Boulton A. A. and Juorio A. V. (1982) Brain Trace Amines, in *Handbook of Neurochemistry* vol. 1 (Lajtha A., ed.), Plenum, New York.

Brands B., Thornhill J. A., Hirst M., and Gowdey C. W. (1979) Suppression of food intake and body weight gain by naloxone in rats. *Life Sci.* **24,** 1773–1778.

Brown D. R. and Holtzman S. G. (1979) Suppression of deprivation-induced food and water intake in rats and mice by naloxone. *Pharmacol. Biochem. Behav.* **11,** 567–573.

Brown D. R. and Holtzman S. G. (1980) Evidence that opiate receptors mediate suppression of hypertonic saline-induced drinking in the mouse by narcotic antagonists. *Life Sci.* **26,** 1543–1550.

Brown D. R. and Holtzman S. G. (1981a) Suppression of drinking by naloxone in the rat: A further characterization. *Eur. J. Pharmacol.* **69,** 331–340.

Brown D. R. and Holtzman S. G. (1981b) Narcotic antagonists attenuate drinking induced by water deprivation in a primate. *Life Sci.* **28,** 1287–1294.

Brown D. R. and Holtzman S. G. (1981c) Opiate antagonists: Central sites of action in suppressing water intake of the rat. *Brain Res.* **221,** 432–436.

Buggy J., Fink G. D., Johnson A. K., and Brody M. J. (1977) Prevention of the development of renal hypertension by anteroventral third ventricular tissue lesions. *Circ. Res.* Suppl. I **40,** 110–117.

Cappell H. and Le Blanc A. E. (1973) Punishment of saccharin drinking by amphetamine in rats and its reversal by chlordiazepoxide. *J. Comp. Physiol. Psychol.* **85,** 97–104.

Chavkin C., James I. F., and Goldstein A. (1982) Dynorphin is a specific endogenous ligand of the κ opioid receptor. *Science* **215,** 413–415.

Cole S. O. (1983) Combined effects of chlordiazepoxide treatment and food deprivation on concurrent measures of feeding and activity. *Pharmacol. Biochem. Behav.* **18,** 369–372.

Coons E. E. and Cruce J. A. F. (1968) Lateral hypothalamus: Food current intensity in maintaining self-stimulation of hunger. *Science* **159,** 1117–1119.

Cooper S. J. (1980a) Benzodiazepines as appetite enhancing compounds *Appetite* **1,** 7–19.

Cooper S. J. (1980b) Naloxone: Effects on food and water consumption in the non-deprived and deprived rat. *Psychopharmacology* **71,** 1–6.

Cooper S. J. (1981) Prefrontal Cortex, Benzodiazepines and Opiates: Case Studies in Motivation and Behaviour Analysis, in *Theory in Psychopharmacology* vol. 1 (Cooper S. J., ed.), Academic, London.

Cooper S. J. (1982a) Specific benzodiazepine antagonist Ro 15-1788 and thirst-induced drinking in the rat. *Neuropharmacology* **21,** 483–486.

Cooper S. J. (1982b) Benzodiazepine mechanisms and drinking in the water-deprived rat. *Neuropharmacology* **21,** 775–780.

Cooper S. J. (1983a) Effects of chlordiazepoxide on drinking compared in rats challenged with hypertonic saline, isoproterenol or polyethylene glycol. *Life Sci.* **32,** 2453–2459.

Cooper S. J. (1983b) Effects of opiate agonists and antagonists on fluid intake and saccharin choice in the rat. *Neuropharmacology* **22,** 323–328.

Cooper S. J. (1985) Neuropeptides and Food and Water Intake, in *Psychopharmacology and Food* (Sandler M. and Silverstone T., eds.), Oxford University, Oxford, UK.

Cooper S. J. and Dourish C. T. (1984) Hypodipsia, stereotypy and hyperactivity induced by β-phenylethylamine in the water-deprived rat. *Pharmacol. Biochem. Behav.* **20,** 1–7.

Cooper S. J. and Estall L. B. (1985) Behavioural pharmacology of food, water and salt intake in relation to drug actions at benzodiazepine receptors. *Neurosci. Biobehav. Rev.* **9,** 5–19.

Cooper S. J. and Francis R. L. (1979) Feeding parameters with two food textures after chlordiazepoxide administration, alone or in combination with *d*-amphetamine or fenfluramine. *Psychopharmacology* **62,** 253–259.

Cooper S. J. and Gilbert D. B. (1985) Clonazepam-induced hyperphagia in nondeprived rats, tests of pharmacological specificity with Ro 5-4864, Ro 5-3663, Ro 15-1788 and CGS 9896. *Pharmacol. Biochem. Behav.* **22,** 753–760.

Cooper S. J. and Holtzman S. G. (1983) Patterns of drinking in the rat following the administration of opiate antagonists. *Pharmacol. Biochem. Behav.* **19,** 505–511.

Cooper S. J. and Turkish S. (1981) Food and water intake in the non-deprived pigeon after morphine or naloxone administration. *Neuropharmacology* **20,** 1053–1058.

Cooper A. J., Jackson A., Morgan R., and Carter R. (1985) Evidence for opiate receptor involvement in the consumption of a high palatability diet in nondeprived rats. *Neuropeptides* **5,** 345–348.

Corey D. T. (1978) The determinants of exploration and neophobia. *Neurosci. Biobehav. Rev.* **2,** 235–253.

Czech D. A. and Stein E. A. (1980) Naloxone depresses osmoregulatory drinking in rats. *Pharmacol. Biochem. Behav.* **12,** 987–989.

Czech D. A., Stein E. A., and Blake M. J. (1983) Naloxone-induced hypodipsia: A CNS mapping study. *Life Sci.* **33,** 797–803.

Davies R. F., Rossi J., Panksepp J., Bean N. J., and Zolovick A. J. (1983) Fenfluramine anorexia: A peripheral locus of action. *Physiol. Behav.* **80,** 723–730.

de Caro G., Massi M., and Micossi L. G. (1978) Antidipsogenic effect of intracranial injections of substance P in rats. *J. Physiol.* **279,** 133–140.

Deutsch J. A. (1978) The stomach in food satiation and the regulation of appetite. *Prog. Neurobiol.* **10,** 135–153.

Deutsch J. A. and Hardy W. T. (1977) Cholecystokinin produces bait shyness in rats. *Nature* **266,** 196.

Epstein A. N. (1959) Suppression of eating and drinking by amphetamine and other drugs in normal and hyperphagic rats. *J. Comp. Physiol. Psychol.* **52,** 37–45.

Epstein A. N. and Hsiao S. (1975) Angiotensin as a Dipsogen, in *Control Mechanisms of Drinking* (Peters G., Fitzsimons J. T., and Peters-Haefeli L., eds.), Springer, Berlin.

Epstein A. N., Fitzsimons J. T., and Rolls B. J. (1970) Drinking induced by injection of angiotensin into the brain of the rat. *J. Physiol.* (Lond.) **210,** 457–474.

Ernits T. and Corbit J. D. (1973) Taste as a dipsogenic stimulus. *J. Comp. Physiol. Psychol.* **83,** 27–31.

Falk J. L. (1961) Production of polydipsia in normal rats by an intermittent food schedule. *Science* **133,** 195–196.

Falk J. L. (1971) Determining Changes in Vital Functions: Ingestion, in *Methods in Psychobiology* vol. 1 (Myers R. D., ed.), Academic, New York.

Falk J. L. and Burnidge G. K. (1970) Fluid intake and punishment-attenuating drugs. *Physiol. Behav.* **5**, 199–202.

Falk J. L. and Tang M. (1984) Chlordiazepoxide elevates the NaCl solution acceptance-rejection function. *Pharmacol. Biochem. Behav.* **21**, 449–451.

Fitzsimons J. T. (1966) Hypovolaemic drinking and renin. *J. Physiol.* (Lond.) **186**, 130–131P.

Fitzsimons J. T. (1969) The role of a renal thirst factor in drinking induced by extracellular stimuli. *J. Physiol.* **201**, 349–368.

Fitzsimons J. T. (1979) *The Physiology of Thirst and Sodium Appetite.* Cambridge University, Cambridge.

Fitzsimons J. T. and Simons B. (1969) The effect on drinking in the rat of intravenous angiotensin, given alone or in combination with other stimuli of thirst. *J. Physiol.* (Lond.) **203**, 45–47.

Foster J. A., Morrison M., Dean S. J., Hill M., and Frenk H. (1981) Naloxone suppresses food/water consumption in the deprived cat. *Pharmacol. Biochem. Behav.* **14**, 419–421.

Fregly M. J., Connor T. M., Kitka D. C., and Threatte R. M. (1980) Dipsogenic effect of *L*-5-hydroxytryptophan in rats. *Brain Res. Bull.* **5**, 719–729.

Garcia J., Kimeldorf D. J., and Koelling R. A. (1955) A conditioned aversion towards saccharin resulting from exposure to gamma radiation. *Science* **122**, 157–159.

Gibbs J., Young R. C., and Smith G. P. (1973) Cholecystokinin decreases food intake in rats. *J. Comp. Physiol. Psychol.* **84**, 488–495.

Grossman S. P. (1962a) Direct adrenergic and cholinergic stimulation of hypothalamic mechanisms. *Am. J. Physiol.* **202**, 872–882.

Grossman S. P. (1962b) Effects of adrenergic and cholinergic blocking agents on hypothalamic mechanisms. *Am. J. Physiol.* **202**, 1230–1236.

Gutman Y. and Krausz M. (1973) Drinking induced by dextran and histamine: Relation to kidneys and renin. *Eur. J. Pharmacol.* **23**, 256–263.

Herman B. H. and Holtzman S. G. (1984) Repeated administration of naltrexone and diprenorphine decreases food intake and body weight in squirrel monkeys. *Life Sci.* **34**, 1–12.

Hoebel B. G. (1977) the Psychopharmacology of Feeding, in *Handbook of Psychopharmacology* vol. 8 (Iversen L. L., Iversen S. D., and Snyder S. H., eds.), Plenum, New York.

Hoffman W. E. and Phillips M. I. (1976) The effect of subfornical organ lesions and ventricular blockage on drinking induced by angiotensin II. *Brain Res.* **108,** 59–73.

Holtzman S. G. (1974) Behavioral effects of separate and combined administration of naloxone and *d*-amphetamine. *J. Pharmacol. Exp. Ther.* **189,** 51–60.

Houpt K. A. and Epstein A. N. (1971) The complete dependence of beta-adrenergic drinking on the renal dipsogen. *Physiol. Behav.* **7,** 897–902.

Hsiao S., Wang C. H., and Schallert T. (1979) Cholecystokinin, meal pattern and the intermeal interval: Can eating be stopped before it starts? *Physiol. Behav.* **23,** 909–914.

Huidobro-Toro J. P., Yoshimura K., Lee N. M., Loh H. H., and Way E. L. (1981) Dynorphin interaction at the kappa-opiate site. *Eur. J. Pharmacol.* **72,** 265–267.

Jalowiec J. E., Panksepp J., Zolovick A. J., Najam N., and Herman B. H. (1981) Opioid modulation of ingestive behavior. *Pharmacol. Biochem. Behav.* **15,** 477–484.

Kikta D. C., Threatte R. M., Barney C. C., Fegly M. J. and Greenleaf J. E. (1981) Peripheral conversion of *L*-5-Hydroxytryptophan to 5-HT induces drinking in rats. *Pharmacol. Biochem. Behav.* **14,** 889–893.

Kikta D. C., Barney C. C., Threatte R. M., Fregly M. J., Rowland N. E., and Greenleaf J. E. (1983) On the mechanism of serotonin induced dipsogenesis in the rat. *Pharmacol. Biochem. Behav.* **19,** 519–525.

Kissileff H. R. (1970) Free feeding in normal and "recovered lateral" rats monitored by a pellet-sensing eatometer. *Physiol. Behav.* **5,** 163–173.

Kissileff H. R., Pi-Sunyer F. X., Thornton J., and Smith G. P. (1981) C-terminal octapeptide of cholecystokinin decreases food intake in man. *Am. J. Clin. Nutr.* **34,** 154–160.

Kraly F. S. (1983) Histamine plays a part in induction of drinking by food intake. *Nature* **301,** 65–66.

Kraly F. S. (1984) A preabsorptive pregastric vagally-mediated histaminergic component of drinking elicited by eating in the rat. *Behav. Neurosci.* **98,** 349–353.

Kraly F. S. and Blass E. M. (1976) Increased Feeding in Rats in a Low Ambient Temperature, in *Hunger: Basic Mechanisms and Clinical Implications* (Novin D., Wyrwicka W., and Bray G., eds.), Raven, New York.

Kraly F. S. and Specht S. M. (1984) Histamine plays a major role for drinking elicited by spontaneous eating in rats. *Physiol. Behav.* **33,** 611–614.

Leander J. D. (1983) Effects of punishment-attenuating drugs on deprivation-induced drinking: Implications for conflict procedures. *Drug Dev. Res.* **3,** 185–191.

Leander J. D. (1984) Kappa-opioid agonists and antagonists: Effects on drinking and urinary output. *Appetite* **5,** 7–14.

Leander J. D. and Hynes M. D. (1983) Opioid antagonists and drinking: Evidence of kappa-receptor involvement. *Eur. J. Pharmacol.* **87,** 481–484.

Ledingham J. G. G., Morton J. J., Phillips P. A., and Rolls B. J. (1983) Effects of hypertonic saline and angiotensin (AII) on thirst in man. *J. Physiol.* (Lond.) **345,** 114P.

Lehr D. and Goldman W. (1973) Continued pharmacologic analysis of consummatory behavior in the albino rat. *Eur. J. Pharmacol.* **23,** 197–210.

Lehr D., Mallow J., and Kurkowski M. (1967) Copious drinking and simultaneous inhibition of urine flow elicited by beta-adrenergic stimulation and contrary effect of alpha-adrenergic stimulation. *J. Pharmacol. Exp. Ther.* **158,** 150–163.

Leibowitz S. F. (1973a) Brain Norepinephrine and Ingestive Behaviour, in *Frontiers in Catecholamine Research* (Usdin E. and Snyder S., eds.), Pergamon, Oxford.

Leibowitz S. F. (1973b) Histamine: A stimulatory effect on drinking behavior in the rat. *Brain Res.* **63,** 440–444.

Leibowitz S. F. (1975a) Amphetamine: Possible site and mode of action for producing anorexia in the rat. *Brain Res.* **84,** 160–167.

Liebowitz S. F. (1975b) Catecholaminergic mechanisms of the lateral hypothalamus: Their role in the mediation of amphetamine anorexia. *Brain Res.* **98,** 529–545.

Leibowitz S. F. (1978a) Paraventricular nucleus: A primary site mediating adrenergic stimulation of feeding and drinking. *Pharmacol. Biochem. Behav.* **8,** 163–175.

Liebowitz S. F. (1978b) Adrenergic stimulation of the paraventricular nucleus and its effects on ingestive behavior as a function of drug dose and time of injection in the light–dark cycle. *Brain Res. Bull.* **3,** 357–363.

Leibowitz S. F. (1979) Histamine: Modification of Behavioral and

Physiological Components of Body Fluid Homeostasis, in *Histamine Receptors* (Yellin T. O., ed.), SP Medical & Scientific, New York.

Leibowitz S. F. (1980) Neurochemical Systems of the Hypothalamus: Control of Feeding and Drinking Behavior and Water-Electrolyte Excretion, in *Handbook of the Hypothalamus* vol. 3, part A, (Morgane P. J. and Panksepp J., eds.), Dekker, New York.

Leibowitz S. F. and Papadakos P. J. (1978) Serotonin–norepinephrine interaction in the paraventricular nucleus: Antagonistic effects on feeding behavior in the rat. *Neurosci. Abstr.* **4,** 542.

Liebowitz S. F. and Rossakis C. (1978) Analysis of feeding suppression produced by perifornical hypothalamic injection of catecholamines, amphetamines, and mazindol. *Eur. J. Pharmacol.* **53,** 69–81.

Leibowitz S. F., Hammer N. J., and Chang K. (1981) Hypothalamic paraventricular nucleus lesions produce overeating and obesity in the rat. *Physiol. Behav.* **27,** 1031–1040.

Leibowitz S. F., Hammer N. J., and Chang K. (1983) Feeding behavior induced by central norephinephrine injection is attenuated by discrete lesions in the hypothalamic paraventricular nucleus. *Pharmacol. Biochem. Behav.* **19,** 945–950.

Le Magnen J., Marfaing-Jallat P., Miceli D., and Devos M. (1980) Pain modulating and reward systems: A single brain mechanism? *Pharmacol. Biochem. Behav.* **12,** 729–733.

Lind R. W. and Johnson A. K. (1981) Periventricular preoptic-hypothalamic lesions: Effects on isoproterenol-induced thirst. *Pharmacol. Biochem. Behav.* **15,** 563–565.

Locke K. W., Brown D. R., and Holtzman S. G. (1982) Effects of opiate antagonists and putative mu- and kappa-agonists on milk intake in rat and squirrel monkey. *Pharmacol. Biochem. Behav.* **17,** 1275–1279.

Lynch W. C. and Libby L. (1983) Naloxone suppresses intake of highly preferred saccharin solutions in food deprived and sated rats. *Life Sci.* **33,** 1909–1914.

Maickel R. P. and Maloney G. J. (1973) Effects of various depressant drugs on deprivation-induced water consumption. *Neuropharmacology* **12,** 777–782.

Maickel R. P. and Webb R. W. (1972) Taste phenomena and drug effects on thirst-induced fluid consumption by rats. *Neuropharmacology* **11**, 283–290.

Maickel R. P. and Zabik J. E. (1977) Minireview. The pharmacology of anorexigenesis. *Life Sci.* **21**, 173–180.

Margules D. L., Moisset B., Lewis M. J., Shibuya H., and Pert C. B. (1978) Beta-endorphin is associated with overeating in genetically obese mice (ob/ob) and rats (fa/fa). *Science* **202**, 988–991.

Martin W. R., Eades C. G., Thompson J. A. Huppler R. E., and Gilbert P. E. (1976) The effects of morphine- and nalorphine-like drugs in the non-dependent and morphine-dependent chronic spinal dog. *J. Pharmacol. Exp. Ther.* **197**, 517–532.

Miller N. E. (1956) Effects of drugs on motivation: The value of using a variety of measures. *Ann. NY Acad. Sci.* **65**, 318–333.

Mogenson G. J. and Stevenson J. A. F. (1967) Drinking induced by electrical stimulation of the lateral hypothalamus. *Exp. Neurol.* **17**, 119–127.

Morley J. E. and Levine A. S. (1981) Dynorphin-(1-13) induces spontaneous feeding in rats. *Life Sci.* **29**, 1901–1903.

Morley J. E. and Levine A. S. (1982) Opiates, Dopamine and Feeding, in *The Neural Basis of Feeding and Reward* (Hoebel B. G. and Novin D., eds.), Haer Institute, Brunswick, Maine.

Morley J. E. and Levine A. S. (1983) Involvement of dynorphin and the kappa opioid receptor in feeding. *Peptides* **4**, 797–800.

Morley J. E., Levine A. S., Gosnell B. A., and Billington C. J. (1984) Which opioid receptor mechanism modulates feeding? *Appetite* **5**, 61–68.

Morley J. E., Levine A. S., Grace M., and Kneip J. (1982a) An investigation of the role of kappa opiate receptor agonists in the initiation of feeding. *Life Sci.* **31**, 2617–2626.

Morley J. E., Levine A. S., Grace M., and Kneip J. (1982b) Dynorphin-(1-13), dopamine and feeding in rats. *Pharmacol. Biochem. Behav.* **16**, 701–705.

Morley J. E., Levine A. S., Yim G. K., and Lowy M. T. (1983) Opioid modulation of appetite. *Neurosci. Biobehav. Rev.* **7**, 281–305.

Neill D. B. and Grossman S. P. (1971) Interaction of the effects of reserpine and amphetamine on food and water intake. *J. Comp. Physiol. Psychol.* **76**, 327–336.

Nielsen E. B. and Lyon M. (1973) Drinking behaviour and brain dopamine: Antagonistic effect of two neuroleptic drugs (pimozide and spiramide) upon amphetamine- or apomorphine-induced hypodipsia. *Psychopharmacologia* **33**, 299–308.

Nieto J. and Posadas-Andrews A. (1984) Effects of chlordiazepoxide on food anticipation, drinking and other behaviors in food-deprived and satiated rats. *Pharmacol. Biochem. Behav.* **20**, 39–44.

Phillips M. I., Quinlan J., Keyser C., and Phipps J. (1978) Organum vasculosum of the lamina terminalis (OVLT) as a receptor site for ADH release, drinking, and blood pressure responses to angiotensin II (AII). *Fed. Proc.* **38**, 438–442.

Pi-Sunyer X., Kissileff H. R., Thornton J., and Smith G. P. (1982) C-terminal octapaptide of cholecystokinin decreases food intake in obese men. *Physiol. Behav.* **29**, 627–630.

Porter J. H., Goldsmith P. A., McDonough J. J., Heath G. F., and Johnson D. N. (1984) Differential effects of dopamine blockers on the acquisition of schedule-induced drinking and deprivation-induced drinking. *Physiol. Psychol.* **12**, 302–306.

Randall L. O., Schallek W., Heise G. A., Keith E. F., and Bagdon R. E. (1960) The psychosedative properties of methaminodiazepoxide. *J. Pharmacol. Exp. Ther.* **129**, 163–197.

Rettig R., Ganten D., and Johnson A. K. (1981) Isoproterenol-induced thirst: Renal and extrarenal mechanisms. *Am. J. Physiol.* **241**, R152–R157.

Robbins T. W. and Fray P. J. (1980) Stress-induced eating: Fact, fiction or misunderstanding? *Appetite* **1**, 103–133.

Rogers P. J. and Blundell J. E. (1979) Effect of anorexic drugs on food intake and the micro-structure of eating in human subjects. *Psychopharmacology* **66**, 159–165.

Rolls B. J., Woods R. J., and Stevens R. M. (1978) Effects of palatability on body fluid homeostasis. *Physiol. Behav.* **20**, 15–19.

Rowland N. (1982) Comparison of the suppression by naloxone of water intake induced in rats by hyperosmolarity, hypovolemia, and angiotensin. *Pharmacol. Biochem. Behav.* **16**, 87–91.

Sahakian B. J., Winn P., Robbins T. W., Deeley R. J., Everitt B. J., Dunn L. T., Wallace M., and James W. P. T. (1983) Changes in body weight and food-related behaviour induced by destruction of the ventral or dorsal noradrenergic bundle in the rat. *Neuroscience* **10**, 1405–1420.

Samanin R. and Garattini S. (1982) Neuropharmacology of Feeding, in *Drugs and Appetite* (Silverstone T., ed.), Academic, London.

Sanger D. J. (1981) Endorphinergic mechanisms in the control of food and water intake. *Appetite: J. Intake Res.* **2,** 193–208.

Sanger D. J. (1983) Opiates and Ingestive Behaviour, in *Theory in Psychopharmacology* vol. 2, (Cooper S. J., ed.), Academic, London.

Sanger D. J. and McCarthy P. S. (1981) Increased food and water intake produced in rats by opiate receptor agonists. *Psychopharmacology* **74,** 217–220.

Sanger D. J. and McCarthy P. S. (1982) The anorectic action of naloxone is attenuated by adaptation to a food-deprivation schedule. *Psychopharmacology* **77,** 336–338.

Schulz R., Wuster M., and Herz A. (1980) Interaction of amphetamine and naloxone in feeding behavior in guinea pigs. *Eur. J. Pharmacol.* **63,** 313–319.

Silverstone T. and Kyriakides M. (1982) Clinical Pharmacology of Appetite, in *Drugs and Appetite* (Silverstone T., ed.), Academic, London.

Simpson J. B. and Routtenberg A. (1973) Subfornical organ: site of drinking elicitation by angiotensin II. *Science* **818,** 1172–1174.

Simpson J. B., Epstein A. N., and Camardo J. S. (1978) Localization of receptors for the dipsogenic action of angiotensin II in the subfornical organ of the rat. *J. Comp. Physiol. Psychol.* **92,** 581–608.

Siviy S. M. and Reid L. R. (1983) Endorphinergic modulation of acceptability of putative reinforcers. *Appetite* **4,** 249–257.

Siviy S. M., Calcagnetti D. J., and Reid L. D. (1982) A temporal analysis of naloxone's suppressant effect on drinking. *Pharmacol. Biochem. Behav.* **16,** 173–175.

Slizgi G. R. and Ludens J. H. (1982) Studies on the nature and mechanism of the diuretic activity of the opioid analgesic ethylketazocine. *J. Pharmacol. Exp. Ther.* **220,** 585–591.

Smith G. P. and Gibbs J. (1979) Postprandial Satiety, in *Progress in Psychobiology and Physiological Psychology* vol. 8, (Sprague J. M. and Epstein A. N., eds.), Academic, New York.

Soulairac A. and Soulairac M. -L. (1970) Effects of Amphetamine-Like Substances and L-DOPA on Thirst, Water Intake and

Diuresis, in *Amphetamines and Related Compounds* (Costa E. and Garattini S., eds.), Raven, New York.

Stanley B. G. and Leibowitz S. F. (1985) Neuropeptide Y injected into the paraventricular hypothalamus: A powerful stimulant of feeding behavior. *Proc. Natl. Acad. Sci. USA* **82,** 3940–3943.

Stolerman I. P. and D'Mello G. D. (1978) Amphetamine-induced hypodipsia and its implications for conditioned taste aversion in rats. *Pharmacol. Biochem. Behav.* **8,** 333–338.

Swerdlow N. R., van der Kooy D., Koob G. F., and Wenger J. R. (1983) Cholecystokinin produces conditioned place-aversions, not place preferences, in food-deprived rats: Evidence against involvement in satiety. *Life Sci.* **32,** 2087–2093.

Tatemoto K. (1982) Neuropeptide Y: Complete amino acid sequence of the brain peptide. *Proc. Natl. Acad. Sci. USA* **79,** 5485–5489.

Thompson D. A., Welle S. L., Lilavivat U., Penicaud L., and Campbell R. H. (1982) Opiate receptor blockade in man reduced 2-deoxy-*d*-glucose induced food intake, but not hunger, thirst and hypothermia. *Life Sci.* **31,** 847–852.

Threatte R. M., Fregly M. J., Connor T. M., and Kikta D. C. (1981) *L*-5-hydroxytryptophan-induced drinking in rats: Possible mechanisms for induction. *Pharmacol. Biochem. Behav.* **14,** 385–391.

Tordoff, M. G., Hopfenbeck, J., Butcher L. L., and Novin D. (1982) A peripheral locus for amphetamine anorexia. *Nature* **297,** 148–150.

Trenchard E. and Silverstone T. (1983) Naloxone reduces the food intake of normal volunteers. *Appetite: J. Intake Res.* **4,** 43–50.

Turkish S. and Cooper S. J. (1984a) Enhancement of saline consumption by chlordiazepoxide in thirsty rats: Antagonism by Ro15-1788. *Pharmacol. Biochem. Behav.* **20,** 869–873.

Turkish S. and Cooper S. J. (1984b) Effects of a kappa receptor agonist, ethylketocyclazocine, on water consumption in water-deprived and nondeprived rats in diurnal and nocturnal tests. *Pharmacol. Biochem. Behav.* **21,** 47–51.

Valenstein E. S., Cox, V. C., and Kakolewski J. W. (1969) The Hypothalamus and Motivated Behavior, in *Reinforcement and Behavior* (Tapp J. T., ed.), Academic, New York.

von Voigtlander P. F., Lahti R. A., and Ludens J. H. (1983) U-50,488H: A selective and structurally novel non-mu (kappa) opioid agonist. *J. Pharmacol. Exp. Ther.* **87,** 481–484.

Weiner I. H. and Stellar E. (1951) Salt preference determined by a single-stimulus method. *J. Comp. Physiol. Psychol.* **44,** 394–401.

West D. B., Fey D., and Woods S. C. (1984) Cholecystokinin persistently suppresses meal size, but not food intake in free-feeding rats. *Am. J. Physiol.* **246,** R776–787.

Wise R. A. (1974) Lateral hypothalamic electrical stimulation: Does it make animals "hungry?" *Brain Res.* **67,** 187–209.

Effects of Drugs on Spontaneous Motor Activity

Colin T. Dourish

1. Introduction

The assessment of drug effects on spontaneous motor activity is of major importance in experimental psychopharmacology. At the simplest level, accurate and reliable measurement of animal movement is clearly necessary to detect potential stimulant and depressant properties of drugs. However, as outlined in subsequent chapters of this volume, the routine monitoring of changes in spontaneous motor activity is also an important requirement in the accurate assessment of drug effects on a wide range of other behavioral parameters, including feeding and drinking, aggression and social behavior, and various forms of conditioned behavior. During the development of experimental psychopharmacology, a large variety of methods has been used to monitor spontaneous motor activity and drug-induced alterations of it. These methods have encompassed techniques adapted from a number of established scientific disciplines, including ethology, neurology, physics, psychology, and pharmacology. The techniques used fall into one of two categories—those that require direct observation of the animal (with or without the aid of video or movie recording) and automatic measures that do not require a human observer. The first section of this chapter reviews the utility and limitations of the methods that are currently available to assess the effects of drugs in small animals. The techniques outlined are used principally to monitor the activity of small rodents, although similar procedures have been successfully adopted to measure the activity of avian species and primates (Dewhurst and Marley, 1965; Scraggs and Ridley, 1978).

The principal concern of this chapter is the assessment of drug effects on locomotor activity *per se* and, therefore, the influence of drugs on exploration and habituation will not be considered in any detail (for recent reviews of these latter topics, *see* Robbins, 1977; File, 1981).

2. Methods Used to Record Spontaneous Motor Activity

2.1. Automatic Measures of Activity

2.1.1. Photocell Devices

The photocell activity cage is by far the most frequently used device for the automatic recording of locomotor activity. Activity is recorded in such a device by the interruption of an infrared photobeam that passes between a light source, on one side of the cage, and a light-activated switch, on the opposite side. Interruption of the beam operates a pulse-forming circuit that, in turn, activates a digital counter. Activity scores from a counter or series of counters can either be read directly by the experimenter or monitored automatically by a computer system.

Photocell devices have been routinely used in the assessment of drug effects on animal movement for the past 30 yr (e.g., Dews, 1953; Krsiak et al., 1970), and increasingly sophisticated systems continue to be developed (Makanjuola et al., 1977; Ljungberg and Ungerstedt, 1978a; Dourish et al., 1983). The earliest devices generally employed a single beam or two horizontal beams arranged at right angles, or in parallel, across one axis of the cage (Robbins, 1977). In contrast, it is commonplace for photocell devices in use today to have as many as 12×12 horizontal photobeams, in addition to being equipped with a separate series of units suspended from the cage walls to measure vertical activity (Dourish et al., 1983). Such devices may also have "built-in" logic circuits that can distinguish between different classes of movement. In a system used by the author, an Opto Varimex Minor (Columbus Inst., USA) was used to make a distinction between whole-body ambulation and photobeam interruptions caused by other movements (*see* Dourish et al., 1983; Dourish and Cooper, 1984b). Total horizontal activity (including locomotion, grooming, scratching, head swaying, tail movements, and so on) was determined by the interruption of any one of 12×12 photobeams in any order. Ambulation, on the other hand, was determined by the interruption of consecutive photobeams. Interruption of any photobeam produced a 1-ms pulse that was counted by a microprocessor/Apple II microcomputer system interfaced to the photocell cages. Using this photocell system, it was shown that when the endogenous amine β-phenylethylamine (PEA) was applied bilaterally to the rat caudate nucleus, the resultant increase in total horizontal activity counts was largely accounted for by an increase in ambulation, rather than the production of stereotyped responses performed in one location (compare Figs. 1 and 2). These photocell-generated data were confirmed by direct observation (Dourish, 1985).

Photobeam systems have also been designed to measure locomotion and exploration. Makanjuola et al. (1977) described a device in which a "hole-board" apparatus had been fitted with photocells to monitor head-dipping automatically. Head-dipping on a hole-board has been proposed to be a valid measure of exploration that is to a large extent independent of locomotion (File and Wardill, 1975). Using computer anaysis, Makanjuola et al. (1977) were able to monitor frequency of head-dipping and its pattern, allowing exploratory head-dipping to be distinguished from stereotyped head-dipping.

To measure locomotion, exploration, and stereotyped behavior, a procedure involving a minicomputer interfaced to a large number of photocells has been described (Ljungberg and Ungerstedt, 1978a). The box consists of a modified open

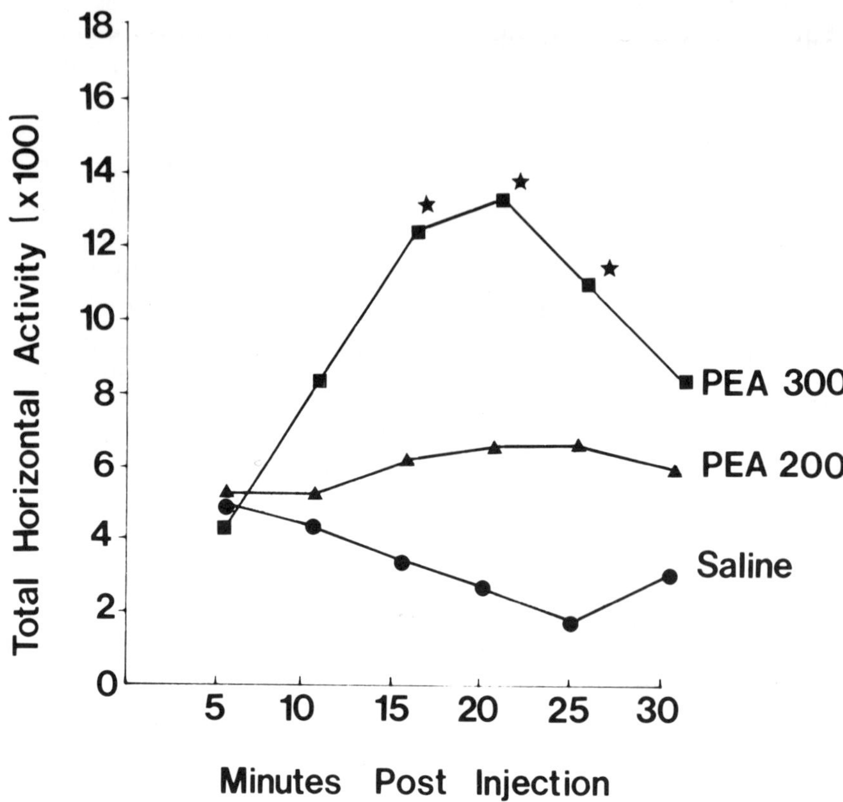

Fig. 1. Time course of the effects of 200 and 300 μg β-phenylethylamine (PEA) injected bilaterally into the caudate nucleus on total horizontal activity in rats ($n = 7$). *$p < 0.05$ drug vs saline treatment [from Dourish (1985), with permission of the publisher].

field enclosure (*see* section 2.2.3), in which the animal can move freely around the periphery but is unable to cross the arena because of a centrally-placed cube of the same height as the walls (*see* Fig. 3). Movements of the animals are detected by interruptions of 10 photobeams placed symmetrically around the arena. Using a logic circuit as described above, ambulation (consecutive beam interruptions) is separated from repetitive interruptions of the same beam. Total locomotion is defined as the number of times the

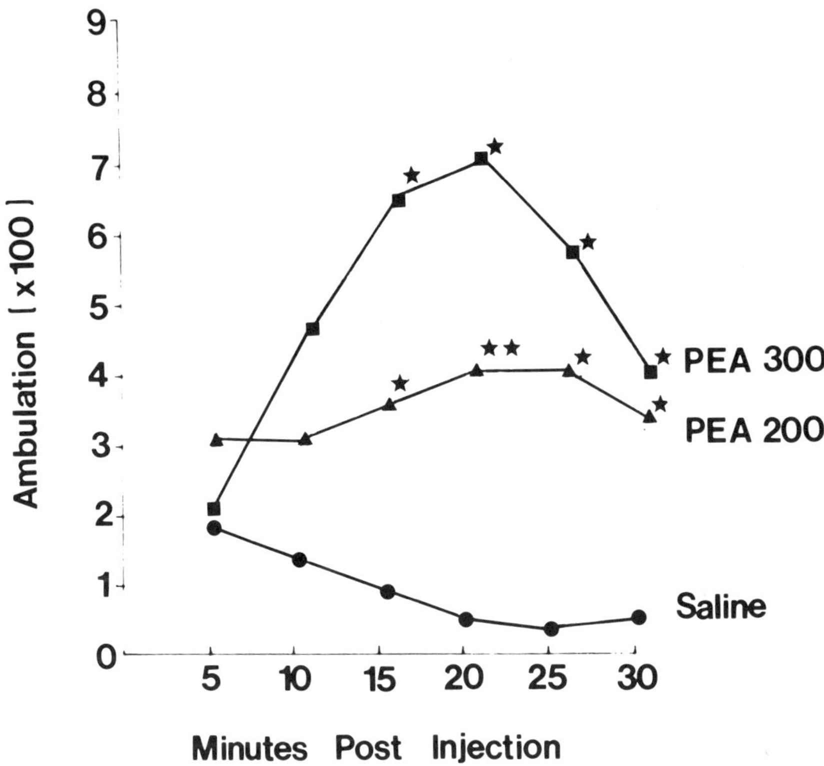

Fig. 2. Time course of the effects of 200 and 300 μg PEA injected bilaterally into the caudate nucleus on ambulation in rats. Data were collected from the same animals as in Fig. 1. Note that an increase in ambulation is responsible for most of the increase in total horizontal activity displayed in Fig. 1 (*see* text for further details). *$p < 0.05$; **$p < 0.01$ vs saline treatment [from Dourish (1985), with permission of the publisher].

animal walks a fixed distance, which is slightly less than the length of the box. Forward locomotion is defined as the number of times the animal walks the same distance but continues from one arm to the next arm (*see* Fig. 3). In addition, head-dipping is measured by photobeams in holes in the floor and gnawing is recorded by a vibration-sensitive plastic block. The apparatus has been used to establish that high doses of apomorphine given sc (subcutaneously) induce two different

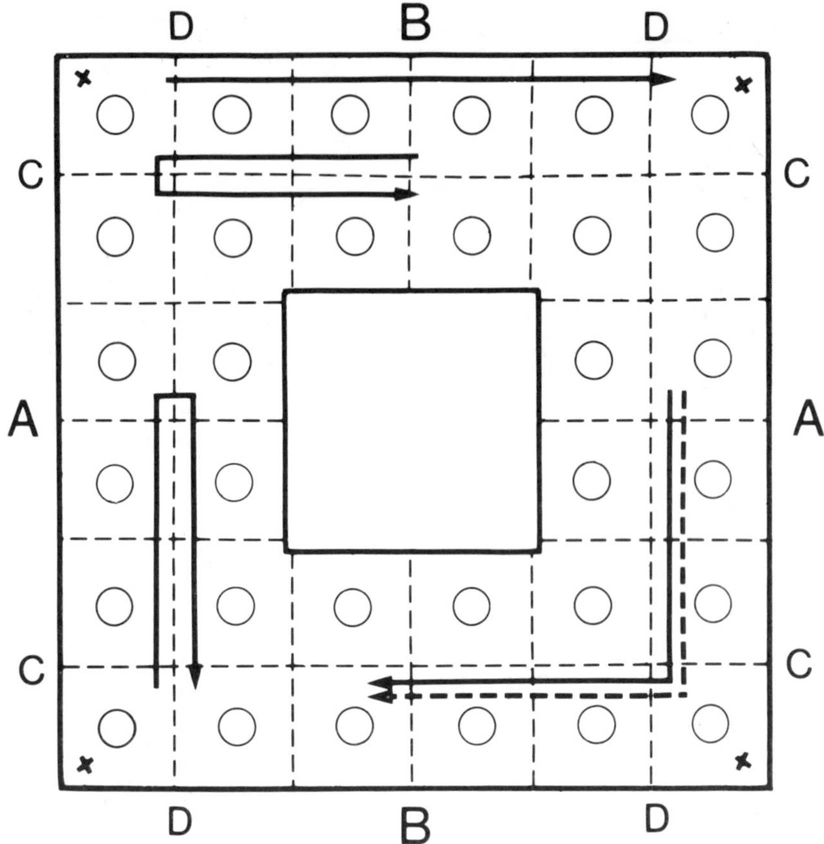

Fig. 3. Schematic illustration of the test box of Ljungberg and Ungerstedt (1978a), which uses a large number of photocells to measure locomotion, exploration, and stereotyped behavior. The box is symmetrically covered by ten photobeams (thin dotted lines). Activity is defined as the number of interruptions of these photobeams. A total locomotion count corresponds to the distance walked by the animal as shown by the solid arrows and a forward locomotion count corresponds to the distance shown by the dotted arrow. These conditions are set by the programming of the digital electronic circuitry. The x in the corner shows the position of the vertical photobeams. Corner count is defined as the number of interruptions of these photobeams and corner time is accumulated time of interruption [from Ljungberg and Ungerstedt (1978a), with permission of the authors and publisher].

types of behavior, one characterized by increased locomotion and the other by strong stereotyped gnawing (Ljungberg and Ungerstedt, 1978b).

2.1.2. Electromagnetic Field Devices

These devices measure activity by continuous monitoring of alterations in electromagnetic wave patterns. The activity cage contains an electromagnetic field that is sensitive to any motion within it. Movement of the animal causes an alteration in the energy of the field that is recorded as a locomotion count.

The first device of this type to become commercially available was the Animex meter (Farad Inc., Sweden), which was initially tested by Svensson and Thieme (1969). The Animex contains a resonating field, produced by a series of inductive coils located beneath the floor of the activity chamber, that can be distorted by animal movement. If the distortion is large enough, it produces a voltage pulse that is recorded as a locomotor count. However, inductive coils produce resonating fields of variable dimensions, and it is possible for rodents to move between the sensing fields without activity being recorded (Tyler and Tessel, 1979). Apparently this problem may be partially resolved by raising field sensitivity and accepting an excess of counts when the animal is directly over a coil to compensate for a lack of counts when the animal moves between fields.

Subsequently, a number of capacitative systems has been developed that, it is claimed, accurately measure vertical motion and can distinguish between different types of movements (Wolthuis et al., 1975; Kameyama and Ukai, 1981).

In a device described by Wolthuis et al. (1975), two capacitor plates are used and the animal moves in a homogenous electric field of which the cage forms a part. Movements of the animal cause changes in the field producing a change in the output signal from the circuit. The largest pulses in the signal correspond to rearing and are counted directly as vertical activity. Smaller signals are filtered (to eliminate noise and drift), classified according to amplitude, and recorded, on four separate counters. One class of signals was caused by the animal breathing, the other three corresponded to horizontal movements (locomotion, grooming, sniffing). It proved difficult to separate different types of horizontal movement in this study (Wolthuis et al., 1975). However, in a more recent study, Kameyama and Ukai (1981) claimed that the Animex II meter, using a similar analysis of the amplitude of signal changes in a capacitance field, was capable of classifying movement as locomotion, rearing, grooming, and tremor.

A more sophisticated capacitative system has been used in an attempt to differentiate between activity counts produced by locomotion and stereotyped behavior. Tyler and Tessel (1979) tested the Varimex meter (Columbus Inst., USA), which used two capacitative sensors to respond to animal-induced changes in a resonating field. The responses of the sensors produced voltage pulses proportional to the amplitude of animal movement. There were two sensitivity measurements, one that corresponded to total horizontal activity and one that represented locomotion (similar to the Opto Varimex photobeam system described by Dourish et al., 1983) (*see* section 2.1.1). Stereotyped responses could be calculated by subtracting locomotor counts from total horizontal counts. However, at high doses of amphetamine, this device miscounted stereotypy (of large amplitude) as locomotion (Tyler and Tessel, 1979).

The use of Doppler-shift radar to measure animal movement was reported by two groups in 1979 (Vanuytven et al., 1979; Marsden and King, 1979). The most sophisticated system was that described by Marsden and King (1979), which operated on the principle of monitoring changes in the signal of a low-energy microwave field caused by movement of an animal. The frequency of the signal was linearly related to the speed of movement and its amplitude proportional to the body area involved. Two frequency bands were used—one that measured low-speed activity consisting of head and body movements without locomotion, and one that measured high-speed activity, consisting of movement around the cage. Thus, it was claimed to be possible to distinguish between drug-induced locomotion and stereotyped behavior performed in one location.

2.1.3. Video-Based Tracking Systems (x−y Plotters)

The video-based tracking system is, in effect, an automated open field (*see* section 2.2.3) that provides a record of both the amount and pattern of locomotion of a test subject. One of the first attempts to monitor rodent activity in this type of device was reported by Tanger et al. (1978). Their apparatus consisted of an open field painted black that was constantly scanned by a television camera. Any white spot or animal of sufficient size against the black background caused a change in the camera output voltages when the spot was scanned by the camera beam. Two output voltages were produced that corresponded to the position of the rat with respect to the left side of the area scanned (*x*-coordinate) and the position of the rat with respect to the upper side of the area scanned (*y*-coordinate). Subsequently, this type of apparatus has been used successfully to examine the changes in activity patterns produced by amphetamine and apomorphine (Strombom, 1979; Nickolson, 1981). It is apparent from Fig. 4 that apomorphine produced distinctive changes in the pattern of rat locomotion that were dependent on dose. A lose dose (0.02 mg/kg) of apomorphine reduced locomotion and inhibited movement across the inner field (*see* middle section of Fig. 4). In contrast, a higher dose of the drug (0.5 mg/kg) increased locomotion and produced stereotyped movement patterns (*see* lower section of Fig. 4). In addition to tracing the pattern of locomotion in an open field, the *x−y* plotter can also be used to assess drug effects on a number of other parameters, including the number of entries into the inner field, the number of stops and starts, and the speed of movements (Nickolson, 1981).

2.1.4. Digitized Videodisplays

One of the most recent developments in automatic activity measurement is the use of a microcomputer to analyze pictures obtained from a video camera (Spruijt and Gispen, 1983). This procedure is made possible by the use of a videodigitizer that is interfaced to the microcomputer. The interface is connected to a video camera and, every few seconds, generates digitized pictures of the display on the

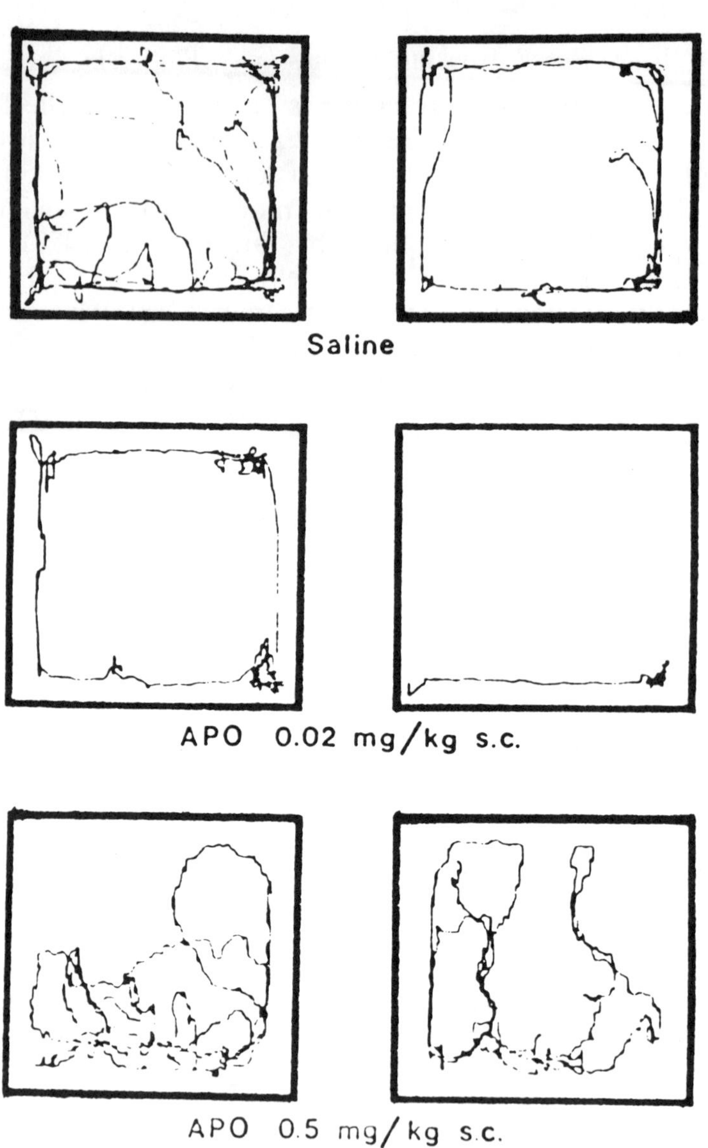

Fig. 4. Walking patterns, as plotted by an *x-y* recorder, of rats treated with either saline (upper row), 0.02 mg/kg of apomorphine (middle row), or 0.5 mg/kg of apomorphine (lower row), given 5 min before exposure to an open field. Patterns on the left were obtained during the first 5 min of testing, patterns on the right were obtained during the second 5 min of testing [from Nickolson (1981), with permission of the author and publisher].

camera screen. The pictures generated are stored in the computer's memory for future analysis. Spruijt and Gispen (1983) have written and tested software that can distinguish between different behavioral categories using the digitized pictures. The program uses the height and width of various animal postures to characterize rearing, sleeping, sitting, and grooming. A study was performed in which the computer had to distinguish between rats treated with adrenocorticotrophic hormone (ACTH) or saline. ACTH treatment is known to elicit a syndrome of yawning, stretching, and excessive grooming in rats (Gispen and Isaacson, 1981). Although the computer analysis was able to successfully distinguish between rearing and lying down, errors became apparent when grooming, performed in one location, was interpreted as sitting (Spruijt and Gispen, 1983). Although this type of automated analysis is presently in its infancy, it seems to hold considerable promise for the future. The automated measurement of individual elements of behavior by microcomputer may eventually provide an accurate, quantitative, and unbiased record of spontaneous behavior.

2.1.5. *Other Automatic Measures*

The devices described above are immobile, with activity counts being produced by movement of the animal. In contrast, devices have been used in the past that record activity by virtue of movement of the environment as a function of animal motion. Such devices, which include running wheels, tilt cages, and stabilimeters, are now rarely used in the study of drug effects and, therefore, will be considered only briefly (for a more detailed discussion of such devices, the reader is referred to Robbins, 1977).

2.1.5.1. *Running Wheels.* The running wheel monitors activity by rotating about its axis as the animal moves. Thus, activity is measured as the number of complete revolutions of the wheel that is recorded on a counter. Since wheel-running is not a natural rodent behavior, the device requires considerable habituation to establish a stable baseline of activity (Finger, 1972). Consequently, it could be argued that a habituated animal has learned to run in the wheel and, therefore, is not exhibiting spontaneous motor activity. This problem is further confounded by large individual differences in the wheel running response.

2.1.5.2. *Stabilimeters, Jiggle Cages, and Tilt Cages.*   These devices record activity by being tilted or displaced (horizontally or vertically) when the animal moves within the device. Activity is recorded as the number of tilts or displacements of the apparatus. There have been numerous criticisms of this type of apparatus, of which the most serious appear to be the measurement of tremor in addition to movement, and the finding that the motion of the cage produces feedback stimuli that affect the activity of the subject.

2.2. Observational Measures of Activity

There is a number of general points to consider regarding observation of animal behavior prior to discussing specific methods that are available. First, and perhaps most importantly, observation should be unobtrusive. Thus, when and where possible, the observer should use a vantage point that is remote from the animal being studied and connected via a one-way mirror or television monitoring system. If observation must be conducted in the test room, then red-light illumination and noise (e.g., from a fan or ventilation system) may be necessary to mask the investigator's presence.

Second, observation should be "blind" (i.e., the observer should be unaware of the experimental treatment), and the reliability of the classification and recording system being used should be checked by employing several observers and calculating the correlation between their data. In many cases, it is not possible for practical reasons to run a completely "blind" study. For example, a drug may induce a clearly visible side effect that is obvious even to an untrained observer. In such a situation, observation of the variable of interest cannot be truly "blind." In other cases, however, in which the use of several "blind" observers is precluded for reasons of unavailability of sufficient personnel, a useful alternative may be to employ one "blind" observer in addition to one or more "nonblind" observers. If there is a sufficiently high concordance between the ratings of all the observers, this "semiblind" method would be acceptable.

Ideally, the animal should be observed continuously during the course of an investigation, although this may be a rather monotonous process. The monotony can be reduced by either using video recordings, or by observing the animal at preselected intervals (time sampling). Time sampling can be a useful and informative procedure, but has the disadvantage of being dependent on frequency measures. This could be an important drawback if a drug of interest has a specific effect on response duration, but does not produce a corresponding change in response frequency.

2.2.1. *Rating Scales and All-or-None Procedures*

Rating scales and all-or-none procedures have been the most widely used observational measures in psychopharmacological studies for many years. Unfortunately, they are also the least informative and most suspect observational measures available (*see* sections 3.3 and 4.2). Rating scales are used to quantify a variety of drug-induced behavioral syndromes, some of which are routinely employed as screening tests by pharmaceutical companies in the development of new drugs. Such syndromes include various forms of drug-induced stereotypy, sedation, and catalepsy. The scale that is probably most familiar to psychopharmacologists is the stereotypy rating scale. A variety of complex stereotypy rating systems are currently used, most of which are derived from that of Quinton and Halliwell (1963). A representative example, used by Borison et al. (1977) to quantify amphetamine- and PEA-induced stereotypy, is illustrated in Table 1.

Similar types of scale have been used to measure drug-induced sedation and catalepsy (Papeschi and Randrup, 1973; Dourish and Cooper, 1982). This type of rating scale is developed from extensive pilot studies in which animals are exposed to a wide range of doses of the drug (or drugs) of interest. However, in order to use such a rating measure, the experimenter assumes that the scale is rating a monotonic continuum of behavior and that the rank intensity is valid.

Table 1
A Stereotypy Rating Scale[a]

Score	Description of stereotyped behavior
0	No stereotyped behavior
+1	Increased exploratory activity, continuous sniffing
+2	Occasional side-to-side head-bobbing; licking, or gnawing at cage floor grid; easily distracted by ambient auditory stimuli
+3	Continuous head-bobbing; remains in one location for as long as 5 min; distracted only by loud auditory stimuli
+4	Continuous head-bobbing; remains in one location for more than 5 min; not distracted by loud auditory stimuli

[a] Scale adapted from Borison et al. (1977).

Such assumptions are not invariably correct (*see* sections 3.3 and 4.2).

An alternative method of quantifying a drug-induced behavioral syndrome is the all-or-none procedure. This procedure has been extensively used in the investigation of the so-called "serotonin syndrome" (Jacobs, 1976). The serotonin syndrome is a characteristic behavioral pattern that can be elicited in rats by a variety of 5-HT precursors, releasers, or receptor agonists. The syndrome is considered to be present in an all-or-none fashion if rats simultaneously exhibit at least four of the six component signs, listed in Table 2, at any time during the observation period (e.g., Trulson and Jacobs, 1976; Sloviter et al., 1978). Other investigators have used a slight variation of this procedure in which components of the syndrome are assessed separately at 5-min intervals (and scored 0 for absent and 1 for present) and summed at the end of the experiment to give an overall score (e.g., Fernando et al., 1980).

Table 2
The Serotonin Syndrome[a]

Component	Description
Resting tremor	Shaking, particularly of head and forelimbs
Rigidity	Assessed both by grasping the rat around the torso and by passively extending and flexing the hindlimbs
Forepaw padding	Rhythmic dorsoventral forelimb movements
Hindlimb abduction	A dramatic splaying out of the hindlimbs
Straub tail	Tail erect
Lateral head weaving	Slow side-to-side head movements

[a] Adapted from Jacobs (1976).

2.2.2. *Ethological Analysis of Behavioral Elements*

Ethological techniques have made an important contribution to the study of the effect of drugs on spontaneous motor activity (*see* review by Mackintosh et al., 1977). The ethological approach to the examination of drug effects involves recording behavior as it occurs in terms of a relatively large number of variables that are observed directly. An assumption of ethological analysis is that animal behavior is not amorphous and infinitely flexible, but is constructed of identifiable elements (Mackintosh et al., 1977). Thus, the investigator can generate a checklist of behavioral items of interest for subsequent observation. An example of the type of checklist that could be used to examine drug effects on spontaneous motor activity is shown in Table 3. A cursory examination of the contents of Table 3 (it should be noted that this is not an exhaustive checklist) should give the reader some impression of the large amount of data that a checklist experiment (using either continuous observation or time sam-

Table 3
An Ethological Checklist of Behavioral Elements That
Could Be Used to Examine Drug Effects[a]

Element	Description
Sniff	Distinctive pattern of air inspiration accompanied by vibrissae movements
Rear	Stand on hind legs
Scan	A combination of rear and sniff
Walk[b]	
Explore	Investigation of surroundings
Genital groom[b]	
Self groom and scratch[b]	
Wash	Forepaws groom face
Displacement groom	Abbreviated face washing
Crouch[b]	
Straight legs	Standing with legs extended
Freeze	Complete cessation of movement
Chatter	Teeth chattering
Tail up	Tail held vertically
Head shake[b]	
Gnaw	Bite cage bars or floor
Dig	Sawdust scraped back with forepaws and kicked with hindpaws
Push dig	Sawdust pushed forward with forepaws
Kick	Kicking movements with hindleg
On bars	Climbing on bars of cage
Off bars	Climbing off bars on cage
Flop	Lying flat

[a] Adapted from Mackintosh et al. (1977).
[b] These elements are self explanatory.

pling) can generate. The accumulation of data, however, is only the first stage in an ethological study. Subsequent data analysis may include identification of elements or groups of elements of behavior that occur together frequently, or in sequence, and which may be functionally related within pathways of behavior (*see* Mackintosh et al., 1977, for further details). Unfortunately, as pointed out by Krsiak and Borgošová (1972), such detailed studies of the effects of drugs on spontaneous motor activity are very rare. The reason for this situation appears to relate to a number of factors: i.e., the data-accumulation process is monotonous and time-consuming and, when the study is complete, the data analysis may be extremely difficult and complex (Mackintosh et al., 1977). Despite this, abbreviated forms of checklist analysis of behavioral elements have been developed and used with considerable success in psychopharmacology. For example, Taylor et al. (1974) developed an abbreviated checklist, as an alternative to a stereotypy rating scale, to examine the CNS effects of a number of anorectic agents. At 5-min intervals, an observer recorded the presence or absence of the following six categories of behavior in an all-or-none fashion: rearing, forward walking, immobility, backward walking, circling, and head swaying. Since this system was designed to examine stereotypy and abnormal behavior, it is not exhaustive and excludes some behavioral patterns that are common in undrugged animals (e.g., grooming, sniffing). However, a more comprehensive checklist analysis of behavior was described and used in earlier studies by this group (Taylor et al., 1971). More recently, Fray et al. (1980) have used an abbreviated checklist (of ten items) and an all-or-none time sampling procedure to compare and contrast the stimulant and stereotypic effects of amphetamine and apomorphine in rats.

Similarly, I have used a list of 13 categories to record the behavioral effects of PEA in mice (*see* Table 4). This analysis used a time-sampling procedure in combination with a five-point rating scale for intensity of each behavioral element (0 = absent; 1 = mild intensity or present 1–2 times during observation period; 2 = moderate intensity or present 3–4

Table 4
Abbreviated Checklist Used to Assess the Stimulant and Stereotypic Effects of PEA in Mice[a]

Behavioral Category	Description
Freezing	Inactive in one location
Forward walking	Coordinated locomotor activity in a forward direction
Rearing	Standing on hind legs
Grooming	Body cleaning and washing
Sniffing	Distinctive pattern of air inspiration accompanied by vibrissae movements
Backward walking	Backward locomotion or backward circling
Headweaving	Repetitive, fast, side-to-side head movements
Padding	Repetitive up-and-down placing movements of the forepaws
Hyperreactivity	Exaggerated startle response
Tremor[b]	
Jumping[b]	
Licking	Licking or biting cage floor or walls
Vocalization[b]	

[a] Adapted from Dourish (1982a).
[b] These items are self explanatory.

times; 3 = high intensity or present 5 or more times; 4 = severe or present for prolonged periods). Abbreviated checklists such as those described above are generally developed (after a series of preliminary studies) for use specifically in the assessment of the effects of a certain drug or class of drugs in rats or mice. Thus, they may not be applicable for use with certain other drug classes or in a different species. In contrast, the ethological checklist (Table 3) has a wider range of applications, and with the addition of relevant categories can be used to examine drug effects on exploration, social behavior, sexual behavior, and aggression.

2.2.3. Open-Field Techniques

Open-field studies involve the direct observation and recording of animal behavior in an enclosure larger than the home cage, using techniques such as an ethological checklist or movement notation (*see* sections 2.2.2 and 2.2.5). The open field is generally a uniform, circular enclosure of 2–3 ft in diameter that has a floor marked in coded squares. Locomotion is assessed by counting the number of times an animal enters a square. By using the code, it is possible for an investigator to trace the animal's path during the course of an experiment. Although open-field studies yield valuable information regarding drug effects on locomotion, they are somewhat rare in psychopharmacology. In this respect, use of the open field appears to be unpopular for the same reasons as comprehensive ethological analysis (see previous section). However, it should be noted that the open field is frequently employed in studies of drug effects on exploration and emotionality in rodents (*see* Robbins, 1977, for further discussion).

2.2.4. Video Recording and Microcomputer Encoding

An increasingly popular alternative to monotonous hours of animal observation is the use of video recording of behavior with subsequent microcomputer encoding of data. Video recording is unobtrusive and can be used to monitor animal behavior for long periods. Subsequently, the recorded tapes are played back and the investigator can encode various behavioral events by pressing the keys of a microcomputer that has been appropriately programmed.

At first, it may appear that the investigator has simply replaced long hours of animal observation with long hours of videotape viewing. However, this is not necessarily the case, for a number of reasons. First, tape recordings can be examined in "search" mode, which allows rapid examination of tapes to locate areas of interest. If the investigator discovers a section of the tape on which the animal is inactive (e.g., sleeping), then the tape can be quickly moved onto a new section. The investigator also has the option of time-sampling from the recording at appropriate intervals.

An additional advantage of video recording is that the same sequence of animal behavior can be observed and analyzed by a number of observers at their leisure. Further, when subsequent microcomputer encoding is used, the investigator can generate quantitative parametric data, including latency, frequency, and duration measures of the behavioral categories of interest. This is generally accomplished with computer programs by pressing the appropriate input key for each specific behavioral category (*see* Hendrie and Bennett, 1983). The first key press will record latency to onset of the first response in that category, and duration may be recorded by depressing the carriage return key at the end of the response. (Note: A real-time clock in the computer is necessary for this procedure.) The computer will sum key presses to provide a frequency measure. If a number of responses of interest occur simultaneously, it is possible to repeat the playback and encoding sequence several times.

The video recording/microcomputer-encoding procedure is now used routinely in many behavioral laboratories and has yielded important information regarding drug effects on locomotor activity. For example, the use of this procedure has enabled Nielsen et al (1980, 1983) to demonstrate that chronic amphetamine intoxication in rats and monkeys appears to produce hallucinatory-specific behavior (limb flicks, shaking, excessive grooming) that may be a useful animal model of psychosis.

Similar methods have been used to study rodent aggression and social behavior (Hendrie and Bennett, 1983), and feeding, drinking, and stereotypy (Dourish et al., 1985a, 1986).

One major disadvantage of computer-encoding procedures is the need for transcription of data for processing and statistical analysis. However, recent software developments, such as those described by DePaulis (1983) and Hendrie and Bennett (1984), that allow rapid encoding, processing of data and statistical analysis of results using a single program may overcome this problem.

2.2.5. *Eshkol-Wachmann Movement Notation*

Perhaps the most important recent development in the analysis of spontaneous motor activity has been the use of Eshkol-Wachmann movement notation to study animal movement. This system, which has been pioneered by Golani, Teitelbaum, and colleagues (Golani et al., 1979; Schallert et al., 1980; Teitelbaum et al., 1982) is used to record movement either from direct observation, or, more commonly, from video tape or movie frames. Analysis of the "natural geometry" of movement (Golani et al., 1979) has provided remarkable insights into various forms of natural rodent locomotion and exploration (Teitelbaum et al., 1982). More importantly for psychopharmacologists, movement notation studies have profoundly increased our conceptual understanding of drug-induced and lesion-induced effects on spontaneous motor activity. For example, movement notation studies have made it possible to explain discrepant findings on stereotyped behavior induced by dopamine agonists (*see* section 4.2.2)

Movement notation describes the motion of the animal as a whole within spherical coordinate systems and, at a finer level, can be used to describe the motion of particular limbs and parts of the body. The animal's body is thought of as a system of straight rods connected by joints (illustrated as bars superimposed in Fig. 5). Thus, bodily movement of the animal is seen as the sum of the movement of these rods that represent particular limb and body segments. As illustrated in Fig. 5, Golani et al. (1979) have considered the body as consisting of the following segments: head, neck, upper torso, middle torso, and lower torso. Each leg is also considered a separate segment. The circles and numerals within them in Fig. 5 describe the position of each segment, bodywise in relation to the next proximal segment in both the vertical (bottom) and horizontal (top) planes. For example, in Fig. 5 the position of the head would be notated as (1)[0], meaning the head is in line with the neck in the horizontal plane and

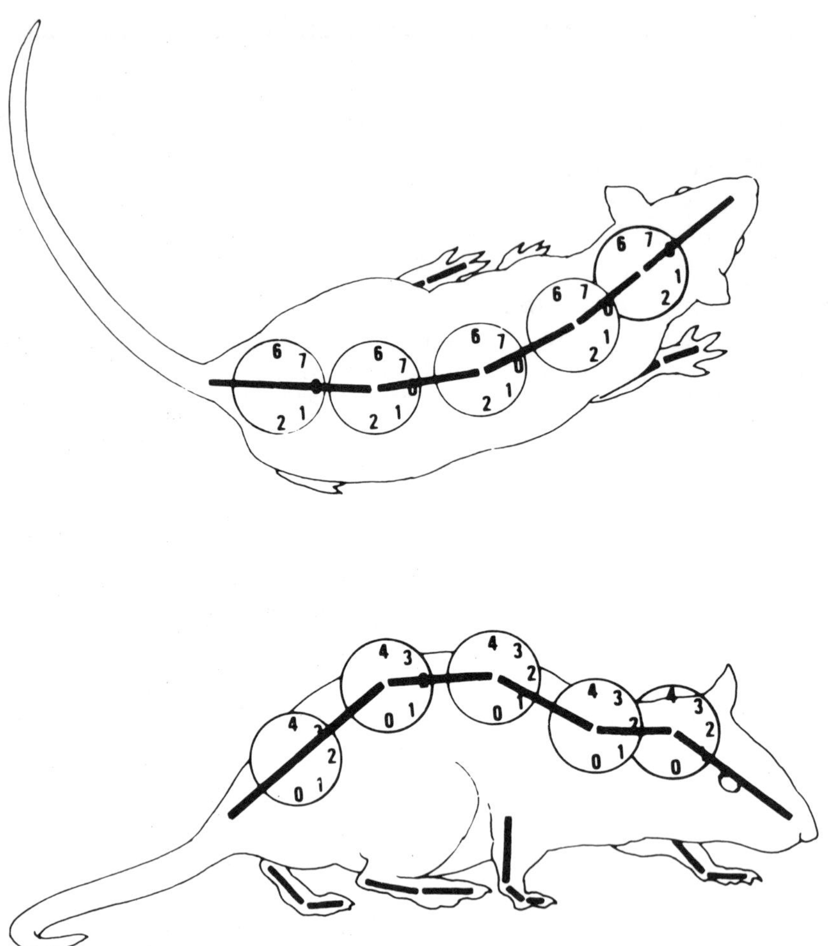

Fig. 5. Schematic illustration of some of the mechanics of Eshkol-Wachmann movement notation. The drawings represent a side and top view of a rat during locomotion. The superimposed bars indicate the body parts considered as separate limb segments. The circles and numerals within them give a side and top view of the spherical coordinate system and coordinates, in relation to which the position of the head was notated as (1)[0], which reads [0] horizontal; that is, in one line with the neck, and (1) vertical; that is, 45° away from vertical, counterclockwise [from Golani et al. (1979), with permission of the authors and publisher].

one unit (45°) counterclockwise away in the vertical plane. A movement is described in terms of the initial and final positions of the bodily segments and the trajectory between them. The trajectory of movement is defined in terms of two factors: (a) clockwise or counterclockwise, and (b) the angle between the axis of the limb segment and the axis of symmetry of movement. Thus, three kinds of movement are described:

1. Rotatory movements, in which the axis of the limb and the axis of the movement coincide.
2. Conical movements, in which the angle of movement is any angle less than 90° and greater than 0°.
3. Plane movements, in which the angle of movement is 90°.

The various limb and body segments are represented on a score page by a series of horizontal lines, and columns represent units of time. In addition to the notation of movement in relation to body segments, activity of the animal is described in terms of three other frames of reference: (1) snout trajectory; (2) elevation (postural support) of the body in space; and (3) contact with surfaces. By reading the notation in all four frames of reference, an experienced observer can accurately visualize the behavior of the animal without having seen it (for further details, *see* Golani et al., 1979; Szechtman et al., 1985).

Movement notation has proved particularly valuable in the investigation of the akinetic and cataleptic state, known as "the lateral hypothalamic syndrome," which can be induced by either large bilateral electrolytic lesions of the lateral hypothalamus (LH), or bilateral 6-hydroxydopamine lesions of the ascending nigrostriatal dopamine neurons (Teitelbaum et al., 1982). These studies have revealed that, in LH-lesioned animals, head, limb, and body movement recovers along specific dimensions. Lateral movement recovers first and lesioned animals exhibit progressively larger-amplitude horizontal lateral head-scanning movements during successive phases of recovery (*see* Fig. 6). Subsequently, longitudinal snout movements and vertical movements appear. Postural

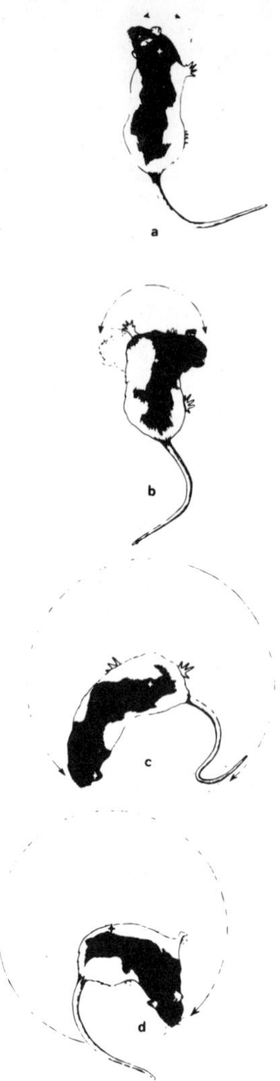

Fig. 6. Schematic drawing illustrating how movement notation
has been used to describe recovery from the akinesia caused by
severe bilateral lateral hypothalamic damage in rats. The drawing
shows the top view of a rat performing increasingly larger amplitude horizontal lateral movements during four successive phases of
recovery. Broken line and full line drawings indicate the extreme
positions that the rat assumes during each phase. The arrows indicate the amplitude of the movements. The + sign indicates the
root of the movement, beyond which there is practically no recruit-
ment of limb and body segments for movement. During increasingly larger lateral movements (b–d), the limb and body segments
are recruited in a cephalocaudal order. Drawings were traced from
individual movie frames [from Golani et al. (1979), with permission of the authors and publisher].

body support recovers concurrently but independently of lateral, horizontal, and vertical movement. Movement notation has also been employed, with considerable success, in the analysis of drug-induced behavioral stereotypy and catalepsy. For instance, apomorphine-induced stereotyped behavior has been described in terms of a behavioral regression that occurs in a sequence that is opposite to the sequence of neurological recovery in LH-lesioned animals (Szechtman et al., 1980, 1985). This hypothesis is discussed in detail below (*see* section 4.2.2). In the case of drug-induced catalepsy, it has been possible to distinguish between two forms of a cataleptic state induced by morphine and haloperidol (DeRyck et al., 1980). Teitelbaum and colleagues have demonstrated that haloperidol-treated rats exhibit a crouched standing posture with broad-based support of the body. This posture enables the rat to respond with a resistant bracing reaction when the experimenter attempts to move the animal. In contrast, morphine-treated rats show a loss of limb support, together with a rigid lying posture, and allow themselves to be easily displaced and rolled over (DeRyck et al., 1980).

3. Utility and Limitations of the Methods Available to Measure Activity

3.1. General Considerations

When using any of the methods described in the preceding pages to measure locomotor activity, there is a number of important factors that must be considered in the design of an experimental study and subsequent analysis of the data collected. Such factors include determination of baseline activity, diurnal rhythms, consideration of internal factors (e.g., age, sex, species, strain, availability of food and water), and previous experience of the subject and determination of appropriate statistical analysis procedures. These factors are considered in detail below.

3.1.1. Determination of Baselines

Baseline locomotor activity may be defined as that exhibited by an animal under control conditions (generally after treatment with saline or drug vehicle). Baseline activity is influenced by a multitude of variables, many of which are discussed in the subsequent sections of this chapter (e.g., age, sex, time of day, and so on). In addition, it is possible for the investigator to manipulate baseline activity to best suit the purpose of a particular experiment. For example, it would be difficult to identify a sedative effect induced by a drug if animals are tested in a familiar or home-cage environment (particularly during the daytime) where baseline activity is low (that is, there may be a "floor effect"). Thus, it is best to test for a sedative effect in a situation in which the animal will reliably exhibit high baseline activity. An example is when an animal is exposed to a novel cage and spends long periods of time engaging in locomotion and exploration. Conversely, if an experiment is designed to examine the locomotor stimulant properties of a drug, high baseline activity could obscure a drug action by producing a "ceiling effect." Consequently, an appropriate test for drug-induced locomotor stimulation requires habituating the animals to the test cage, or conducting the experiment in the home cage. In both of these situations, the animal should display a low activity baseline. Various forms of habituation are possible and include: (a) daily exposure to the test environment; (b) exposure of the animal to the test environment for a long period, such as overnight; and (c) introduction of the animal to the environment for a short period prior to testing. A reliable procedure is to use either (a) or (b) in combination with (c).

It should be stressed that the reliable assessment of baseline activity in any drug study is of vital importance in determining the nature of a drug effect (Robbins, 1977).

3.1.2. Diurnal Rhythms and Illumination

Despite the fact that most rodent species are nocturnal and therefore inactive during the daylight hours, the majority of studies of drug effects on locomotion are conducted during the day. There have been few investigations into the role of circadian rhythms in determining an animal's response to drugs. Recently, however, a few experiments have been reported in which a significant influence of diurnal rhythms on drug-induced locomotion and stereotyped behavior was observed (Nakano et al., 1980; Itoh et al., 1981; Decoursey, 1982; Marzullo and Friedhoff, 1982). In addition to assessing the influence of the day/night cycle on drug response, it is clearly of considerable physiological importance to examine the motor activity of awake rodents rather than the behavior of rodents that have been disturbed from sleeping (i.e., to test during the night rather than during the day). This can be achieved, with minimum inconvenience to the investigator, by adapting the rodents to a "reversed light cycle" in a room in which light and dark periods can be programmed. Thus, testing can be conducted under "red bulb" illumination (to which rats are relatively insensitive) during the animals' night phase and the investigators' daytime. Despite the availability of this simple procedure, however, relatively few drug studies on locomotor activity are conducted using a reversed light cycle.

3.1.3. Age

The age of an animal has a profound effect on its locomotor responses to drug treatment. Developing rats pass through a phase of hyperreactivity to stimulant drugs before acquiring the inhibitory controls that are characteristic of adult animals (Spear, 1979). Thus, the dose–response curve for amphetamine-induced locomotor stimulation, measured by photocells, is significantly different in neonatal and adult rats (Campbell et al., 1969). Similarly, sedation which is evident in adult rats treated with low doses of the dopamine agonists apomorphine and piribedil is absent in rats that are 4 wk old or younger (Shalaby and Spear, 1980; Dourish and Cooper, 1984a). Furthermore, aged rats exhibit supersensitive responses to stimulants compared to their younger counterparts (e.g., Smith et al., 1978; Roffman et al., 1980), an effect that may be analogous to the supersensitivity induced by monoamine-depleting brain lesions (Severson and Finch, 1980).

3.1.4. Sex

Male rats are more frequently used in studies of drug effects on locomotor activity than female rats. This is probably because of reports that activity levels are influenced by the estrus cycle (Wang, 1923). However, it is important to note that the question of whether males or females are employed in a particular study is relatively unimportant provided that exclusively male or female groups are used. It is unwise to assess drug effects in groups of mixed gender, since drug and sex interactions can occur that may influence results. For example, Stretch (1963) has reported that gender can influence the locomotor response to amphetamine and barbiturates.

3.1.5. Appetite

The availability of food and water (before and during testing) influences the locomotor response of an animal to drug treatment. Thus, food deprivation potentiates the locomotor stimulant effect of amphetamine and apomorphine in the rat (Campbell and Fibiger, 1973; Sahakian and Robbins, 1975). Water deprivation alters the locomotor depressant action of low doses of apomorphine and piribedil in the same species (Dourish and Cooper, 1981a,b).

Nutritional interactions with drug effects on locomotion may arise, at least in part, from a change in the availability of dietary amino acids such as Trp and Tyr, which are the precursors of 5-HT and the catecholamines, respectively. In this regard, it is known that alteration of the brain concentrations of Trp and Tyr can modify the behavioral syndrome elicited by large doses of amphetamine and fenfluramine (Fernando and Curzon, 1981).

3.1.6. Species Variations

There are numerous reports of species differences in locomotor responses to drug treatment, which underscores the importance of examining drug responses in a variety of different species. Too often, unfortunately, a result obtained in one species (usually the rat) may be generalized to other rodent species and even to higher mammals and humans. That such extrapolation is unwise is illustrated by the following example. In rats, PEA given in large doses produces stereotyped behavior that consists of head-weaving, forepaw padding, and sniffing. Grooming is abolished and gnawing or licking is never observed (Dourish, 1984). In complete contrast, large doses of PEA in mice elicit compulsive grooming, gnawing, and licking (Dourish 1982a).

3.1.7. Strain Variations

The demonstration of significant differences in response to drug treatment between different strains of the same species places further constraints on the generality of results. Strain differences in mice in response to drugs have been widely documented (e.g., Sansone et al., 1981; Kendler and Davis, 1984). Reports of strain differences in rats are less frequent, but do exist. For example, a number of recent studies have demonstrated differences in the response of two albino rat strains (Wistar and Sprague-Dawley) to drug treatments that alter central 5-HT levels (Emery and Larsson, 1979; Jones and Dourish, 1982; Dourish and Dewar, 1982). These strain variations in behavioral response may arise from reported differences in endogenous 5-HT concentrations between Wistar and Sprague-Dawley rats (Jones and Dourish, 1982).

3.1.8. Previous Experience

The previous experience of drug or test situation by an animal can modify the subsequent response of the animal to the same test situation, in a drugged or undrugged state. For example, Rushton et al. (1963) showed that a single drug experience in a Y-maze apparatus significantly modified the subsequent response (up to 3 mo later) when the animal was given an amphetamine/barbiturate mixture in the same test apparatus. The importance of environmental influences on drug response has been repeatedly demonstrated in numerous subsequent studies (e.g., Einon and Sahakian, 1979; Mumford et al., 1979; Dourish and Cooper, 1984b). Experience of certain drugs may increase or decrease the response of an animal to subsequent drug treatments (that is, produce tolerance). Conversely, repeated treatment with other drugs may increase certain behavioral responses (that is, produce reverse-tolerance or sensitization). These phenomena have obvious implications for the use of repeated-measures testing in drug experiments. In a repeated-measures study, an animal is generally tested after saline treatment and after different doses of a drug (or drugs), on separate occasions. Thus, the animal acts as its own control, which tends to reduce error variance and is a good economic measure. However, care must be taken in such studies to control for the development of drug tolerance or sensitization. The development of tolerance or sensitization to the locomotoor stimulant and stereotypic effects of various stimulant compounds has been well documented and will be discussed in detail later (*see* section 4.2.3).

3.1.9. Effect of Maintenance and Test Conditions

Social isolation in animals induces dramatic changes in behavior and brain biochemistry. Thus, male mice (and male rats of certain strains) that have been isolated for 3–4 wk exhibit persistent and compulsive aggressive behavior. In the brain, isolation causes decreases in the turnover of 5-HT and noradrenaline, and an increase in dopamine turnover (Valzelli, 1981). It is not surprising, therefore, that drug responses are influenced by housing conditions. For example, social isolation prior to testing enhances the stereotypic effects of amphetamine and apomorphine in rats (Sahakian et al., 1975). Test conditions also modify drug response, and different drug effects may be observed when animals are tested individually and in groups. A familiar example is the enhancement of amphetamine toxicity in group-tested mice, first reported by Gunn and Gurd (1940). More recently, it has been shown that test conditions can influence the locomotor stimulant and stereotypic effects of a psychomotor stimulant. Thus, the predominant feature of PEA treatment in mice tested individually is a compulsive grooming response. However, these animals are also hyperreactive and, when tested in groups, the exaggerated startle responses of running, jumping, and vocalization inhibit the development of stereotyped behavior (Dourish, 1982a).

3.1.10. Statistical Methods

The choice of an appropriate statistical test for the analysis of data collected in an activity study is problematic because of the large variety of methods used to measure locomotion. Statistical tests that are available for the analysis of activity data can be broadly classified into parametric and nonparametric procedures. Parametric tests should be used to analyze normally distributed interval or ratio data of relativity homogenous variance generated by automatic activity measures, such as photocell cages, or by observational techniques, such as video recording and microcomputer encoding. Appropriate statistical treatment of such data involves the use of factorial analysis of variance (ANOVA or *F* test), as required by the experimental design. (*Note:* In cases in which only two groups are being compared, the Student's *t*-test will produce the same result as ANOVA.) If ANOVA yields a significant result, a variety of *post hoc* tests is available that can be used to locate specific between-group differences. Examples are the Scheffé test, Tukey test, Dunnett test, and Newman-Keuls test (*see* Winer, 1971, for further discussion of the use of ANOVA and other parametric tests).

Ranked scores generated by the use of rating procedures do not constitute interval or ratio data and should be analyzed by nonparametric statistical procedures. Nonparametric tests can also be employed in the analysis of parametric data that are not normally distributed or severely skewed, or where the sample size is small. Suitable nonparametric tests for comparing two groups of ranked data include the Mann Whitney U test (independent groups) and the Wilcoxon test (correlated groups). These tests are the nonparametric equivalents of the Student's *t*-test.

When more than two groups of ranked data are being analyzed, there are a number of available procedures and choice is dependent on experimental design. In a simple one-factor experiment with independent groups, the Kruskal Wallis ANOVA can be used. Where the ANOVA yields a significant result, between-groups comparisons can be carried out using the Mann Whitney U test. In multifactorial studies, or in studies using repeated measures, statistical analysis may be carried out using contingency tables. Suitable tests include the chi-Square test (*see* Siegel, 1956; Winer, 1971, for further details). The chi-Square test is hampered by the requirement for five or more observations in each cell of the matrix and, therefore, Robbins (1977) has advocated the use of an analogous test called the information statistic, which is not constrained by small cell frequencies.

In cases in which all-or-none procedures are used and data are classified in the form of either 0 (absent) or 1 (present) (e.g., the serotonin syndrome described in section 2.2), appropriate statistical tests are the Q statistic (Cochran, 1950) or Fisher's exact probability test.

3.2. A Critique of Automatic Measures of Activity

There have been numerous important studies on the reliability of various automatic devices for the assessment of drug effects on activity. Krsiak et al. (1970) compared and contrasted the data generated by photocell cages and direct observation using two "standard" drugs, amphetamine and amylobarbitone (and combinations of these two). They found that, in undrugged animals, photocell counts correlated well with observational data for walking ($r = 0.77$) and rearing ($r = 0.8$, $p < 0.001$ in both cases), but that there was no correlation with grooming ($r = -0.15$). However, when rats were treated with increasing doses of amphetamine, the correlation between rearing and photocell counts was reduced. In contrast, photocell counts exaggerated the stimulant effect of amphetamine on walking and increased the correlation between photocell counts and walking. Interestingly, amylobarbitone did not significantly alter the correlations from those obtained in undrugged rats. These data illustrate how photocell cages, if used in isolation, may generate misleading information on drug effects. Krsiak et al. (1970) concluded that observational procedures will yield more meaningful data than photocell cages. This view is shared by Ljungberg (1978), who compared results obtained from two different types of activity box (a photocell device and an Animex, resonating field device) with data obtained by direct observation. Rats were tested after saline, apomorphine, phenoxybenzamine, clozapine, reserpine, and various combinations of these drugs. There was no correlation between the results obtained with the Animex and the results obtained with the photocell cage. Thus, it would appear that locomotor activity recorded using the Animex is different from locomotor activity counted by photocells. For example, direct observation revealed that 1 mg/kg apomorphine produced slow forward walking with continuous sniffing of the floor. This behavior was recorded as a significant increase in the Animex high sensitivity counts, no change in the Animex low sensitivity counts, and a significant decrease in photocell counts, compared to saline controls. These data from Ljungberg's (1978) drug studies are consistent with the findings of Tapp et al. (1968), who demonstrated that different types of activity devices generate results that are essentially independent of each other, in undrugged animals. Similarly, Ljungberg confirmed the results of Krsiak et al. (1970) that observational changes in behavior are not invariably correlated with changes in automatic activity recordings. Furthermore, increases or decreases in automatic activity counts were not always related to particular changes in observed behavior. Thus, it was shown that locomotor activity cannot be considered a single homogenous behavior. Instead, it should be regarded as a complex phenomenon consisting of various components such as walking, rearing, sniffing, and so on (Ljungberg, 1978). A limitation of automatic activity devices is that they do not appear to be equally sensitive to all of the various components of spontaneous motor activity.

Another major disadvantage of many automatic devices (particularly photocell cages) is their inability to differentiate between locomotion and stereotyped responding performed in one location (*see* Fig. 7). As noted above (*see* section 2.1),. attempts have been made to overcome this problem with logic circuits that discriminate between multiple interruptions of a single photobeam and consecutive photobeam interruptions. Similarly, x–y plotters have been used to trace patterns of locomotion. Despite these recent developments, however, automatic devices are unable to record individual components of activity (e.g., walking, grooming, licking, head movements) that may be differentially altered by drug treatment. For example, photocell cage studies indicated that low doses of

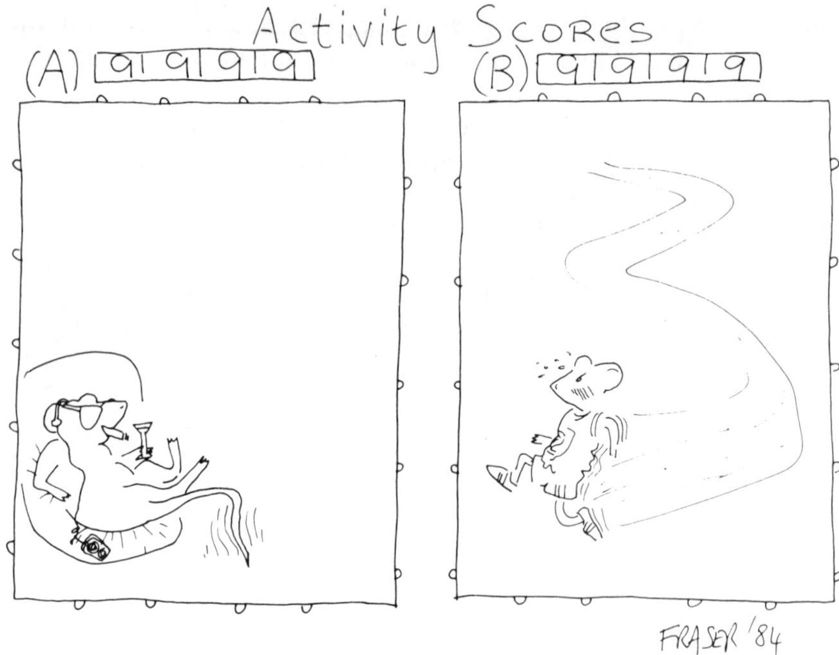

Fig. 7. Cartoon illustrating how photocell cages can generate misleading results in studies of locomotion. The rat in Cage A is relaxing, while listening to a personal stereo, and interrupting photobeams by tail movements only. In contrast, the rat in Cage B is a marathon runner and is extremely active. However, it is apparent that both rats have the same activity score generated by photobeam interruptions.

apomorphine reduced locomotor activity in rodents (Strombom, 1975). This "crude" finding was elaborated upon by subsequent observational analysis that showed that low-dose apomorphine treatment produced a reduction in locomotion accompanied by recurrent episodes of yawning, stretching, chewing, penile grooming, erection, and ejaculation (Mogilnicka and Klimek, 1977; Yamada and Furukawa, 1980; Dourish et al., 1985b). Thus, although the photocell counts indicated that the drug reduced locomotion, they provided no indication of the concurrent increase in various other components of activity (i.e., grooming, yawning, stretching).

Furthermore, automated devices do not provide information regarding the qualitative nature of drug-induced locomotion. The importance of this limitation may be illustrated by recent studies in which observation revealed that apomorphine-induced walking is directed by continual snout contact with the floor surface (snout contact fixation) (Szechtman et al., 1982, 1985).

3.3. *A Critique of Observational Measures of Activity*

Various forms of rating scales are routinely employed to assess the effect of drugs on activity (*see* section 2.2.1). The advantage of a global rating method is that it is simple to use and provides a straightforward quantitative ranking of drug response. However, it has become apparent that the numerous disadvantages of rating scales generally outweigh these advantages. This may be illustrated by considering a stereotypy rating scale (*see* Table 1).

Stereotypy is a descriptive term that refers to behavioral responses, or sequences of behavior, that are continually repeated, relatively fixed in form, and not goal-directed. In the rat, stereotyped behavior may take the form of locomotion along a fixed path, repetitive movement of the head up and down (head-bobbing), or repetitive gnawing on the bars of the cage. The use of a rating scale tends to confound the measurement of stereotypy (Fray et al., 1980), which is the description of the nature of a response, with identification of different responses (e.g., head-bobbing, gnawing). Intensity of stereotypy on a rating scale is often judged by the transition from one type of response to another. For example, in Table 1 continuous head-bobbing ($+4$ on the scale) is judged to be representative of more intense stereotyped behavior than increased exploration and discontinuous sniffing ($+1$ on the scale). However, there is considerable evidence that suggests that stereotyped behavior does not follow such a monotonic dose–response curve, and that various stereotyped responses may exhibit different temporal parameters and possess separate neurochemical substrates (Fray et al., 1980; Dourish, 1984). Thus, ip injection of 75–100 mg/kg PEA in mice elicits a syndrome of stereotyped behavior (Dourish, 1982a) that 5–20 min after injection consists of repetitive grooming, head movements, and forepaw padding, but 20–45 min after injection, changes to repetitive locomotion, rearing, gnawing, and licking. How would an investigator use a stereotypy rating scale to rank the intensity of this syndrome? Since gnawing and licking are often taken as being representative of "high-intensity" stereotypy (Creese and Iversen, 1973; Costall and Naylor, 1975), the gnawing/licking response may be ranked as more intense on the rating scale than the grooming/forepaw padding response. However, as Teitelbaum has remarked, this type of scoring is like comparing apples with oranges (Teitelbaum et al., 1982). The responses being compared are qualitatively and temporally distinct and, with the aid of ethological checklist analysis, have been shown to be mediated by different neurochemical mechanisms (Dourish, 1982b). The use of a rating procedure to assess stereotypy (or sedation and catalepsy) implies that any change in the qualitative nature of the behavior simply represents a shift in intensity along a unidimensional scale. This assumption, in the light of recent evidence, would generally appear to be untenable (Robbins, 1977; Fray et al., 1980; Teitelbaum et al., 1982).

The use of all-or-none procedures has limitations similar to those described above in relation to rating scales. This method, which is commonly used to assess the serotonin syndrome (*see* section 2.2.1), can obscure drug effects on specific components of this complex behavioral pattern (Andrews et al., 1982; Curzon, 1986). Thus, in a comparison of the all-or-none procedure with separate assessment of individual behavioral components (e.g., forepaw padding, head-weaving), Dickinson et al. (1983) demonstrated that the use of these different methods would lead to quite different conclusions.

The alternative to using global rating scales in the assessment of drug effects on activity is to employ ethological analysis or movement notation (*see* section 2.2). Ethological checklist techniques have been used for many years by ethologists, zoologists, and psychologists to study animal behavior.

The application of these techniques in psychopharmacology (via direct observation or video recording/microcomputer encoding) allows assessment of drug effects on individual components of spontaneous motor activity. Similarly, the introduction of movement notation in the study of drug effects on activity enables the investigator to isolate and identify pharmacological actions on specific movement subsystems.

Recently, the use of ethological component analysis and movement notation has yielded important insights into the mechanism of action of various psychomotor stimulants (e.g., Fray et al., 1980; Nielsen et al., 1980; Szechtman et al., 1982; 1985) (*see* section 4.2).

The major disadvantages of these detailed observational methods as compared to global rating methods are: (1) they take longer to learn; (2) they require that the investigator spends long periods of time observing animal behavior directly or from video recordings or movie frames; and (3) they require relatively complex data analysis. Notwithstanding these requirements, there is little advantage in using a quick and easy global rating scale if it is impossible to decide what the results mean.

3.4. Conclusions

It is clear from the preceding discussion that a wide variety of automatic and observational methods exists for recording spontaneous motor activity in rodents. With such a wide choice available, the obvious question for the investigator is: Which is the best method to use in examining drug effects on spontaneous motor activity? The answer to this question will depend, to a large extent, on the priorities of the investigator (e.g., neurochemical, pharmacological, behavioral), and some methods may be more suitable in certain situations than others. However, a number of general points should be considered. I strongly believe that automatic activity-recording devices are of limited value and are only useful for providing a crude assessment of a drug effect. Furthermore, it is likely that the use of such devices without concurrent observation of the animal will produce misleading results and conclusions. This concurs with the views of a number of other authors (e.g., Krsiak et al., 1970; Ljungberg, 1978; Robbins, 1977). A related point, put forward by Robbins (1977), is that a useful research strategy is to employ more than one measurement technique in examining drug effects on activity. Therefore, photocell counts can be useful for identifying a gross drug effect on locomotion, which should be confirmed and extended using reliable observational methods (*see* section 2.1.1). Reliable observational methods include various forms of ethological checklist analysis (e.g., open-field, video recording/microcomputer encoding) and movement-notation techniques. Global rating scales are of limited value since they lose valuable information about response patterns and often generate misleading results. Although it is unwise to use automatic activity measures without concurrent observation of the animal (see above), the converse is not necessarily true. Thus, automatic devices are unlikely to yield any important additional information about a drug effect on activity that has already been assessed by ethological checklist analysis or movement notation.

Finally, it is important to consider the relative cost and benefit of the various methods available to record spontaneous motor activity. Many of the automatic devices described above (e.g., multiple photobeam systems incorporating logic circuits, Doppler-shift devices, capacitative systems, $x-y$ plotters) necessitate a considerable financial investment on the part of the investigator. In contrast, informative observational methods, such as ethological checklist analysis and movement notation, require only video equipment and/or microcomputer facilities that are normally standard equipment in a behavioral laboratory (Note: If the laboratory budget is very limited, ethological analysis and movement notation can also be carried out using direct observation of the animal without employing video or computer facilities.)

In industrial settings, automation is of considerable importance in cost/benefit analysis. Therefore, the use of automatic activity devices is likely to be continued for the purpose of routine drug screening. Nevertheless, considering the serious limitations of automatic devices, there seems to be little benefit for the individual investigator of purchasing a sophisticated (but expensive) automatic activity system. At best, automatic devices provide only a crude assessment of a drug effect and, therefore, a simple, inexpensive photocell cage (with one or two photocells) used in conjunction with a reliable observational method is likely to be a good choice.

4. Assessment of Drug Effects on Spontaneous Motor Activity: A Case Study of Stereotypy

4.1. Introduction

The development of increasingly sophisticated methods for recording spontaneous motor activity in animals (outlined in the preceding sections) has led to the accumulation of an enormous wealth of data concerning the effects of drugs on movement. Consequently, the precise interpretation of the data generated by these various methods is a difficult problem for the investigator. In the concluding section of this chapter, I shall attempt to illustrate the complex nature of the analysis of drug effects on activity using a specific example—drug-induced stereotyped behavior. I have chosen this particular example because stereotypy is a behavioral pattern that has been frequently ill-defined, misinterpreted, and misunderstood in the psychopharmacology literature. As will become apparent from the ensuing discussion, the all-too-frequent misinterpretation of data from experimental studies of stereotyped behavior has resulted, in part, from crude measurement of activity and from a misunderstanding or misinterpretation of the nature of stereotypy.

4.2. Drug-Induced Stereotyped Behavior

4.2.1. What Is Stereotyped Behavior?

As defined earlier in this chapter, stereotypy is a term that refers to behavioral response patterns that are continually repeated, are invariant in form, and are apparently purposeless. Stereotyped behavior has been observed in all mammalian species studied, including humans, and amphetamine-induced stereotypy has been proposed by Snyder et al. (1974) as a useful animal model of schizophrenia. Although recent evidence (see below) has cast doubt on this schizophrenia model, the study of stereotypy in animals continues to be relevant to stereotyped behavior associated with childhood autism, mental retardation, and organic brain damage (Robbins and Sahakian, 1981; Cooper and Dourish, 1986).

Recent studies have demonstrated that the stereotyping of behavior can occur in a wide variety of forms and can be elicited by a range of pharmacological agents or environmental circumstances or a combination of both (see below). Therefore, it is particularly unfortunate that the term stereotypy has to a large extent become synonymous with a particular pattern of rat behavior that is produced by large doses of dopamine agonists and consists of sniffing, head movements, gnawing, and licking (Robbins and Sahakian, 1981). Numerous other forms of stereotyped behavior have been observed in rats. For example, low doses of dopamine agonists, muscarinic agonists,and ACTH and related peptides elicit repetitive stretching, chewing, yawning, and grooming (Gessa et al., 1967; Urba-Holmgren et al., 1977; Mogilnicka and Klimek, 1977). Stereotyped shaking behavior (termed wet-dog shakes in rats or head twitches in mice) can be produced by 5-HT agonists or morphine withdrawal (Bedard and Pycock, 1977; Wei, 1983). Similarly, drugs that increase central 5-HT transmission induce a stereotyped syndrome of head movements, forepaw padding, and tremor (Gerson and Baldessarini, 1980; Curzon, 1986). Learned responses can also become stereotyped, as illustrated in an experiment by Robbins (1980), in which apomorphine elicited stereotyped lever-pressing in hungry rats working under a random sequence of food delivery. Rats had to press two levers to obtain food and under control conditions quickly learned the appropriate response sequence. However, when treated with apomorphine the animals continually responded at a high rate on one lever, which resulted in no food being delivered.

Stereotyped behavior can be produced by nonpharmacological means such as isolation rearing or environmental restriction. Dogs reared in isolation exhibit stereotyped pacing and whirling and isolated monkeys engage in body rocking, head rolling, and swaying (Melzack, 1954; Berkson et al., 1963). Similarly, there is documented evidence of stereotyped head banging and body rocking in children raised in almost total isolation (Davis, 1940). Cage stereotypies have also been reported in which confined circus or farm animals have been observed to engage in head rolling and abnormal licking and chewing (Holzapfel, 1939; Sharman, 1978).

In this brief overview, only a few selected examples of stereotyped behavior are considered. For a more comprehensive treatment of this topic, the reader is referred to recent reviews by Robbins and Sakahian (1981), Lewis and Baumeister (1982), Ridley and Baker (1983), and Cooper and Dourish (1986).

4.2.2. Assessment of Stereotypy: From Rating Scales to Fractionation of Components

The most influential early studies on pharmacological stereotypies were performed by Randrup and Munkvad (1966, 1967) and Ernst (1967), who drew attention to the repetitive behavior that could be induced by amphetamine and apomorphine in both animals and humans. These findings stimulated a worldwide interest in the study of stereotyped behavior, particularly in relation to certain psychiatric conditions (in which stereotypy was often a symptom), which to a large extent resulted in the formulation of the dopamine hypothesis of schizophrenia (Snyder, 1973; Snyder et al., 1974). Schizophrenia was postulated to result from an overactivation of brain dopamine neurotransmission, which was modeled by amphetamine-induced stereotypies in rodents. The dopamine hypothesis was supported by the discovery that most clinically effective neuroleptic drugs were potent antagonists of amphetamine- and apomorphine-induced stereotypy. Consequently, stereotyped behavior induced by these drugs in rodents was adopted as a screening test for pharmacological agents with potential antischizophrenic properties (Janssen et al., 1967). With the emergence of stereotypy as a routine drug-screening procedure came the need for a method to measure intensity of stereotypy. The method employed for this purpose was the stereotypy rating scale, which has been useful but suffers from a number of disadvantages (considered in detail in sections 2.2.1 and 3.3). Subsequently, automated devices were designed to measure stereotyped gnawing (Moss et al., 1980; Redgrave et al., 1982). However, these devices have similar limitations to other automatic activity recording devices (*see* section 3.2).

The most important developments in the understanding of stereotyped behavior have resulted from the recent application of ethological analysis and movement notation to the study of the effect of drugs on components and subsystems of spontaneous motor activity (*see* section 2.2). Thus, checklist analysis has revealed important differences in the stereotyped behavior induced in rats by the two reference dopamine agonists, amphetamine and apomorphine (Fray et al., 1980). Amphetamine increased locomotion, rearing, and sniffing at particular doses, but rarely induced licking or gnawing. In contrast, apomorphine increased locomotion, sniffing, licking, and gnawing, but did not increase rearing. The different behavioral elements measured also had different threshold doses and exhibited different temporal parameters. These findings contrast with earlier reports from studies using rating scales or informal observation that amphetamine reliably induces gnawing (Creese and Iversen, 1973; Randrup and Munkvad, 1967).

Apomorphine-induced stereotypy has been described in various studies as consisting of either sniffing, licking, and gnawing (Ernst, 1967; Costall and Naylor, 1973) or rearing and climbing (Protais et al., 1976; Decsi et al., 1979). Until recently, the reason for the induction of these two different types of stereotyped response pattern by the same doses of apomorphine was unclear. However, experiments in which apomorphine stereotypy was examined using movement notation analysis appear to have identified a number of fundamental factors that control drug responses (Szechtman et al., 1980, 1982, 1985). It has been proposed that apomorphine induces a sequence of behavioral regression which is opposite to the sequence of neurological recovery that occurs following LH lesions (Szechtman et al., 1980, 1985). Thus, apomorphine progressively shuts down various components of exploratory locomotion (*see* Fig. 8). In the apomorphine-treated rat, long forward-locomotion trajectories predominate at first. These forward movements progressively shrink as lateral turning appears to grow in amplitude until gradually the animal begins to engage in tight circling without any forward locomotion at all. Eventually, the hindlegs become relatively immobile and side-to-side movements of the head and forequarters predominate. This regression sequence identified by movement notation bears certain similarities to the hypothesis of Lyon and Robbins (1975) regarding stereotyped behavior. They proposed that drug-induced stereotypy could be described as an increased response frequency in a decreased number of response categories. As stereotypy emerged, only simple motor responses were performed and complex patterns of behavior (e.g., feeding, social interaction) disappeared.

In the apomorphine-treated rat, as in the LH-lesioned animal, all of the head trajectories are strongly influenced by snout contact with surfaces (Golani et al., 1979; Szechtman et al., 1982, 1985). Consequently, if an apomorphine-treated rat is placed in a small, high-walled enclosure, forward movement is directed upward, guided by snout contact along the vertical surfaces, and the animal engages in rearing and climbing (Szechtman et al., 1982, 1985). Alternatively, if a wire mesh floor is available, gnawing may dominate other forms of activity. Such data illustrate the importance of environmental influences on stereotyped behavior, a factor that has been previously noted by others (Einon and Sahakian, 1979; Mumford et al., 1979). An extreme example of environmental control of stereotypy has been revealed in movement notation analysis of stereotypy induced by the anticholinergic drug atropine (Schallert et al., 1980). When an animal under the influence of atropine encounters the blind end of an alley it repetitively scans along or up and down the surfaces with its snout for long periods. Undrugged animals scan briefly and turn around to escape through the open end of the alley. The atropine-treated animal appears to be

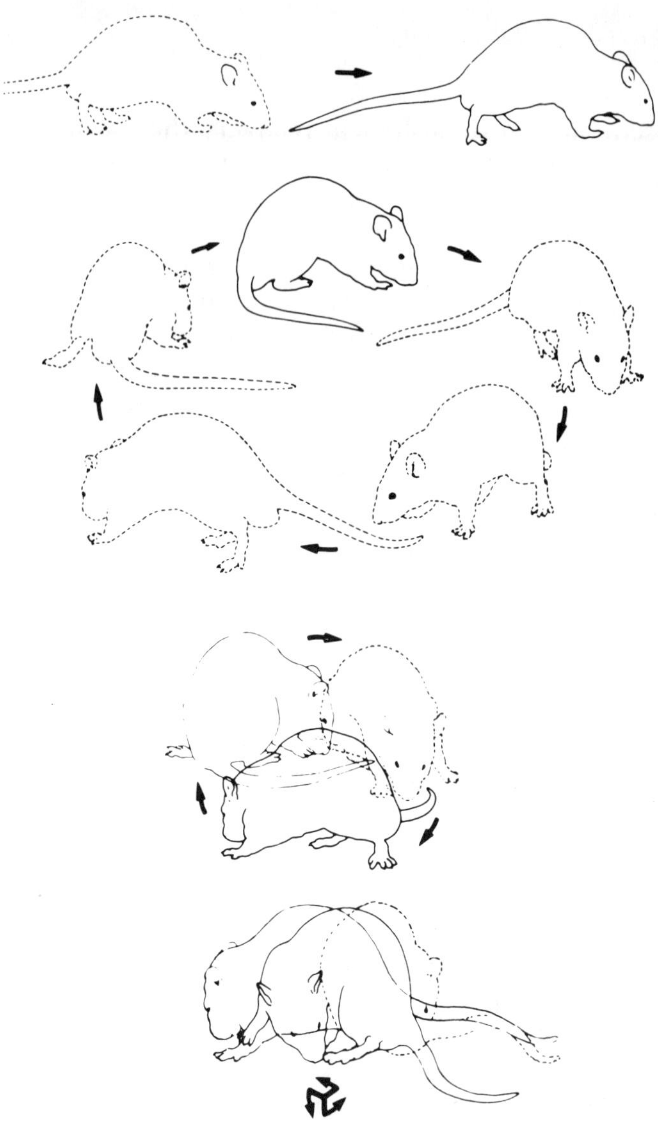

Fig. 8. Schematic drawing illustrating how movement notation has been used to describe the effects of apomorphine on locomotion in rats. In the first few minutes after injection (top drawings), only forward locomotion in long trajectories is seen. Then forward longitudinal movement shrinks as lateral turning movements emerge and grow in amplitude. Their algebraic interaction produces tighter and tighter circling as longitudinal forward locomotion becomes less and less. Note how movement is strongly controlled by snout contact [from Teitelbaum et al. (1982), with permission of the authors and publisher].

trapped in this environment by the sensory input from the snout (Schallert et al., 1980).

4.2.3. Influence of Previous Drug Experience

As noted earlier in this chapter (*see* section 3.1.8), previous drug experience of the animal has a strong influence on drug response. There is considerable interest in the effect of chronic administration of psychostimulant drugs on animal behavior (Segal, 1975), which arises in part from reports that chronic amphetamine abuse in humans can cause a toxic pyschosis (Connell, 1958). However, there have been conflicting findings regarding the effects of repeated amphetamine administration on stereotyped behavior in animals. A particular problem is the interaction of drug effects with environmental variables. Thus, Tilson and Rech (1973) have demonstrated that it is possible for repeated amphetamine administration to result in increased motor activity that is conditioned to neutral stimuli associated with drug treatment. The result is an apparent progressive augmentation in amphetamine's stimulant effects on locomotion. A further confounding factor is the variety of methods employed to assess the stimulant and stereotypic effects of amphetamine, many of which involve the use of photocell devices and stereotypy rating scales. The disadvantages of employing these methods have already been considered in detail (*see* sections 3.2 and 3.3). In addition, different modes of drug administration (e.g., various routes of injection, implanted pellet, osmotic minipump) have resulted in different effects on behavior.

Two major types of effect on motor activity have been reported following various regimens of chronic amphetamine administration, i.e., augmentation of locomotion and stereotypy or the description of "emergent" behaviors. Segal and Schuckit (1983) have described a dose-related augmentation of locomotion and certain aspects of stereotypy that occurs with repeated daily injections of constant doses of amphetamine. Low doses (0.5–2.5 mg/kg) initially enhance locomotion as the predominant response and chronic treatment results in a gradual increase in intensity and duration of the locomotor stimulation. At moderate doses (1.5–2.5 mg/kg) the initial locomotor stimulant effect is replaced over time by progressively longer episodes of stereotyped behavior. Repeated injections of high doses (2.5–7.5 mg/kg) reduce the latency to onset of stereotyped behavior and augment a long latency locomotor-stimulant effect.

The observation of emergent behavior produced by chronic amphetamine treatment has been reported in cats by Trulson and Jacobs (1979) and in rats and monkeys by Ellison et al. (1978) and Nielsen et al. (1980, 1983). The latter group administered amphetamine via slow-release silicone pellets that release the drug for periods of up to 14 d when implanted subcutaneously (Nielsen et al., 1983). Continuous video monitoring of animals revealed that various behavioral stages were evident during amphetamine administration. Initially, rats exhibited increased locomotion and exploration that by the second day was replaced by stereotyped sniffing, head movements, and oral behavior. However, after 4–5 d, these stereotypies declined and were replaced by newly emergent stereotyped responses consisting of intense grooming, body-shaking, and limb flicking. A similar pattern of emergent behavior was observed in monkeys implanted with amphetamine pellets (Nielsen et al., 1983). Nielsen and Ellison (1980) have proposed that these emergent stereotypies may be a more relevant model of schizophrenia than the acute amphetamine stereotypies of sniffing, licking, and head movements (Nielsen et al., 1983). However, as Segal and Schuckit (1983) have pointed out, an important criterion for the development of an animal model of psychosis is the demonstration that the proposed behaviors are antagonized by neuroleptics. Amphetamine-induced sniffing, head movements, licking, and so on are inhibited by neuroleptics (Janssen et al., 1967), but it remains to be seen whether antipsychotics antagonize the emergent behavioral stereotypies of grooming, shaking, and limb flicking. Further studies, incorporating movement notation analysis of emergent stereotypies induced by chronic amphetamine intoxication, seem likely to yield valuable information on amphetamine psychosis, schizophrenia, and the neural basis of stereotyped behavior.

5. Summary

This chapter outlines the methods available for recording drug effects on spontaneous motor activity in rodents. The utility and limitations of various automatic devices and observational techniques are compared and contrasted. It is concluded that the use of automatic activity measurement devices in isolation (i.e., without observation of the animal) is likely to produce misleading data regarding drug effects. It is, therefore, recommended that a study of drug action on locomotor activity should involve the use of a reliable observational measure of activity. Suitable observational techniques include ethological checklist analysis and movement notation, both of which may be carried out by direct observation or from video recordings. The use of global rating scales is not advised (unless supplemented by one of the latter techniques), since these methods lose valuable information by lumping unrelated responses together and may generate misleading data regarding intensity of response by ranking behavior on a unidimensional scale. Some of the problems of data interpretation that may be encountered by an investigator examining drug effects on locomotor activity are outlined with particular reference to stereotyped behavior. It is emphasized that stereotypy refers to the description of the nature of a response or group of responses, rather than the indentification of particular responses themselves. In this regard, the inaccurate association of the term stereotypy exclusively with dopamine agonist-induced sniffing, head-bobbing, and licking is highlighted. It is emphasized that the methods used to assess drug-induced stereotypy can profoundly influence the outcome of a particular study and the subsequent interpretation of results. Therefore, recent advances in our understanding of the nature of stereotypy, made possible by the use of powerful observational techniques such as ethological analysis and movement notation, are highlighted. Finally, the importance of the environment and past experience of the animal in shaping the drug response is discussed.

Acknowledgments

The author wishes to thank Professor A. A. Boulton for encouragement, and Dr. S. J. Cooper for helpful comments on an earlier draft of the manuscript, and Ms. N. McLaren and Ms. R. James who patiently typed the manuscript at short notice. Professor P. Teitelbaum and Dr. T. Ljungberg kindly provided photographic prints of figures. Also, thanks to Ian Fraser for the artwork in Fig. 7. Previously unpublished data were collected with the aid of financial support from the Medical Research Council of Canada and Saskatchewan Health. This chapter is dedicated to my mother, Mona J. Dourish, who died during the course of its preparation.

References

Andrews C. D., Fernando J. C. R., and Curzon G. (1982) Differential involvement of dopamine-containing tracts in 5-hydroxytryptamine-dependent behaviours caused by amphetamine in large doses. *Neuropharmacology* **21**, 63–68.

Bedard P. and Pycock C. J. (1977) "Wet dog" shake behaviour in the rat: A possible quantitative model of central 5-hydroxytryptamine activity. *Neuropharmacology* **16**, 663–670.

Berkson G., Mason W. A., and Saxon S. V. (1963) Situation and stimulus effects on stereotyped behaviour of chimpanzees. *J. Comp. Physiol. Psychol.* **56**, 786–792.

Borison R. L., Havdala H. S., and Diamond B. I. (1977) Chronic phenylethylamine stereotypy in rats: A new animal model for schizophrenia? *Life Sci.* **21**, 117–122.

Campbell B. A. and Fibiger H. C. (1973) Potentiation of amphetamine-induced arousal by starvation. *Nature* **233**, 424–425.

Campbell B. A., Lytle L. D., and Fibiger H. C. (1969) Ontogeny of adrenergic arousal and cholinergic inhibitory mechanisms in the rat. *Science* **166**, 635–637.

Cochran W. G. (1950) The comparison of percentages in matched samples. *Biometrika* **37**, 256–266.

Connell P. H. (1958) *Amphetamine Psychosis.* Maudsley Monographs, No. 5, Oxford University Press, Oxford.

Cooper S. J. and Dourish C. T. (1986) *Neurobiology of Behavioural Stereotypy.* Oxford University Press, Oxford, in press.

Costall B. and Naylor R. J. (1973) The role of telencephalic dopaminergic systems in the mediation of apomorphine-stereotyped behaviour. *Eur. J. Pharmacol.* **24,** 8–24.

Costall B. and Naylor R. J. (1975) Action of Dopaminergic Agonists on Motor Function, in *Advances in Neurology,* vol. 9, (Calne D. B., Chase T. N., and Barbeau A., eds.), Raven, New York.

Creese I. and Iversen S. D. (1973) Blockage of amphetamine induced motor stimulation and stereotypy in the adult rat following neonatal treatment with 6-hydroxydopamine. *Brain Res.* **55,** 369–382.

Curzon G. (1986) Stereotypical and Other Motor Responses to 5-Hydroxytryptamine Receptor Activation, in *Neurobiology of Behavioural Stereotypy* (Cooper S. J. and Dourish C. T., eds.), Oxford University Press, Oxford, in press.

Davis K. (1940) Extreme isolation of a child. *Am. J. Sociol.* **45,** 554–565.

Decoursey P. J. (1982) Lighting schedule effects on entrainment and moduation of circadian free-running rhythms of locomotor activity in two nocturnal rodents. *Am. Zool.* **22,** 932.

Decsi L., Gacs E., Zambo K., and Nagy J. (1979) Simple device to measure stereotyped rearing of the rat in an objective and quantitative way. *Neuropharmacology* **18,** 723–727.

DePaulis A. (1983) A microcomputer method for behavioural data acquisition and subsequent analysis. *Pharmacol. Biochem. Behav.* **19,** 729–732.

DeRyck M., Schallert T., and Teitelbaum P. (1980) Morphine versus haloperidol catalepsy in the rat: A behavioural analysis of postural support mechanisms. *Brain Res.* **201,** 143–172.

Dewhurst W. G. and Marley E. (1965) Action of sympathomimetic and allied amines of noradrenaline, phenylethylamine and tryptamine on the central nervous system of the chicken. *Br. J. Pharmacol.* **25,** 705–727.

Dews P. B. (1953) The measurement of the influence of drugs on voluntary activity in mice. *Br. J. Pharmacol.* **8,** 46–48.

Dickinson S. L., Jackson A., and Curzon G. (1983) Effect of apomorphine on behaviour induced by 5-methoxy-*N*, *N*-Dimethyltryptamine: 3 different scoring methods give 3 different conclusions. *Psychopharmacology* **80**, 196–197.

Dourish C. T. (1982a) An observational analysis of the behavioural effects of β-phenylethylamine in isolated and grouped mice. *Prog. Neuropsychopharmacol. Biol. Psychiat.* **6**, 143–158.

Dourish C. T. (1982b) A pharmacological analysis of the hyperactivity syndrome induced by β-phenylethylamine in the mouse. *Br. J. Pharmacol.* **77**, 129–139.

Dourish C. T. (1984) Studies on the Mechanism of Action of β-Phenylethylamine Stereotypy in Rodents: Implications for a β-Phenylethylamine Animal Model of Schizophrenia, in *Neurobiology of the Trace Amines*, (Boulton A. A., Baker G. B., Dewhurst W. G., and Sandler M., eds.), Humana, New Jersey.

Dourish C. T. (1985) Local application of β-phenylethylamine to the caudate nucleus of the rat elicits locomotor stimulation. *Pharmacol. Biochem. Behav.* **22**, 159–162.

Dourish C. T. and Cooper S. J. (1981a) Effects of acute or chronic administration of low doses of a dopamine agonist on drinking and locomotor activity in the rat. *Psychopharmacology* **72**, 197–202.

Dourish C. T. and Cooper S. J. (1981b) Single or repeated administration of small doses of apomorphine on water intake and activity in water-deprived rats. *Neuropharmacology* **20**, 257–260.

Dourish C. T. and Cooper S. J. (1982) Suppression of drinking and induction of sedation by a dopamine agonist is blocked by small doses of spiperone. *Neuropharmacology* **21**, 69–72.

Dourish C. T. and Cooper S. J. (1984a) Effects of piribedil and of *d*-amphetamine on locomotor activity in immature rats. *Prog. Neuropsychopharmacol. Biol. Psychiat.* **8**, 249–255.

Dourish C. T. and Cooper S. J. (1984b) Environmental experience produces qualitative changes in the stimulant effects of β-phenylethylamine in rats. *Psychopharmacology* **84**, 132–135.

Dourish D. T. and Dewar K. M. (1982) Behavioural variations in response to β-phenylethylamine administration in three rat strains. *IRCS Med. Sci.* **10**, 56–57.

Dourish C. T., Dewar K. M., Dyck L. E., and Boulton A. A. (1983)

Potentiation of the behavioural effects of the antidepressant phenelzine by deuterium substitution. *Psychopharmacology* **81**, 122–125.

Dourish C. T., Hutson P. H., and Curzon G. (1985a) Low doses of the putative serotonin agonist 8-hydroxy-2-(di-*n*-propylamino)tetralin (8-OH-DPAT) elicit feeding in the rat. *Psychopharmacology* **86**, 197–204.

Dourish C. T., Cooper S. J., and Philips S. R. (1985b) Yawning elicited by systemic and intrastriatal injection of piribedil and apomorphine in the rat. *Psychopharmacology* **86**, 175–181.

Dourish C. T., Hutson P. H., and Curzon G. (1986) Parachlorophenylalanine prevents feeding induced by the serotonin agonist 8-hydroxy-2-(di-*n*-propylamino) tetralin (8-OH-DPAT). *Psychopharmacology* **89**, 467–471.

Einon D. F. and Sahakian B. J. (1979) Environmentally induced differences in susceptibility of rats to CNS stimulants and CNS depressants: Evidence against a unitary explanation. *Psychopharmacology* **61**, 299–307.

Ellison G. D., Eison M., and Huberman H. (1978) Stages of constant amphetamine intoxication: Delayed appearance of abnormal social behaviours in rat colonies. *Psychopharmacology* **56**, 293–299.

Emery D. E. and Larson K. (1979) Rat strain differences in copulatory behaviour after *para*-chlorophenylalanine and hormone treatment. *J. Comp. Physiol. Psychol.* **93**, 1067–1084.

Ernst A. M. (1967) Mode of action of apomorphine and *d*-amphetamine on gnawing compulsion in rats. *Psychopharmacologia* **10**, 316–323.

Fernando J. C. R. and Curzon G. (1981) Behavioural responses to drugs releasing 5-hydroxytryptamine and catecholamines: Effects of treatments altering precursor concentration in brain. *Neuropharmacology* **20**, 115–122.

Fernando J. C. R., Lees A. J., and Curzon G. (1980) Differential antagonism by neuroleptics of backward-walking and other behaviours caused by amphetamine at high dosage. *Neuropharmacology* **19**, 549–553.

File S. E. (1981) Pharmacological Manipulations of Responses to Novelty and Their Habituation, in *Theory in Psychopharmacology*, vol. 1, (Cooper S. J., ed.), Academic, London.

File S. E. and Wardill A. G. (1975) Validity of head-dipping as a measure of exploration in a modified holeboard. *Psychopharmacologia* **44**, 53–59.

Finger F. W. (1972) Measuring Behavioural Activity, in *Methods in Psychobiology*, vol. 2, (Myers R. D., ed.), Academic, London.

Fray P. J., Sahakian B. J., Robbins T. W., Koob G. F., and Iversen S. D. (1980) An observational method for quantifying the behavioural effects of dopamine agonists: Contrasting effects of *d*-amphetamine and apomorphine. *Psychopharmacology* **69**, 253–259.

Gerson S. C. and Baldessarini R. J. (1980) Motor effects of serotonin in the central nervous system. *Life Sci.* **27**, 1435–1451.

Gessa G. L., Pisano M., Vargiu L., Crabai F., and Ferrari W. (1967) Stretching and yawning movements after intracerebral injection of ACTH. *Rev. Can. Biol.* **26**, 229–236.

Gispen W. H. and Isaacson R. L. (1981) ACTH-induced excessive grooming in the rat. *Pharmacol. Ther.* **12**, 209–246.

Golani I., Wolgin D. L., and Teitelbaum P. (1979) A proposed natural geometry of recovery from akinesia in the lateral hypothalamic rat. *Brain Res.* **164**, 237–267.

Gunn J. A. and Gurd M. R. (1940) The action of some amines related to adrenalinecyclohexylkylamines. *J. Physiol.* (Lond.) **97**, 453–470.

Hendrie C. A. and Bennett S. (1983) A microcomputer technique for the detailed analysis of animal behaviour. *Physiol. Behav.* **30**, 233–235.

Hendrie C. A. and Bennett S. (1984) A microcomputer technique for the detailed behavioural and automatic statistical analysis of animal behaviour. *Physiol. Behav.* **32**, 865–870.

Holzapfel M. (1939) The formation of several stereotyped movements in captive mammals and birds. *Rev. Suisse Zool.* **46**, 567–580.

Itoh S., Katsunra I., and Hirota R. (1981) Diminished circadian rhythm of locomotor activity after vagotomy in rats. *Jpn. J. Physiol.* **31**, 957–961.

Jacobs B. L. (1976) Minireview: An animal behaviour model for studying central serotonergic synapses. *Life Sci.* **19**, 777–786.

Janssen P. A. J., Niemegeers C. J. E., Schellekens K. H. L., and Lenaerts F. M. (1967) Is it possible to predict the clinical effects of neuroleptic drugs (major tranquilizers) from animal data? *Arzneimittelforsch* **17**, 841–854.

Jones R. S. G. and Dourish C. T. (1982) Variation in response to stimulation of central 5-hydroxytryptamine mechanisms in two strains of albino rat. *Brain Res.* **247**, 172–176.

Kameyama J. and Ukai M. (1981) Multi-dimensional analyses of behaviour in mice treated with alpha-endorphin. *Neuropharmacology* **20**, 247–250.

Kendler K. S. and Davis K. L. (1984) Genetic control of apomorphine-induced climbing behaviour in two inbred mouse strains. *Brain Res.* **293**, 343–351.

Krsiak H. M. and Borgošová M. (1972) Drugs and spontaneous behaviour: Why are detailed studies still so rare? *Acta Nerv. Sup. Praha.* **14**, 285–293.

Krsiak H. M., Steinberg H., and Stolerman I. P. (1970) Uses and limitations of photocell activity cages for assessing effects of drugs. *Psychopharmacologia* **17**, 285–274.

Lewis M. H. and Baumeister A. A. (1982) Stereotyped Mannerisms in Mentally Retarded Persons: Animal Models and Theoretical Analyses, in *International Review of Research in Mental Retardation,* vol. 11, (Ellis N. R., ed.), Academic, London.

Ljungberg T. (1978) Reliability of two activity boxes commonly used to assess drug-induced behavioural changes. *Pharmacol. Biochem. Behav.* **8**, 191–195.

Ljungberg T. and Ungerstedt U. (1978a) A method for simultaneous registration of 8 behavioural parameters related to monoamine neurotransmission. *Pharmacol. Biochem. Behav.* **8**, 483–489.

Ljungberg T. and Ungerstedt U. (1978b) Classification of neuroleptic drugs according to their ability to inhibit apomorphine-induced locomotion and gnawing: Evidence for 2 different mechanisms of action. *Psychopharmacology* **56**, 239–247.

Lyon M. and Robbins T. W. (1975) The Action of CNS Stimulant Drugs: A General Theory Concerning Amphetamine Effects, in *Current Developments in Psychopharmacology* (Essman W. B. and Valzelli L., eds.), vol. 2, Wiley, New York.

Mackintosh J. H., Chance M. R. A., and Silverman A. P. (1977) The Contribution of Ethological Techniques to the Study of Drug Effects, in *Handbook of Psychopharmacology,* vol. 7,

(Iversen L. L., Iversen S. D., and Snyder S. H., eds.), Plenum, New York.

Makanjuola R. O. A., Hill G., Maben I., Dow R. C., and Ashcroft G. W. (1977) An automated method for studying exploratory and stereotyped behaviour in rats. *Psychopharmacology* **52,** 271–277.

Marsden C. A. and King B. (1979) The use of doppler shift radar to monitor physiological and drug induced activity patterns of the rat. *Pharmacol. Biochem. Behav.* **10,** 631–635.

Marzullo G. and Friedhoff A. J. (1982) Apomorphine-induced pecking in young chicks: Diurnal cycles. *Soc. Neurosci. Abstr.* **8,** 394.

Melzak R. (1954) The genesis of emotional behaviour: An experimental study of the dog. *J. Comp. Physiol. Psychol.* **47,** 166– 168.

Mogilnicka E. and Klimek V. (1977) Drugs affecting dopamine neurons and yawning behaviour. *Pharmacol. Biochem. Behav.* **7,** 303–305.

Moss D. E., McMaster S. B., Castaneda E., and Johnson R. L. (1980) An automated method for studying stereotyped gnawing. *Psychopharmacology* **69,** 267–269.

Mumford L., Teixeira A. R., and Kumar R. (1979) Sources of variation in locomotor activity and stereotypy in rats treated with d-amphetamine. *Psychopharmacology* **62,** 241–245.

Nakano S., Hara C., and Ogawa N. (1980) Circadian rhythm of apomorphine-induced stereotypy in rats. *Pharmacol. Biochem. Behav.* **12,** 459–461.

Nickolson V. J. (1981) Detailed analysis of the effects of apomorphine and *d*-amphetamine on spontaneous locomotor behaviour of rats as measured in a TV-based automated open-field system. *Eur. J. Pharmacol.* **72,** 45–56.

Nielsen E. G., Lee T., and Ellison G. (1980) Following several days of continuous administration *d*-amphetamine acquires hallucinogen-like properties. *Psychopharmacology* **68,** 197–200.

Nielsen E. G., Lyon M., and Ellison G. (1983) Apparent hallucinations in monkeys during around-the-clock amphetamine for seven to fourteen days. *J. Nerv. Ment. Dis.* **171,** 222–233.

Papeschi R. and Randrup A. (1973) Catalepsy, sedation and hypothermia induced by alpha-methyl-*p*-tyrosine in the rat.

An ideal tool for screening of drugs active on central catecholaminergic receptors. *Pharmacopsychiatry* **6**, 137–157.

Protais P., Costentin J., and Schwartz J. C. (1976) Climbing behaviour induced by apomorphine in mice: A simple test for the study of dopamine receptors in striatum. *Psychopharmacologia* **50**, 1–6.

Quinton R. and Halliwell G. (1963) Effects of α-methyl dopa and dopa on the amphetamine excitatory response in reserpinized rats. *Nature* **200**, 178–179.

Randrup A. and Munkvad I. (1966) Dopa and other naturally occurring substances as causes of stereotypy and rage in rats. *Acta Psychiat. Scand.* (Suppl) **191**, 193–199.

Randrup A. and Munkvad I. (1967) Stereotyped activities produced by amphetamine in several animal species and man. *Psychopharmacologia* **11**, 300–310.

Redgrave P., Dean P., and Lewis G. (1982) A quantitative analysis of stereotyped gnawing induced by apomorphine. *Pharmacol. Biochem. Behav.* **17**, 873–876.

Ridley R. M. and Baker H. F. (1983) Is There a Relationship Between Social Isolation, Cognitive Inflexibility and Behavioural Stereotypy? an Analysis of the Effects of Amphetamine in the Marmoset, in *Ethopharmacology: Primate Models of Neuropsychiatric Disorders,* (Miczek K. A., Kruk M. R., and Olivier B., eds.), Alan R. Liss, New York.

Robbins T. W. (1977) A Critique of the Methods Available for the Measurement of Spontaneous Motor Activity, in *Handbook of Psychopharmacology,* vol. 7, (Iversen L. L., Iversen S. D., and Snyder S. H., eds.), Plenum, New York.

Robbins T. W. (1980) Stereotypy of a learned response after apomorphine. *Br. J. Pharmacol.* **69**, 275–276.

Robbins T. W. and Sahakian B. J. (1981) Behavioural and Neurochemical Determinants of Drug-Induced Stereotypy, in *Metabolic Disorders of The Nervous System,* (Rose F. C., ed.), Pitman, London.

Roffman M., Cordasco F., and Kling A. (1980) Apomorphine-induced stereotypy in mature and senescent rats following cessation of chronic haloperidol treatment. *Comm. Psychopharmacol.* **4**, 283–286.

Rushton R., Steinberg H., and Tinson C. (1963) Effects of a single expeience on subsequent reactions to drugs. *Br. J. Pharmacol. Chemother.* **20**, 99–105.

Sahakian B. J. and Robbins T. W. (1975) Potentiation of locomotor activity and modifiction of stereotypy by starvation in apomorphine treated rats. *Neuropharmacology* **14**, 251–257.

Sahakian B. J., Robbins T. W., Morgan M. J., and Iversen S. D. (1975) The effects of psychomotor stimulants on stereotypy and locomotor activity in socially deprived and control rats. *Brain Res.* **84**, 195–205.

Sansone M., Ammassari-Teule M., Renzi R., and Oliverio A. (1981) Different effects of apomorphine on locomotor activity in C57BL/6 and DBA/2 mice. *Pharmacol. Biochem. Behav.* **14**, 741–743.

Schallert T., DeRyck M., Wishaw I. Q., Ramirez V. D., and Teitelbaum P. (1980) Atropine stereotypy as a behavioural trap: A movement subsystem and EEG analysis. *J. Comp. Physiol. Psychol.* **94**, 1–24.

Scraggs P. R. and Ridley R. M. (1978) Behavioural effects of amphetamine in a small primate: Relative potencies of the *d*- and *l*-isomers. *Psychopharmacology* **59**, 243–245.

Segal D. S. (1975) Behavioural and Neurochemical Correlates of Repeated *d*-amphetamine Administration, in *Advances in Biochemical Psychopharmacology*, vol. 13, (Mandel A. J., ed.), Raven, New York.

Segal D. S. and Schuckit M. A. (1983) Animal Models of Stimulant-Induced Psychosis in *Stimulants: Neurochemical, Behavioural and Clinical Perspectives*, (Creese I., ed.), Raven, New York.

Severson J. A. and Finch C. E. (1980) Reduced dopaminergic binding during aging in the rodent striatum. *Brain Res.* **192**, 147–162.

Shalaby I. A. and Spear L. P. (1980) Psychopharmacological effects of low and high doses of apomorphine during ontogeny. *Eur. J. Pharmacol.* **67**, 451–459.

Sharman D. F. (1978) Brain Dopamine Metabolism and Behavioural Problems of Farm Animals, in *Advances in Biochemical Psychopharmacology*, vol. 19, (Roberts P. J., Woodruff G. N., and Iversen L. L., eds.), Raven, New York.

Siegel S. (1956) *Non-Parametric Statistics for the Behavioural Sciences,* McGraw-Hill, New York.

Sloviter R. S., Drust E. G., and Connor J. D. (1978) Specificity of a rat behavioural model for serotonin receptor activation. *J. Pharmacol. Exp. Ther.* **206**, 339–347.

Smith R. C., Leelavathi D. E., and Lauritzen M. R. (1978) Behavioural effects of a dopamine agonist increase with age. *Commun. Psychopharmacol.* **2**, 39–43.

Snyder S. H. (1973) Amphetamine psychosis: A "model" schizophrenia mediated by catecholamines. *Am. J. Psychiat.* **130**, 61–67.

Snyder S. H., Banerjee S. P., Yamamura H. I., and Greenberg D. (1974) Drugs, neurotransmitters and schizophrenia. *Science* **184**, 1243–1253.

Spear L. P. (1979) The Use of Psychopharmacological Procedures to Analyse the Ontogeny of Learning and Retention: Issues and Concerns, in *Ontogeny of Learning and Memory,* (Spear N. E. and Campbell B. A., eds.), Lawrence Erbbaum, New Jersey.

Spruijt B. M. and Gispen W. G. (1983) Prolonged animal observation by use of digitized videodisplays. *Pharmacol. Biochem. Behav.* **19**, 765–769.

Stretch R. (1963) Effects of amphetamine and pentobarbitone on exploratory behaviour in rats. *Nature* **199**, 787–789.

Strombom U. (1975) Effects of low doses of catecholamine receptor agonists on locomotor activity in mice. *Acta Physiol. Scand.* (Suppl) **431**, 3–43.

Strombom U. (1979) Qualitative aspects of motility changes in mice induced by low doses of apomorphine and clonidine. *J. Neural Trans.* **45**, 129–137.

Svensson T. G. and Thieme G. (1969) An investigation of a new instrument to measure motor activity of small animals. *Psychopharmacologia* **14**, 157–163.

Szechtman H., Ornstein K., Hofstein R., Teitelbaum P., and Golani I. (1980) Apomorphine Induces Behavioural Regression: A Sequence That is the Opposite of Neurological Recovery, in *Enzymes and Neurotransmitters in Mental Disease* (Usdin E., Sourkes T. L., and Youdim M. B. H., eds.), Wiley, New York.

Szechtman H., Ornstein K., Teitelbaum P., and Golani I. (1982) Snout contact fixation, climbing, and gnawing during apomorphine stereotypy in rats from two substrains. *Eur. J. Pharmacol.* **80**, 385–392.

Szechtman H., Ornstein K., Teitelbaum P., and Golani I. (1985) The morphogenesis of stereotyped behaviour induced by the dopamine receptor agonist apomorphine in the laboratory rat.*Neuroscience* **14**, 783–798.

Tanger H. J., Vanwersch R. A. P., and Wolthuis O. L. (1978) Automated TV-based system for open field studies: Effects of methamphetamine. *Pharmacol. Biochem. Behav.* **9**, 555–557.

Tapp J. T., Zimmerman R. S., and D'Encarnacao P. S. (1968) Intercorrelational analysis of some common measures of rat activity. *Psychol. Rep.* **23**, 1047–1050.

Taylor M., Goudie A. J., Mortimore S., and Wheeler T. J. (1974) Comparison between behaviours elicited by high doses of amphetamine and fenfluramine: Implications for the concept of stereotypy. *Psychopharmacologia* **40**, 249–258.

Taylor M., Livesey J., Dempster T., and Bunce R. (1971) The effects of acutely administered fenfluramine on activity and eating behaviour. *Psychopharmacologia* **21**, 165–173.

Teitelbaum P., Szechtman H., Sirkin D. W., and Golani I. (1982) Dimensions of Movement, Movement Subsystems and Local Reflexes in the Dopaminergic Systems Underlying Exploratory Locomotion, in *Behavioural Models and the Analysis of Drug Action*, (Spiegelstein M. Y. and Levy A., eds.), Elsevier, Amsterdam.

Tilson H. A. and Rech R. H. (1973) Conditioned drug effects and absence of tolerance to *d*-amphetamine induced motor activity. *Pharmacol. Biochem. Behav.* **1**, 149–153.

Trulson M. E. and Jacobs B. L. (1976) Behavioural evidence for the rapid release of CNS serotonin by PCA and fenfluramine. *Eur. J. Pharmacol.* **36**, 149–154.

Trulson M. E. and Jacobs B. L. (1979) Long-term amphetamine treatment decreases brain serotonin metabolism. *Science* **205**, 1295–1297.

Tyler T. D. and Tessel R. E. (1979) A new device for the simultaneous measurement of locomotor and stereotypic frequency in mice. *Psychopharmacology* **64**, 285–290.

Urba-Holmgren R., Gonzalez R. M., and Holmgren B. (1977) Is yawning a cholinergic response? *Nature* **267**, 261–262.

Valzelli L. (1981) *Psychobiology of Aggression and Violence*, Raven, New York.

Vanuytven M., Vermeire J., and Niemegeers C. J. E. (1979) A new motility meter based on the Doppler principle. *Psychopharmacology* **64,** 333–336.

Wang G. H. (1923) Relation between "spontaneous" activity and oestrus cycle in the white rat. *Comp. Psychol. Monogr. Ser.* **6,** 2.

Wei E. T. (1983) Inhibition of shaking movements in rats by central administration of cholinergic and adrenergic agents. *Psychopharmacology* **81,** 111–114.

Winer B. J. (1971) *Statistical Principles in Experimental Design,* McGraw-Hill, New York.

Wolthuis O. L., De Vroome, H., and Vanwersch R. A. P. (1975) Automatically determined effects of lithium, scopolamine and methamphetamine on motor activity of rats. *Pharmacol. Biochem. Behav.* **3,** 515–518.

Yamada K. and Furukawa T. (1980) Direct evidence for involvement of dopaminergic inhibition and cholinergic activation in yawning. *Psychopharmacology* **67,** 39–43.

Effects of Drugs on Schedule-Controlled Behavior

David J. Sanger

1. Introduction to Operant and Schedule-Controlled Behavior

One of the major preoccupations of experimental psychology has always been the study of learning, probably because of interest in the undeniable flexibility of human behavior. Thus, many investigations of the behavior of rats and other laboratory animals use methods for inducing specific patterns of learned or conditioned behavior. Skinner (1938) drew the distinction between two forms of learning that he referred to as respondent conditioning, which was exemplified by the studies of Pavlov (1927), and operant (or instrumental) conditioning, which was initially studied by North American researchers, such as Thorndike (1911) and Skinner himself. Although there has been much controversy about the relationship between behaviors conditioned by respondent and operant procedures, the distinction remains an important one for experimental psychologists (Mackintosh, 1974).

Operant behavior is simply behavior that operates on the environment in the sense that it produces a particular environmental change or consequence. Operant conditioning is the process by which a particular response becomes strengthened because of the consequence of this response. Thus, if an experimenter arranges for a paticular response of a hungry rat to result in the delivery of a small pellet of food, it is likely that the animal will repeat the response. This simple observation forms the basis of operant conditioning. Because the animal will work for food, the food is said to be a reinforcer, and the process by which the response is strengthened by food delivery is referred to as positive reinforcement. Negative reinforcement refers to the process by which responses that lead to avoidance of, or escape from, noxious events are strengthened. Operant conditioning is thus a process by which behavior can be changed or controlled by the environment. Furthermore, if an experimenter arranges certain relationships between a rat's response and the consequence of the response, it is possible to induce the animal to emit a variety of quite predictable temporal patterns of responding. As we shall see, this behavior, which is called schedule-controlled, can be changed in predictable ways by drug administration.

The relationship between responses and reinforcers arranged by the experimenter is called the schedule of reinforcement. Schedules can take many forms, and a number were described in a standard text by Ferster and Skinner (1957). The two basic types of schedule are: (1) ratio schedules, in which reinforcers may be obtained after a certain number of responses, and (2) interval schedules, in which a response may be reinforced after a certain time period has elapsed. Response requirements or time periods can be fixed or variable to give rise to fixed- or variable-ratio (FR, VR), and fixed- or variable-interval (FI, VI) schedules. Table 1 shows the characteristics of several simple reinforcement schedules. By arranging for responses to be repeatedly reinforced after certain periods of time or after certain response requirements have been satisfied, it is possible to maintain highly predictable patterns of responding over long periods of time. The extent to which such behavior is changed by drug administration can then be easily investigated with an individual animal providing both control data and information about drug action, perhaps at several doses. It is also possible

Table 1
Some Basic Schedules of Reinforcement

Schedule name	Abbreviation	Characteristics
Continuous reinforcement	CRF or FR 1	Every response is reinforced
Fixed ratio	FR	A reinforcer is delivered after a certain fixed number of responses, e.g., FR 10: Every 10th response is reinforced.
Variable ratio	VR	A reinforcer is delivered after a number of responses, which varies and is usually defined by a mean and range. e.g., VR 10: On average, one reinforcer is obtained for every 10 responses.
Fixed interval	FI	A reinforcer is delivered for a response that is emitted after a certain fixed time has elapsed. e.g., FI 1-min: The first response after 1 min is reinforced.
Variable interval	VI	A reinforcer is delivered for a response that is emitted after a variable time period has elapsed. e.g., VI 1-min: Reinforcers can be obtained every 1 min on average
Differential reinforcement of low rate	DRL	A reinforcer is delivered for a response emitted after a certain fixed delay. Responses emitted during this delay cause the clock to reset. e.g., DRL 10-sec: A response is reinforced if it occurs at least 20 sec after the preceding response
Differential reinforcement of high rate	DRH	A reinforcer is delivered for a response emitted before a certain fixed time since the preceding response. e.g., DRH 1-sec: A response produces a reinforcer only if the response occurs less than 1 sec after the preceding response

with such techniques to induce similar patterns of behavior in a variety of species, and the effects of many drugs have been studied on the schedule-controlled behavior of mice, rats, pigeons, and monkeys, often showing similar effects in different species. Of course, such interspecies comparisons make it more likely that laboratory studies with animals will have some relevance to drug action in man. It seems unlikely that the study of any other type of behavior can provide such effective comparisons across species. More thorough descriptions of the characteristics of schedule-controlled behavior have been provided in a number of useful books and articles at both relatively basic (e.g., Blackman, 1974) and more advanced (Rachlin, 1976) levels.

2. Operant Behavior in the Pharmacology Laboratory

Probably the first studies to systematically investigate the effects of drugs on the reactions of laboratory animals under quite closely controlled experimental conditions were carried out in Pavlov's laboratory (Laties, 1979). In the 1920s, several investigators in North America also initiated experimental studies, although using techniques such as maze learning in rats, which were much more within the North American tradition of experimental psychology (e.g., Macht, 1924). However, it is certainly to an article by Skinner and Heron, published in 1937, that we can look for the first report of a study using techniques essentially similar to those popular today.

Skinner and Heron noted that, at that time, " . . . sensitive indicators of the effects of drugs on behavior (*were*) rare" and they carried out a study in which the effects of caffeine and benzedrine on the rate of schedule-controlled lever pressing in rats were investigated. Food-deprived rats were trained during daily sessions to obtain food pellets by lever-pressing on a FI 4-min schedule. Thus, the first lever-press to be emitted after each 4-min period since the preceding reinforcer, was reinforced. Having established a reliable behavioral baseline, the researchers studied the effects of drug injections and found that rates of lever-pressing were increased. The results of this study are not particularly striking in relation to more recent investigations of the behavioral effects of stimulant drugs, and the authors chose to discuss their results in terms that would not be acceptable today. However, this study is of considerable importance because it introduced a powerful new methodology which is characterized by several important factors.

(1) The experiment established a predictable pattern of behavior, or behavioral baseline, in individual animals, and each animal was used as its own control, providing data for both drug and control sessions. This, of course, is not a unique feature of schedule-controlled behavior; it is possible to repeatedly test subjects in other procedures to attempt to establish predictable patterns of behavior that may be changed by drug administration. Nevertheless, this experimental design has become associated with studies of schedule-controlled behavior more than with any other method.

(2) The important behavioral variable measured by Skinner and Heron was rate of lever-pressing. Response rate has always been emphasized by researchers interested in operant behavior, and it has recently become clear that it can be an extremely important variable in behavioral pharmacology.

(3) The data obtained in this study were presented for individual animals on single days. This also is an aspect that has become characteristic of behavioral pharmacological studies using schedule-controlled behavior.

Following this seminal publication by Skinner and Heron, only a few similar studies were reported (e.g., Wentink, 1938) during the subsequent decade and a half. Of course, research was being carried out during this time involving the action of drugs on animal behavior, but much of this was interwoven with motivational or cognitive theorizing, such as the research of Masserman (e.g., Masserman and

Yum, 1946) on the effects of drugs on experimental neuroses in cats, and was thus in a different tradition of experimental psychology and used different techniques. It was in the 1950s, however, that Dews began to carry out and publish his pioneering studies demonstrating that schedule-controlled behavior could not only provide convenient behavioral baselines for studying drug action, but that, in addition, the results of such studies could provide important insights into the mechanisms of drug action on a strictly behavioral level of analysis.

Dews (1978a) has more recently provided an illuminating account of how he, and other researchers, began using schedule-controlled behavior for investigating drug action. He describes how, when visiting Skinner's laboratory, he saw the cumulative records showing the operant behavior of experimental animals. He was struck by their similarity in principle to the pen recordings traditionally used by pharmacologists in studying the effects of drugs on the "behavior" of pieces of isolated tissue in organ baths. In both cases it was possible to study the ongoing behavior of a "preparation" and thus, to note changes in the temporal patterning of this activity after drug administration. Dews began to make use of these operant techniques, and the results of his earlier studies were published in a series of articles (Dews, 1955a,b, 1958a), some of which will be described in a later section. These studies showed the utility of operant techniques because they demonstrated the specificity of drug action. Thus, drugs from different pharmacological classes were found to produce different changes in similar patterns of behavior, and different patterns of schedule-controlled responding could be differentially affected by a single drug.

3. Advantages of Schedule-Controlled Behavior in Psychopharmacology

In the years since Dews began his studies, the operant and schedule-controlled behavior of laboratory animals has become one of the most popular methods for investigating behavioral effects of drugs. This is demonstrated by the large number of articles regularly published describing the use of these techniques. The practical advantages of this methodology can be briefly listed as follows:

(1) Schedule-controlled behavior provides predictable patterns of responding that may be emitted at relatively stable rates for long periods and over many sessions. Thus, patterns of responding that occur after drug administration can be compared easily with control patterns. Furthermore, by manipulating the parameters of the reinforcement schedule, a variety of different patterns of responding can be induced.

(2) Individual animals can be studied in detail and provide both control data and data obtained after drug administration. In this way it may be possible to minimize the significance of individual variation that can often complicate the interpretation of behavioral studies. Of course, it is also possible to use experimental designs involving comparisons between groups of animals receiving different pharmacological treatments. Indeed, such designs may be essential in some studies, such as those involving repeated drug administration or the effects of drugs with irreversible actions.

(3) Similar patterns of schedule-controlled responding can be obtained in a variety of different species, thus facilitating cross-species comparisons (Dews, 1976).

(4) A variety of different reinforcing events (e.g., food, water, electrical stimulation of the brain, and escape from, or avoidance of, aversive stimuli, such as electric shocks) can be used to maintain schedule-controlled behavior. This enables analysis of the significance of such motivational factors in determining drug action.

Thus, there are several important factors that have led to the popularity of operant behavior in psychopharmacology. It has also frequently been observed that schedule-controlled behavior can be very sensitive to the action of drugs, exhibiting highly specific changes after relatively low doses. The effects of anxiolytic drugs on punished responding (*see* chapter by Dantzer in this volume) provide an example of this. However, it must not be assumed that such exquisite sensitivity is always observed. Indeed, it is often found that some patterns of responding may be very insensitive to change after drug administration, and that animals that are clearly debilitated after a drug may continue to respond as usual once placed in an operant test chamber. Also, the advantages of schedule-controlled operant behavior noted above are gained at the expense of other factors. Such experiments are, in general, very time-consuming, with the animals requiring weeks or months of training before they provide behavioral baselines suitable for drug administration.

4. Schedule-Dependent Drug Effects

The contribution that can be made by schedule-controlled behavior in the analysis of psychoactive drug action became apparent with the results of the first study reported by Dews (1955a). In this experiment four pigeons were trained to peck an illuminated response disk to obtain access to grain. For two birds, the schedule in operation was an FR 50; for the other two it was an FI 15-min. Each bird was given injections of several doses of pentobarbital, and the changes in overall rates of responding were noted. Subsequently, the birds were switched to the alternate schedules, and after performance had stabilized, each received the series of drug treatments a second time.

Under both schedules, pentobarbital produced small increases in responding at lower doses and reductions in responding at higher doses. However, the dose–response curve for pecking under FI control was shifted to the right of the curve obtained for FR pecking. Thus, at certain doses (1–2 mg) pentobarbital reduced rates of pecking maintained by the FI schedule and facilitated rates of the same response maintained by the FR schedule. These differential effects were, of course, obtained in the same birds, which were maintained under the same conditions of food deprivation, tested in the same apparatus, and making the same response.

This result was of great significance for several reasons. First, it demonstrated that schedule-controlled behavior can be sensitive to drug administration, and that drug-induced changes in rates of responding are not necessarily what might be expected on the basis of preconceived notions about the action of a drug. Thus, pentobarbital was, and still is, usually described or classified as a depressant, but Dew's study (and many subsequent experiments) showed that behavioral output could be enhanced by certain doses. Second, the results showed clearly that the effects of pentobarbital on rates of pecking could depend upon the schedule of reinforcement maintaining this behavior.

Such schedule-dependent drug effects indicate the behavioral specificity of drug action and have been observed in many subsequent studies with a variety of drugs and several species. Of course, behavioral specificity of drug action can also be observed with techniques other than those involving schedule-controlled behavior. However, it is with schedule-controlled responding that some of the most striking examples have been found. Furthermore, these techniques provide the possibility of teasing out the precise factors that give rise to the specificity because of the high degree of control that the experimenter can exert over a subject's behavior.

Some of the most important demonstrations of the dependence of drug effects on reinforcement schedules can be observed with multiple schedules. With such procedures, two or more different temporal patterns of responding can be maintained in an individual subject during a single experimental session by arranging for external stimuli to signal the operation of different reinforcement schedules. Drug administration can then be shown to induce apparently different changes in the behavior of a single subject during the different schedule components. for example, multiple schedules with FI and FR components have been used to study the effects of drugs in primates (Byrd, 1973), pigeons

(McMillan, 1968), rats (Clark and Steele, 1966), and mice (Wenger and Dews, 1979). With these procedures, it has often been observed that amphetamines and related drugs can give rise to increases in rates of FI responding and leave unchanged, or even decrease, rates of FR responding.

Several other groups of researchers have made use of a three-component multiple schedule—with periods when responding is reinforced according to a VI schedule; periods when responding is reinforced, but also produces electric shocks (punishment); and periods in which responding has no scheduled consequences (time-out) (Hanson et al., 1967; Miczek, 1973; Tye et al., 1979). In one study (Tye et al., 1979), the effects of several drugs were investigated, and schedule dependence was observed in a number of cases. For example, the benzodiazepines, chlordiazepoxide and diazepam, induced large increases in rates of punished responding, smaller increases in rates of nonreinforced responding during the timeout periods, and had little effect on responding maintained by the VI schedule, except to decrease it at higher doses. In contrast, *d*-amphetamine gave rise to small increases in VI response rates and large increases in responding during the time out periods, but had no effect on punished responding.

5. Principles of Behavioral Pharmacology

The now well-established observation that drug-induced changes in behavior are not immutable properties of particular drugs, but are dependent on aspects of the experimental situation (such as the schedule of reinforcement), can perhaps be thought of as the most fundamental principle in psychopharmacology. However, such vague statements can only be considered the very first stage in a scientific analysis of drug action. In order to more effectively describe, explain, and predict drug effects, considerably greater precision is required. In recent years many studies have investigated the particular factors that give rise to the schedule-dependence of drug action. Although this work has sometimes appeared to progress slowly, and certainly a great deal more research will be necessary, it is now possible to point to several specific elements of any experimental situation that can be of major significance in determining the way in which drugs induce changes in behavior. Following the lead of Barrett (1984), general statements arising from this research will be referred to as behavioral principles. More detailed reviews of this area have been provided by Kelleher and Morse (1968a) and McKearney and Barrett (1978).

5.1. Response Rate

It is now clear that the extent to which a particular behavior is altered in rate by a drug may depend upon the rate at which the behavior occurs under control conditions. A similar principle may apply in many areas of biology and has been referred to as the Law of Initial Values (Wilder, 1967). However, it was once again Dews (1958a,b) who was responsible for first recognizing the importance of response rate as a determinant of the behavioral effects of drugs.

Dews was interested in the effects of methamphetamine on the schedule-controlled key-pecking of pigeons. In these studies he investigated the effects of the drug on relatively high rates of responding maintained by an FR 50 or a VI 1-min schedule and relatively low rates of responding maintained by an FI 15-min or FR 900 schedule. The results showed that although certain doses of methamphetamine would increase rates of key-pecking maintained by the FI 15-min and FR 900 schedules (as would be expected of a drug classed as a stimulant), these same doses had little or no effect on responding maintained by the FR 50 and VI 1-min schedules. Dews considered that the important factor giving rise to the different drug effects was the very different inter-response times produced by the different schedules. More recently, Dews (1981), as well as many other researchers (*see* reviews by Dews and Wenger, 1977; Robbins, 1981; Sanger and Blackman, 1976), have preferred to describe such effects in terms of a principle of rate-dependence. Thus, in Dews' study the effects of methamphetamine were rate-dependent, with low overall response rates being increased by doses that had no effect on high response rates.

Many subsequent studies of operant responding maintained by different schedules have found effects of amphetamine that are rate-dependent. Low response rates maintained by FI, DRL, or shock avoidance schedules are often increased by doses that have little effect on, or even decrease, high response rates maintained by VI or FR schedules. In one study, Heffner et al. (1974) trained rats to lever-press for water, using FI, VI, and FR schedules. The experimenters observed a variety of different rates of responding in their subjects, which were produced by these different schedules. The effects of *d*-amphetamine were found to be dependent on the predrug response rates. Low control rates were increased by doses of the drug that had little effect on intermediate rates and decreased high rates. It has also been reported that the variability in the effects of amphetamine on rates of VI responding in individual members of a group of rats could be accounted for by the different baseline rates shown by different individual animals (Beecher and Jackson, 1976). Dews and Wenger (1977) have furthermore suggested that the operation of rate-dependence can be observed if the effects of amphetamine on the variety of different behaviors, operant and nonoperant, are considered together. Also, rate-dependent effects of amphetamine have been observed in several species.

In addition to the comparison of rates of responding maintained by different reinforcement schedules, a second method has been used to investigate rate-dependent drug effects that involves the detailed analysis of responding under FI schedule control. Such responding is characterized by either a pause and respond or an accelerating temporal pattern between successive reinforcers. If each interval is divided into a number of periods or segments and the average response rate for each segment is computed, a range of different response rates is obtained. These rates can then be compared before and after drug administration, and this is often done by plotting the control and drug rates (or more usually the rates of responding after drug administration expressed as a percentage of control). Such data generally show a linear relationship between control response rates and the effects of amphetamine (e.g. Branch and Gollub, 1974; Leander and McMillan, 1974) as illustrated in Fig. 1. This method of data presentation appears to provide an impressive indication of the importance of control response rates, particularly when it can be shown that data from another schedule, such as an FR schedule forming part of a multiple FI–FR, fit close to the regression line plotted with the FI data. There has, however, been some controversy about the adequacy of this method of data analysis. Some researchers have argued that this method of plotting data is unacceptable (Byrd, 1981; Gonzalez and Byrd, 1977), whereas others have countered that it provides a meaningful description of drug action (Dews, 1978b; Katz and McLeod, 1979; McKearney, 1981).

That amphetamines and similar drugs induce effects that are response-rate dependent, and that this principle can apply across a variety of experimental conditions, is now well established. The extent to which the same principle applies to the effects of drugs from other classes is not yet completely clear. For example, the results of Dews (1955a), described above, show quite different effects of pentobarbital. In this experiment, higher response rates maintained by an FR schedule were less sensitive to the depressant effects of the drug than were lower rates of FI responding. Thus, in this case, if rate-dependence is in operation, the relationship appears to be the inverse of that obtained with amphetamine. Robbins (1981) has summarized much of the relevant data obtained with a number of drug classes, including minor tranquillizers, neuroleptics, and hallucinogens. It seems clear that response rate can also be a significant determinant of the action of these drugs. Thus, patterns of FI responding have been altered in a rate-dependent manner by phenothiazine neuroleptics (Leander, 1975), benzodiazepines (Wuttke and Kelleher, 1970), and barbiturates (Leander and McMillan, 1974). However, in many cases, effects have been observed that cannot be described as rate-dependent, with benzodiazepines, for example, (Sanger and Blackman, 1981) and with hallucinogens (Harris et al., 1978). Although rate of respond-

                                                        Sanger

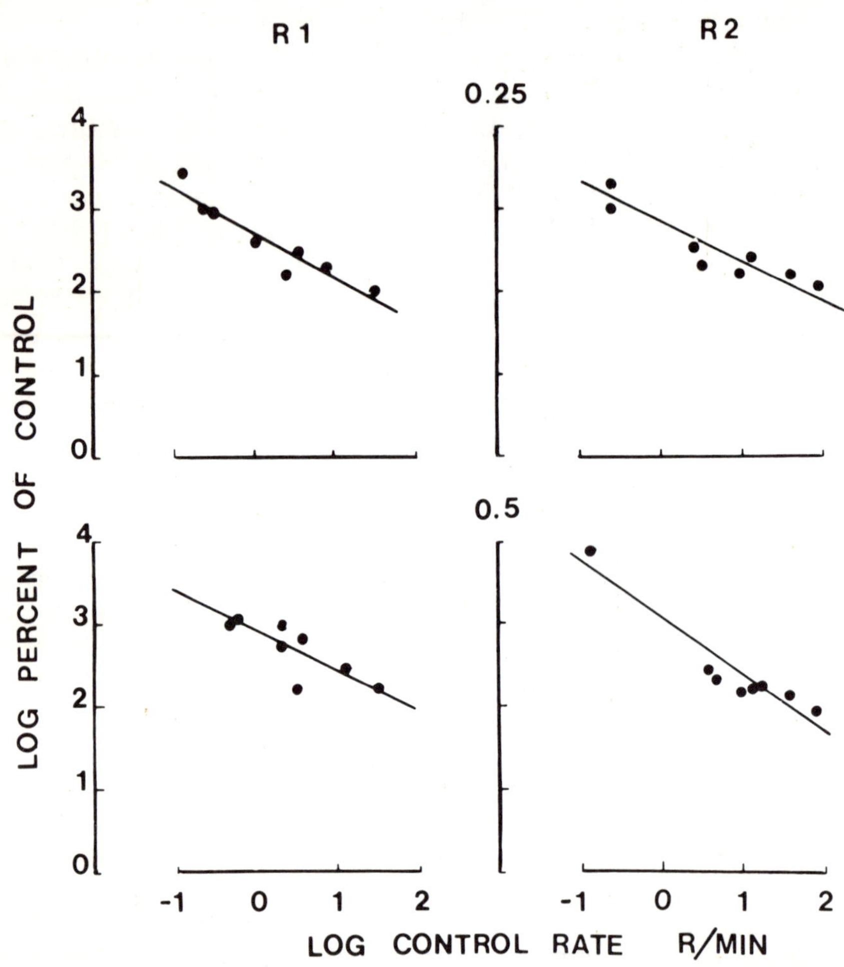

Fig. 1. Rate-dependent effects of two doses (0.25, 0.5 mg/kg) of *d*-amphetamine on the responses of two rats (R1, R2) maintained by a FI 2-min schedule of food reinforcement. Each interval was divided into eight 15-s segments and average rates of responses calculated for each segment in each animal. The regression lines were then obtained by plotting, on logarithmic paper, these response rates during a control session against the same rates after drug administration calculated as a percentage of the corresponding control rates.

ing is probably one of the most important determinants of the effects of amphetamine-like drugs, it is not the only one, as will be described in later sections. It seems likely that with drugs from other classes, response rate may be important in determining their effects, but other factors may be of even greater significance.

The finding that behavioral effects of drugs may be determined by control response rates is of considerable importance for behavioral pharmacology. This principle makes it imperative that all behavioral effects of drugs be assessed with control response rates in mind. Thus, if a drug is found to increase behavioral output in one experimental situation and to decrease output in another, it may be that the drug is producing qualitatively different effects in the two situations (which may, therefore, be mediated by different neurochemical mechanisms). Another possibility, however, is that the two effects may be only quantitatively different, the apparent qualitative difference being accounted for by rate-dependence (McKearney, 1981).

Rate-dependence thus provides a useful descriptive principle in this area of psychopharmacology, bringing together a great deal of apparently disparate data for individual drugs and allowing comparisons between different drugs. A number of researchers, however, have also attempted to go further than this by providing more theoretical accounts of rate-dependence. McKim (1981) has speculated that rate-dependence may represent relatively nonspecific drug action, and Ksir (1981) has used the term rate-convergence to suggest that rate-dependence may be an indication of the tendency for drugs to break down all temporal control of behavior. Other workers (Grilly, 1977; Lyon and Robbins, 1975) have put forward accounts of the rate-dependent effects of amphetamine-like drugs that are concerned with response competition or the ability of these drugs to affect the interactions between operant responding and other behaviors available to an animal in the experimental situation. Also, Seiden and his colleagues (1975) have carried out a number of studies that have attempted to relate rate-dependent effects of amphetamine with the changes in brain catecholamine activity that can be produced by drug administration and certain behavioral and environmental manipulations. Finally, there is some evidence that the behavioral effects of stimulant drugs in humans are also rate-dependent (Robbins and Sahakian, 1979).

5.2. Reinforcement and Punishment

5.2.1. Different Reinforcers

Everyday interpretations of the effects of drugs on behavior have tended to emphasize motivational, emotional, and cognitive explanations. Drugs are said, for example, to affect hunger, anxiety, mood, or ability to think, learn, or concentrate. Researchers in the operant tradition have attempted to redefine such concepts in terms of observable aspects of behavior or the environment. It is possible to investigate the significance of motivational factors in determining the effects of drugs (Miller, 1956) by comparing the effects of drugs on behavior maintained by different reinforcing events. However, in using such a technique, great care must be taken that the patterns and rates of responding maintained by different reinforcers are similar. If this is not done, it is possible that any apparently reinforcer-dependent drug effect is in fact dependent upon some other difference between different experimental situations, such as response rate.

Some of the first studies in contemporary psychopharmacology made use of shock-avoidance procedures with rats to investigate the actions of neuroleptic drugs (Courvoisier et al., 1953). It was believed that such drugs, which at that time were considered to exert tranquilizing effects, could specifically disrupt the ability of an animal to avoid shocks because such behavior was thought to be motivated by fear that was reduced by drug administration. Avoidance techniques remain useful for studying the properties of neuroleptic drugs (Beninger et al., 1980; Sanger 1985), and it has been demonstrated that the effects of these drugs in disrupting this behavior can correlate with their clinical potencies in the treatment of schizophrenia (Kuribara and Tadokoro, 1981). However, as discussed in detail by Carlton (1983), a number of other non-neuroleptic drugs can produce similar disruptions of avoidance behavior. Indeed, this was demonstrated some years ago by Morpurgo (1965). It is interesting to note that recent theoretical accounts of the effects of these drugs (e.g., Wise, 1982) have emphasized drug-induced changes in positively reinforced, rather than negatively reinforced, responding (*see* chapter by Greenshaw and Wishart in this volume).

The earliest studies in which systematic comparisons were made between the effects of drugs on positively and negatively reinforced responding were reported by Cook and Catania (1964), Ray and Bivens (1967), and Kelleher and Morse (1964). In the latter study, squirrel monkeys were trained on multiple FI–FI schedules to either obtain food or avoid electric shocks. The effects of *d*-amphetamine and chlorpromazine were investigated. The results showed that although the observed drug effects were different for each drug and also different for the two schedule components, the reinforcing event (i.e., either food presentation or shock avoidance) appeared not to be a significant determinant of drug action.

The result of this and other similar studies led to the belief that motivational factors were relatively unimportant in determining the behavioral effects of drugs. Several more recent studies, however, have found that, under certain circumstances, some drugs do exert actions that are reinforcer-dependent. A number of researchers have shown that it is possible to maintain responding in monkeys with schedules of electric shock presentation (Kelleher and Morse, 1968b). McKearney (1974) made use of this procedure to compare the effects of several drugs on FI responding maintained by food or shock delivery. It was found that *d*-amphetamine increased rates of responding under both conditions, but that the effects of morphine and chlorpromazine depended on the maintaining event. Morphine increased rates of responding for shock and decreased rates for food, whereas chlorpromazine reduced rates for food and had variable effects on shock-reinforced responding.

Using a similar experimental technique, Barrett (1976) investigated the effects of several other drugs. Like amphetamine, cocaine increased FI response rates maintained by both food and shock presentation. Alcohol, chlordiazepoxide, and pentobarbital increased food-maintained responding and decreased that maintained by shock. In another similar experiment, Branch (1979) confirmed that FI responding for food or shock delivery was similarly affected by acute administration of *d*-amphetamine, but found that the effects of the drug became reinforcer-dependent after repeated administration. Several other studies have compared drug effects on responding maintained by food delivery and shock avoidance. When FR schedules were used, rates of food-maintained and avoidance-maintained responding were reduced by a variety of drugs (Katz and Barrett, 1978; McKearney, 1980). However, when responding was maintined by FI schedules, chlordiazepoxide was found to increase rates of food-reinforced responding and to have little effect on shock avoidance (Ator, 1979; Barrett et al., 1977).

In all the experiments described thus far in the present section, comparisons have been made between responding maintained by food and that maintained by shock delivery or shock avoidance. There has also been a small number of studies that have made direct comparisons between food-reinforced responding and behavior maintained by other events, excluding noxious electric shocks. Hearst (1961) trained rats to obtain food and water by pressing two different levers according to VI schedules. Amphetamine produced similar effects on responding maintained by both reinforcers. Carey and his coworkers (1974), however, found that amphetamine could differentially affect rates of FR lever-pressing maintained by food or electric stimulation of the lateral hypothalamus. Responding maintained by food was decreased, but that maintained by intracranial stimulation was increased by several doses of the drug. Kida et al. (1981) obtained similar results in a study that used a multiple VI schedule of food or electrical brain stimulation, an effect that could not be accounted for in terms of differences in control response rates during the two schedule components. In the same study, however, chlordiazepoxide did not give rise to effects that were consistently reinforcer-dependent.

These and other recent studies have demonstrated that, under circumstances where rates and temporal patterns of responding are kept constant, the effects of some drugs may, in some conditions, be dependent upon the reinforcing event maintaining behavior. Barrett (1984) has suggested that it may be possible to categorize drugs according to their actions on behavior maintained by different events. However, Barrett and Katz (1981), in a thorough review of this research area, have cautioned against drawing conclusions about the effects of drugs on motivational states on the basis of such results. They point out that, although the effects of drugs may be reinforcer-dependent, they may at the same time be schedule-dependent, so that other aspects of the ongoing behavior or of the experimental environment may override the significance of the reinforcer. Thus, although these results provide a second descriptive principle for operant psychopharmacology, that drug action may be reinforcer-dependent, a more theoretical account of this research is not yet available.

5.2.2. *Reinforcement Frequency*

Several groups of researchers have considered the possibility that, in addition to the type of reinforcement, the frequency of reinforcement may be important as a determinant of drug action. Different schedules of reinforcement provide the possibility for subjects to obtain very different numbers of reinforcers, making it possible that some schedule-dependent drug effects may be accounted for in terms of differences in reinforcement rates. Furthermore, since higher response rates are frequently associated with higher reinforcement frequencies, it is possible that apparently rate-dependent drug effects may, in fact, be related to differences in reinforcement frequencies.

A number of studies have attempted to vary independently response rate and reinforcement frequency and to study the effects of drugs on the resulting patterns of schedule-controlled responding (Lucki, 1983; MacPhail and Gollub, 1975; Sanger and Blackman, 1975a; Stitzer and McKearney, 1977). In one of these studies (Sanger and Blackman, 1975a), rats obtained food under either a VI schedule of reinforcement or under a similar VI schedule to which a response pacing requirement had been added. This had the effect of greatly reducing the overall response rates and having little effect on overall reinforcement frequencies. The effects of *d*-amphetamine differed greatly between the two schedules—the low, paced response rates were increased, and the higher, unpaced VI rates decreased. These results suggested that response rate, not reinforcement frequency, was the important determinant of amphetamine's action in this study. Similar results were obtained by MacPhail and Gollub (1975). More recently, Lucki (1983) made use of 12 VI schedules to study the effects of amphetamine on different control response rates and reinforcement frequencies. In this study, it was found that the effects of the drug varied with changes in both response rate and reinforcement frequency, but that response rate was a more effective predictor of amphetamine's action. Lucki and DeLong (1983) obtained similar results using multiple schedules to vary independently response and reinforcement rates.

5.2.3. Punishment

A reinforcer was defined in a preceding section as an event that, when consequent upon a response, leads to the response becoming more frequent. Events that give rise to the opposite effect, reducing the frequency of responses that produce them, are defined as punishers. Punished responding may be very sensitive to drug administration (Houser, 1978; McMillan, 1975). Geller and Seifter (1960) demonstrated that rates of punished lever-pressing in rats could be greatly increased by drugs used clinically for their antianxiety properties, such as barbiturates, benzodiazepines, and meprobamate. Such effects have been confirmed in many experiments (*see* chapter by Dantzer in this volume).

It has been suggested that these antipunishment effects of anxiolytic drugs can be accounted for by rate-dependence, the low punished response rates being particularly sensitive to drug-induced increments (Rawlins et al., 1980; Spealman, 1979; Wuttke and Kelleher, 1970). However, although this question remains controversial, much of the evidence suggests that such drugs exert specific actions on punished responding because low response rates maintained under other conditions are facilitated to a considerably smaller extent (Huppert and Iversen, 1975; Hymowitz and Abramson, 1983; McMillan and Leander, 1975).

The effects of amphetamines on punished responding also cannot be accounted for entirely in terms of rate-dependence. Although alterations in rates of punished responding can, under some circumstances, be described as rate-dependent (Foree et al., 1973), amphetamine does not induce marked increases in overall rates of punished responding. In fact, it may lead to further decreases in response rate (Geller and Seifter, 1960). In recent studies, a number of other drugs have also been reported to further decrease rates of punished responding (Barrett et al., 1985; Feldon et al., 1983; Prado de Carvalho et al., 1983) and it has been suggested that these effects may indicate anxiety-inducing properties of these drugs in humans (Pellow and File, 1984).

5.3. Environmental and Behavioral Context

The preceding sections have described research that has shown that one environmental factor (i.e., type of reinforcer) and one aspect of an organism's ongoing behavior (i.e., response rate) can be important determinants of the behavioral effects of drugs. Studies of schedule-controlled behavior have indicated that other aspects of the complete environment and behavioral context within which a particular behavior occurs can also be of significance. In this section, consideration will be given to two such factors: the extent to which responding is under the control of external stimuli, and the interaction between behavior maintained by different components of multiple schedules.

5.3.1. Stimulus Control

It is possible to bring patterns of schedule-controlled responding under the control of specific external stimuli. This process is described as stimulus control or discrimination, and examples involving multiple schedules have been described earlier. Behavior under such stimulus control can be used to investigate schedule- or rate-dependent drug effects or to study the possibility that drugs may interfere with discrimination (Thompson, 1978). However, a number of studies have also shown that the degree to which behavior is under the control of external stimuli may itself modulate the extent to which drugs induce changes in responding (Laties, 1972; Laties and Weiss, 1966). This is dealt with by Dykstra and Genovese in a later chapter in this volume and thus, will not be discussed here.

5.3.2. *Behavioral Context*

Reference has already been made in the present chapter to the utility of multiple schedules for analyzing the effects of drugs. An implicit assumption of such studies is that the extent to which a schedule-controlled pattern of responding is disrupted by a drug does not depend upon whether or not the schedule forms part of a multiple schedule. Indeed, this is generally the case because, for example, the effects of amphetamine on FI and FR responding do not depend on whether these schedules are in operation individually or form components of a multiple schedule. However, in certain circumstances, complex interactions can occur between behavior during different components of a multiple schedule.

McKearney and Barrett (1975) trained two squirrel monkeys to obtain food on an FI 10-min schedule. Subsequently, this responding was maintained at a low rate by arranging that every 30th response was punished with an electric shock. During the first part of this experiment, this punishment schedule was alternated with periods during which responding had no programmed consequences (timeout period). When *d*-amphetamine was injected, low doses had no effect, whereas the highest dose tested further reduced rates of punished responding. In a second part of the experiment, the timeout period was replaced by a schedule of shock avoidance. When amphetamine was studied under these conditions, not only did it increase rates of avoidance responding, but it also substantially increased rates of punished responding. In a subsequent experiment (Barrett, 1977b), it was also found that amphetamine increased rates of punished responding when the punishment schedule formed part of a multiple schedule that also contained an FI shock presentation component.

The effects of amphetamine on punished responding thus depend on the context in which the punished responding occurs. It is also possible that the actions of this drug on responding that does not involve aversive stimuli may be context-dependent. Numerous experiments have shown that the slow, temporally spaced rates of responding maintained by DRL schedules can be greatly increased by administration of amphetamine (Sidman, 1955; Sanger et al., 1974). However, in one study, *d*-amphetamine was found to have relatively little effect on DRL response rates (Sanger, 1978). In this experiment, rats were trained on a multiple DRL–FI schedule of food reinforcement, with responding during the two schedule components being required on separate levers. During the DRL schedule component, amphetamine had relatively little effect on DRL response rates, but greatly increased response rates on the second (i.e., incorrect) lever. It is possible that this result may be accounted for in terms of effects of the drug on spatial preferences or perseverative responding (*see* Glick and Jerussi, 1974). Whatever the explanation, however, this study provides a further demonstration that drug effects on a particular pattern of schedule-controlled responding may depend on the behavioral context in which this pattern of responding occurs.

5.4. Past Experience

Another factor that is of major significance in determining the form that an individual organism's behavior takes is the past experience or previous history of the organism. As would be expected, past experience can also influence the behavioral effects of drugs. Such experience can conveniently be divided into two categories for the present discussion. First, *pharmacological experience*, which refers to a change in the effect of a drug because of previous administration of the same or a different drug and, second, *behavioral experience*, which may also be important, such that the behavioral effect of a drug can depend upon the behavioral history of an animal (*see* chapter by Dourish in this volume).

5.4.1. Pharmacological Experience

It is a common observation in pharmacology and medicine that after repeated or chronic administration of a drug, the initial effect declines. This effect is described as tolerance. On some occasions the opposite phenomenon may occur, and the effect of a drug becomes larger after repeated administration. Often, tolerance can be a result of dispositional factors, as when induction of the activity of metabolizing enzymes effectively causes less of the drug to reach its sites of action. In such cases it would be expected that all effects of the drug would be altered to a similar degree. However, in psychopharmacology the administration of a single dose of a drug can, of course, produce a variety of behavioral effects, and it is often observed that tolerance or sensitization will occur to some, but not all, of these effects. In fact, there is now substantial evidence to show that complex interactions can occur between repeated drug administration and repeated experience of a particular behavioral test environment (Goudie and Demellweek, 1986).

Because schedules of reinforcement provide relatively stable behavioral baselines over long periods of time, this technique can be used for analyzing changes in drug effects after repeated administration. Many such studies have been carried out, and this research has been described in reviews by Corfield-Summer and Stolerman (1978) and by Demellweek and Goudie (1983b).

As noted earlier, amphetamines can greatly increase the low rates of operant responding maintained by DRL schedules. Schuster and Zimmerman (1961) found that with repeated administration, the increase in operant responding became smaller, indicating tolerance, but there was no tolerance to the increase in locomotor activity induced by the drug. In a further report, Schuster and coworkers (1966) described a study aimed at investigating the behavioral mechanisms responsible for such differential tolerance. In two experiments the effects of repeated administration of amphetamine on the lever-pressing of rats maintained by DRL, FI, and shock avoidance were studied. It was found that when the initial effect of the drug produced a loss of reinforcement, as with an increase in DRL response rate, tolerance developed. However, when the initial effect involved no reinforcement loss, as with increased rates of shock-avoidance responding, no tolerance was observed. Schuster and his colleagues concluded with the hypothesis that tolerance would occur to the effects of amphetamines when the initial administration of the drug " . . . disrupts the organism's behavior in meeting the environmental requirements for reinforcement."

Similar hypotheses emphasizing how tolerance to drug action may occur through behavioral adaptation have been put forward for drugs other than amphetamine, such as marijuana (Ferraro, 1976; Galbicka et al., 1980). Demellweek and Goudie (1983b) have provided a detailed review of the literature concerned with development of tolerance to the behavioral effects of amphetamines and similar drugs. These workers point out that behavioral mechanisms are probably of great importance in the development of tolerance to the anorectic action of amphetamine because rats are able to learn to adapt their behavior to overcome the drug effect when this leads to an overall loss of food or water (Demellweek and Goudie, 1983a). There is also a number of more recent reports of results consistent with those obtained by Schuster et al., and described above, showing that behavioral mechanisms can be important in the development of tolerance to amphetamine-induced changes in schedule-controlled behavior (e.g., Thompson, 1974). However, Demellweek and Goudie (1981; 1983b) suggest that drug-induced changes in reinforcement density do not provide a complete explanation of tolerance development.

It is also sometimes observed that with repeated administration of a drug, the initially small effect may increase. A series of experiments by Wise and coworkers, for example, (Fouriezos and Wise, 1976; Wise, 1982; Wise et al., 1978) has shown that repeated administration of neuroleptic drugs, such as pimozide, to animals responding to obtain food, water, or reinforcing brain stimulation produces what appears to be a gradually accumulating drug effect. This is manifested as a depression of responding so that drug doses that initially have little effect appear, after several injections, to completely suppress responding. This effect occurs only in animals repeatedly tested after drug administration, and is therefore a true drug–behavior interaction and not a result of accumulation of drug in the body. Wise (1982) has interpreted this phenomenon as demonstrating a drug-induced block of the effectiveness of positive reinforcers, which he has termed anhedonia. Thus, the gradual decline in responding after repeated drug administration is equivalent to the decline in responding that occurs when a response is no longer reinforced (i.e., extinction). However, there has been much discussion of this hypothesis, and there are numerous experimental findings with which it cannot easily deal. For example, it has also been demonstrated that repeated administration of neuroleptic drugs can give rise to a gradual decline in rates of shock-avoidance responding (Hayashi et al., 1982; Sanger 1985) (*see* chapter by Greenshaw and Wishart).

5.4.2. *Behavioral Experience*

Many experiments in psychopharmacology have reported that certain types of prior experience without drugs can critically affect the subsequent behavioral actions of some drugs. For example, in a series of studies, Steinberg and her colleagues (1961; also *see* Rushton et al., 1963) showed that a mixture of amphetamine and amylobarbitol produced large increases in the exploratory behavior of rats in a novel Y-shaped maze, but that the same drug mixture had little or no effect on the activity of rats that had previously been exposed to the maze. Although such experiments certainly suggest that behavioral history is a factor of importance in determining drug action, it is sometimes unclear whether differential drug effects after different types of experience are a result of some aspect of the experience itself or of different levels of behavior in animals with different histories. This factor may also be a complication in studies involving schedule-controlled responding (Urbain et al., 1978). However, operant techniques do provide the possibility that drug action can be investigated in animals showing equivalent response baselines, but after different behavioral histories.

Terrace (1963) trained pigeons in a discrimination task, using two training procedures. In one, the birds were prevented from emitting erroneous reponses (errorless training), whereas in the other, condition errors could occur. When the discrimination had been established, Terrace found that chlorpromazine and imipramine increased nonreinforced responding only in the birds trained with errors. More recently, Barrett (1977a) has described an experiment in which monkeys were trained to obtain food on an FI schedule with a superimposed FR-punishment contingency. Injection of *d*-amphetamine had little effect, except to reduce response rates at higher doses, in animals trained only in this procedure. However, in monkeys with prior experience of responding to avoid or produce electric shocks, amphetamine administration increased rates of punished FI responding. Bacotti and McKearney (1979) obtained similar effects with *d*-amphetamine, but found that the response rate-decreasing action of chlorpromazine on punished FI responding was not changed by experience of a shock-avoidance schedule. However, Barrett and Stanley (1983) found that morphine could increase rates of avoidance responding in monkeys with a history of response-produced shock, but not in animals without such a history.

These results are important in showing that a complete understanding of the behavioral effects of drug will not be acquired without taking into account the prior experience of the drugged organism. It is clear, however, that differences in behavioral history do not always give rise to changes in drug effects (Poling et al., 1980). Indeed, if this were so, drug action in man would be almost impossible to predict. Furthermore, the studies described in this section have involved manipulations of only a small number of environmental factors in order to provide different experimental histories in different subjects. It is not yet possible to say which precise types of prior experience will lead to which types of changes in the actions of which drugs. Nor do we have any information about the behavioral mechanisms involved in such effects.

6. Parameters Other Than Operant Response Rate

The studies described and disucssed up to the present point in this chapter have dealt almost exclusively with changes in average rates of schedule-controlled responding produced by drug administration. Response rate is not only a convenient measure of behavioral output to use in assessing drug effects, but also one that has been found to be an important determinant of drug action. Nevertheless, it is not unrealistic to suppose that other aspects of an organism's behavior, even within a typical experiment involving schedule-controlled responding, may also be altered by drug administration in consistent and predictable ways. Thus, in the present section consideration will be given to studies that have assessed drug effects using measures other than response rate. First, several studies will be mentioned that have made use of aspects of operant responding other than response rate, and, second, a short discussion will be presented on the ways in which drugs can change behavior other than the specified operant response, but which may nevertheless occur in predictable patterns during schedules of reinforcement (schedule-induced behavior).

6.1. Response Distribution, Duration, and Force

Operant responding is characterized not only by the overall rate at which the response is emitted, but also by the force of the response, its duration, its location (if there are several locations available), and the time between successive responses (interresponse time: IRT). The use of IRTs for studying drug action has been particularly useful with schedules that provide reinforcement only if a response completes a certain IRT. With DRL schedules, for example, a response is reinforced only if it follows an IRT with a certain minimum duration. Responses after shorter IRTs reset the interval. With this schedule, subjects generally show slow, regularly paced responding, which can be described as timing behavior. As described earlier, a number of drugs will disrupt this behavior, and such drug effects have often been analyzed in terms of IRT distributions. Under control conditions, these distributions show a peak at the approximate value of the minimum reinforced IRT (indicating accurate timing) and often a second peak of very short IRTs (response bursts). Sidman (1955) showed that amphetamine could shift the whole distribution toward shorter IRTs, whereas alcohol did not shift the peak of the distribution, but nevertheless reduced overall rates of responding. More recent studies have also shown that detailed analysis of IRT distributions may be able to distinguish between the effects of different classes of drugs on DRL responding (Ando, 1975; O'Donnell and Seiden, 1983). For example, Sanger et al. (1974) found that both *d*-amphetamine and chlordiazepoxide could increase the overall rate of DRL responding in rats and shift the peak of the IRT distribution to shorter values. However, chlordiazepoxide was also found to consistently increase the proportion of very short IRTs, an effect that may be specific for drugs with clinical anxiolytic properties (Canon and Lippa, 1977; Sanger and Blackman, 1975b).

It is also possible to analyze IRT distributions with schedules other than DRL. Weiss and Gott (1972), for example, investigated the effects of amphetamine, imipramine, and pentobarbital on patterns of IRTs produced by pigeons obtaining food according to an FR-30 schedule. Although amphetamine and imipramine produced relatively selective increases in the duration of the long IRTs that followed reinforcement (postreinforcement pauses), pentobarbital shortened these pauses. This study was followed up by Eckerman and Edwards (1978) using pigeons trained to respond on a multiple FR–FI schedule. These workers also found that postreinforcement pauses during the FR component were increased by amphetamine, but, in contrast, pause durations during the FI component were decreased by the drug. Eckerman and Edwards suggested that the effects of drugs on pause durations may be schedule-dependent, as are effects on overall response rates.

It is possible to arrange an experiment so that operant responding shows a particular geographical distribution, in addition to a temporal distribution, by reinforcing responses in different locations. Response location may also be affected by drug administration. Moerschbaecher et al. (1979) trained monkeys to respond on a multiple FR–FI schedule with six response levers, any one of which could be chosen. After administration of either methamphetamine of scopolamine, the variability of response location was increased. Similarly, Robbins and Watson (1981) found that *d*-amphetamine increased the amount of response switching shown by rats that were required to respond on two levers to obtain reinforcers. However, the extent to which the drug induced this effect was dependent upon the control levels of response repetition that were changed by manipulation of the parameters of the reinforcement schedules in operation.

In an interesting series of studies, Fowler and his colleagues (1977, *see* also Ford et al., 1979; Walker et al., 1981) investigated the actions of several anxiolytic and antipsychotic agents on the durations of operant responses in rats. The animals were required to lever-press to obtain food or water according to FR schedules, and the average duration of responses, as well as average response rates, were measured. In certain experiments the force required in order to register a response was also varied. Generally, the drugs were found to decrease response rates and increase response durations. However, Walker et al., using a sophisticated statistical analysis, concluded that measures of response rate and response duration did not provide the same information. Furthermore, Ford et al. reported that although chlorpromazine and clozapine reduced response rate and peak response force, increases in response durations were seen only under conditions in which rats were required to press a manipulandum with a relatively high force. Such results show that measures of response duration and force can be sensitive to drug administration. It has also been found that response duration may provide a useful measure of the effects of drugs on responding maintained by schedules of brain stimulation (Greenshaw et al., 1983). However, it will require considerably more research to determine whether such measures will provide much more information concerning the mechanisms of drug action than that provided by measures of response rate (*see* chapter by Greenshaw and Wishart in this volume).

6.2. Schedule-Induced Behavior

Every experimenter is aware that during an experiment involving schedule-controlled behavior, an animal may spend a great deal of time behaving in ways other than that explicitly specified by the schedule. Indeed, with certain time-based schedules of reinforcement, the rate and vigor of other behaviors may surpass that of the operant response. It is possible to arrange experimental conditions so that particular behaviors, such as running in a wheel (Skinner and Morse, 1975) or drinking (Falk, 1961), will occur and can be measured, and it has been found that under some circumstances, such behavior can occur with highly predictable patterns.

Falk (1961) was the first to describe high levels of water consumption during a schedule of intermittent food reinforcement, a phenomenon he named schedule-induced polydipsia. Subsequently, many studies have shown that when food-deprived rats or primates receive intermittent deliveries of small food portions, they will drink after each portion despite never having been deprived of water by the experimenter. The characteristics of this behavior have been described in detail by Falk (1971, 1977), who has suggested that this drinking may be one of a variety of patterns of behavior that may occur in similar conditions. He called this behavior schedule-induced or adjunctive. Furthermore, Falk suggests that such behavior may be analogous to certain excessive or pathological patterns of human behavior, including drug abuse (Falk, 1981; 1983). However, the existence of such a category of adjunctive behavior has been subject to some controversy (Roper, 1981; Wetherington, 1982), as has the analogy with drug abuse (Sanger, 1986).

For the present discussion, the question of interest concerns the sensitivity of schedule-induced drinking to drug action. A number of studies have investigated this, and, because this work has been reviewed elsewhere (Sanger and Blackman, 1978), it will be dealt with relatively briefly here. Such research is of interest because it concerns the adequacy of considering schedule-induced behavior as a behavioral category functionally distinct from other categories (e.g., operant and respondent behavior). Also, it is of great interest to determine whether the general descriptive statements referred to above as behavioral principles of drug action apply to schedule-induced, in addition to schedule-controlled, responding.

A number of drugs, including amphetamine, scopolamine, chlorpromazine, and haloperidol, have been shown to reduce or suppress schedule-induced drinking in rats, whereas benzodiazepines, such as chlordiazepoxide and diazepam, can produce small increases (Sanger and Blackman, 1978). These results suggest that drugs affect schedule-induced drinking in much the same manner that they affect water intake induced by other manipulations, such as water deprivation. This, of course, can be investigated either by comparing the effects of a drug on drinking induced by a reinforcement schedule with that induced by other means, or by making comparisons between the effects of a drug on topographically different schedule-induced behaviors. Unfortunately, relatively few studies have made use of either experimental design to date (*see* chapter by Cooper and Turkish in this volume).

It appears, however, that drugs do not necessarily induce similar alterations in schedule-induced and deprivation-induced drinking. Sanger and Corfield-Sumner (1979) investigated the effects of *d*-amphetamine and chlordiazepoxide on similar levels of water intake induced in rats by water deprivation or by a schedule of intermittent food delivery. Amphetamine produced similar reductions in levels of water intake under both conditions, and chlordiazepoxide increased deprivation-induced drinking to a considerably greater extent than schedule-induced drinking. In more recent experiments, it has been shown that the opiate antagonist naloxone, which is known to reduce levels of food and water intake under a variety of circumstances (Sanger, 1981), has no effect on schedule-induced drinking (Brown and Holtzman, 1981; Cooper and Holtzman, 1983).

Fewer experiments have studied other forms of schedule-induced behavior. Smith and Clark (1975) investigated the effects of several drugs on the drinking and wheel-running of rats during a multiple DRL schedule. The results were complex, varying across subjects and experimental conditions. More recently, Williams and White (1984) found that amphetamine and scopolamine each affected schedule-induced drinking and wheel-running in similar ways. Cherek and Thompson (1973) found that, in pigeons, THC produced greater decreases in schedule-induced key-pecking, which provided the opportunity to attack another bird, than in schedule-controlled key-pecking. Such an effect may be caused by either a specific action of the drug on schedule-induced behavior or a specific effect on aggressive responses.

7. Applications of Operant Behavioral Pharmacology

Most of the studies that have been described in the preceding sections of this chapter might be considered academic in nature. The primary purpose of these studies has been to obtain scientific information about behavioral effects of drugs in order to allow general statements to be made about the determinants of such effects. Such an enterprise is, of course, perfectly legitimate as the first step toward a thorough understanding of drug action. However, behavioral techniques can also be used in the more practical matter of searching for novel psychoactive drugs and detecting hazards associated with presently used drugs or other chemicals. Before concluding this account of the importance of schedule-controlled behavior for psychopharmacology, brief mention will be made of these applications of operant methodology.

Schedule-controlled behavior in laboratory animals can be used in the search for new and more effective drugs to be used in the treatment of psychiatric disorders. Attempts to develop animal models of psychiatric disorders have not yet proven to be the most effective means of discovering and evaluating new molecules, not least of all because of the relative lack of knowledge of the biological and environmental causes of these disorders. Thus, pharmacologists searching for new drugs generally proceed by looking for specific behavioral effects of well-known drugs, then by studying the effects of newly synthesized compounds in the same tests. Although this approach has been criticized for only giving rise to "me-too" drugs (Kumar, 1974), it is possible in this way to detect new drugs with pharmacological properties considered desirable and probably relevant to the proposed clinical use, but without certain undesirable effects. To give one example, by using appropriate behavioral tests it should be possible to show that a new drug exerted activities similar to those of anxiolytic agents, but without the myorelaxation and sedation that may be considered undesirable side effects of this class of drugs.

Because of the necessity for synthesizing and testing large numbers of new molecules, schedule-controlled behavior is not a convenient method for use during the early stages of screening for new drugs. However, in later stages of drug selection and development, these methods can be of great importance. It has already been noted that avoidance behavior has played an important part in the development of antipsychotic drugs, although it is now clear that these drugs do not exert specific effects on such behavior. Punishment procedures are also of importance in research aimed at discovering new anxiolytic drugs. Another method involving schedule-controlled behavior, and which has recently become important in drug development, is drug discrimination, as described in the chapter by Järbe in this volume. Also, in the search for drugs that may be effective in treating dementia, operant procedures play their part (e.g. Bartus et al., 1983).

In addition to the search for new drugs, much recent applied behavioral research has been attempting to deal with the problem of detecting and analyzing undesirable behavioral effects of drugs and chemicals, such as food additives and environmental pollutants. This important area of research is now known as behavioral toxicology (Evans and Weiss, 1978). There has been much discussion about the most appropriate tests to be applied in the animal laboratory in order to detect effects considered to indicate behavioral toxicity (Pryor et al., 1983; Sanger et al., 1983). As with the search for new drugs, it is clear that if many substances are to be tested, operant techniques cannot be used in the early stages of screening for behavioral toxicity. However, these methods can be very important in providing more sophisticated and perhaps more sensitive measures of undesirable behavioral actions (Laties, 1978). As examples, it is possible to cite the use of self-administration techniques for evaluating the dependence potential of new drugs (Griffiths et al., 1980; Johanson, 1978) and the sensitivity of psychophysical methods, using operantly conditioned behavior, for detecting impaired sensory function produced by environmental pollutants (Hanson, 1974).

8. Conclusions

The effects of drugs on behavior are complex and varied. Those researchers who hope to find some invariant relationship between the administration of a particular dose of a drug and a change in a certain pattern of behavior will almost certainly be disappointed. If one thing is certain in psychopharmacology, it is that drug effects can depend critically on a variety of aspects of the drugged organism and on a number of environmental variables. This general point is as applicable to animals in a well-controlled laboratory as it is for drug action in humans.

The search for an accurate and useful understanding of drug effects requires the specification of the biological and environmental factors that are important in determining drug action. The present chapter has attempted to show how schedule-controlled behavior of laboratory animals can be used in such research. Although the review of relevant studies has necessarily been selective, and in parts relatively brief, it is to be hoped that the research described has shown that operant methodology can provide powerful techniques for studying drug effects on well-controlled, predictable behavioral baselines.

Studies of the effects of drugs on patterns of schedule-controlled operant responding have demonstrated that several factors can be important in determining drug action. It is not surprising to discover that it is precisely those aspects of an animal's environment, such as type and frequency of reinforcement and punishment, stimulus control, and past experience, that are important in determining the form of behavior that are also significant determinants of drug effects. Probably the attempt to specify a list of behavioral principles for determining drug action is one of the most important current contributions of schedule-controlled behavior to psychopharmacology. In some cases, such as the dependence of the effects of amphetamine-like drugs on baseline response rates, there is general acceptance of the principle. In other cases, as with the importance of behavioral context or past experience, a great deal more information is necessary. Thus, the statement that the effects of some drugs may, under some circumstances, depend on some types of past experience, is so imprecise that it is of little use. It will be necessary to specify which drug effects depend on which types of past experience. Of course, it will not be possible to test all known drugs in all possible experimental situations, and thus, in order to provide very general predictive statements about drug action, the formulation of behavioral theories will be necessary.

References

Ando K. (1975) Profile of drug effects on temporally spaced responding in rats. *Pharmacol. Biochem. Behav.* **3,** 833–841.

Ator N. A. (1979) Differential effects of chlordiazepoxide on comparable rates of responding maintained by food and shock avoidance. *Psychopharmacology* **66,** 222–231.

Bacotti A. V. and McKearney J. W. (1979) Prior and ongoing experience as determinants of the effects of *d*-amphetamine and chlorpromazine on punished behavior. *J. Pharmacol. Exp. Ther.* **211,** 80–85.

Barrett J. E. (1976) Effects of alcohol, chlordiazepoxide, cocaine and pentobarbital on responding maintained under fixed-interval schedules of food or shock presentation. *J. Pharmacol. Exp. Ther.* **196,** 605–615.

Barrett J. E. (1977a) Behavioral history as a determinant of the effects of *d*-amphetamine on punished behavior. *Science* **198,** 67–69.

Barrett J. E. (1977b) Effects of *d*-amphetamine on responding simultaneously maintained and punished by presentation of electric shock. *Psychopharmacology* **54,** 119–124.

Barrett J. E. (1984) Behavioral Principles in Psychopharmacology, in *Aspects of Psychopharmacology* (Sanger D. J. and Blackman D. E., eds.), Methuen, London.

Barrett J. E. and Katz J. L. (1981) Drug Effects on Behaviors Maintained by Different Events, in *Advances in Behavioral Pharmacology* vol. 3, (Thompson T., Dews P. B., and McKim W. A., eds.), Academic, New York.

Barrett J. E. and Stanley J. A. (1983) Prior behavioral experience can reverse the effects of morphine. *Psychopharmacology* **81,** 107–110.

Barrett J. E., Dworkin S. I., and Zuccarelli R. R. (1977) Effects of *d*-amphetamine, chlordiazepoxide and promazine on responding of squirrel monkeys maintained under fixed-interval schedules of food presentation or stimulus-shock termination. *Pharmacol. Biochem. Behav.* **7,** 529–535.

Barrett J. E., Brady L. S., Witkin J. M., Cook J. M., and Larscheid P. (1985) Interactions between the benzodiazepine receptor antagonist RO 15-1788 (flumazepil) and the inverse agonist β-CCE: Behavioral studies with Squirrel monkeys. *Life Sci.* **36,** 1407–1414.

Bartus R. T., Dean R. L., and Beer B. (1983) An evaluation of drugs for improving memory in aged monkeys: Implications for clinical trials in humans. *Psychopharmacol. Bull.* **19,** 168–184.

Beecher M. D. and Jackson D. E. (1976) Rate-dependent effect of ampheatmine in rats: Extension to between-subjects effect. *Psychopharmacologia* **46,** 307–309.

Beninger R. J., Mason S. T., Phillips A. G., and Fibiger H. C. (1980) The use of conditioned suppression to evaluate the nature of neuroleptic-induced avoidance deficits. *J. Pharmacol. Exp. Ther.* **213,** 623–627.

Blackman D. E. (1974) *Operant Conditioning*, Methuen, London.

Branch M. N. (1979) Consequent events as determinants of drug effects on schedule-controlled behavior: Modification of effects of cocaine and *d*-amphetamine following chronic amphetamine administration. *J. Pharmacol. Exp. Ther.* **210**, 354–360.

Branch M. N. and Gollub L. R. (1974) A detailed analysis of the effects of *d*-amphetamine on behavior under fixed-interval schedules. *J. Exp. Anal. Behav.* **21**, 519–539.

Brown D. R. and Holtzman S. G. (1981) Suppression of drinking by naloxone in the rat: A further characterization. *Eur. J. Pharmacol.* **69**, 331–340.

Byrd L. D. (1973) Effects of *d*-amphetamine on schedule-controlled key pressing and drinking in the chimpanzee. *J. Pharmacol. Exp. Ther.* **185**, 633–641.

Byrd L. D. (1981) Quantitation in Behavioral Pharmacology, in *Advances in Behavioral Pharmacology* vol. 3, (Thompson T., Dews P. B., and McKim W. A., eds.), Academic, New York.

Canon J. G. and Lippa A. S. (1977) Use of DRL in differentiating anxiolytic and neuroleptic properties of CNS drugs. *Pharmacol. Biochem. Behav.* **6**, 591–593.

Carey R. J., Goodall E. B., and Procopio G. F. (1974) Differential effects of *d*-amphetamine on fixed ratio 30 performance maintained by food versus brain stimulation reinforcement. *Pharmacol. Biochem. Behav.* **2**, 193–198.

Carlton P. L. (1983) *A primer of behavioral pharmacology*, W. H. Freeman, New York.

Cherek D. R. and Thompson T. (1973) Effects of Δ^9-tetrahydrocannabinol on schedule-induced aggression in pigeons. *Pharmacol. Biochem. Behav.* **1**, 493–500.

Clark F. C. and Steele B. J. (1966) Effects of *d*-amphetamine on performance under a multiple schedule in the rat. *Psychopharmacologia* **9**, 157–169.

Cook L. and Catania A. C. (1964) Effects of drugs on avoidance and escape behavior. *Fed. Proc.* **23**, 818–835.

Cooper S. J. and Holtzman S. G. (1983) Patterns of drinking in the rat following the administration of opiate antagonists. *Pharmacol. Biochem. Behav.* **19**, 505–511.

Corfield-Sumner P. K. and Stolerman I. P. (1978) Behavioral Tolerance, in *Contemporary Research in Behavioral Pharmacology* (Blackman D. E. and Sanger D. J., eds.), Plenum, New York.

Courvoisier S., Fournel J., Ducrot R., Kolsky M., and Koetschet P. (1953) Propriétés pharmacodynamiques du chlorhydrate de chloro-3 (diméthylamino-3′propyl)-10 phénothiazine. *Arch. Int. Pharmacodyn. Ther.* **92,** 305–361.

Demellweek C. and Goudie A. J. (1981) A Molecular Analysis of the Effects of Chronic *d*-Amphetamine Treatment on Fixed Ratio Responding in Rats: Relevance to Theories of Tolerance, in *Quantification of Steady-State Operant Behaviour* (Bradshaw C. M., Szabadi E., and Lowe C. F., eds.), Elsevier/ North Holland Biomedical, Amsterdam.

Demellweek C. and Goudie A. J. (1983a) An analysis of behavioural mechanisms involved in the acquisition of amphetamine anorectic tolerance. *Psychopharmacology* **79,** 58–66.

Demellweek C. and Goudie A. J. (1983b) Behavioural tolerance to amphetamine and other psychostimulants: The case for considering behavioural mechanisms. *Psychopharmacology* **80,** 387–307.

Dews P. B. (1955a) Studies on behavior. I. Differential sensitivity to pentobarbital of pecking performance in pigeons depending on the schedule of reward. *J. Pharmacol. Exp. Ther.* **113,** 393–401.

Dews P. B. (1955b) Studies on behavior. II. The effects of pentobarbital, methamphetamine and scopolamine on performances in pigeons involving discriminations. *J. Pharmacol. Exp. Ther.* **115,** 380–389.

Dews P. B. (1958a) Studies on behavior. IV. Stimulant actions of methamphetamine. *J. Pharmacol. Exp. Ther.* **122,** 137–147.

Dews P. B. (1958b) Analysis of effects of psychopharmacological agents in behavioral terms. *Fed. Proc.* **17,** 1024–1030.

Dews P. B. (1976) Interspecies Differences in Drug Effects: Behavioral, in *Psychotherapeutic Drugs. Part 1, Principles* (Usdin E. and Forrest I. S., eds.), Marcel Dekker, New York.

Dews P. B. (1978a) Origins and future of behavioral pharmacology. *Life Sci.* **22,** 1115–1122.

Dews P. B. (1978b) Rate-dependency hypothesis. *Science* **198,** 1182–1183.

Dews P. B. (1981) History and Present Status of Rate-Dependency Investigations, in *Advances in Behavioral Pharmacology* vol. 3, (Thompson T., Dews P. B., and McKim W. A., eds.), Academic, New York.

Dews P. B. and Wenger G. R. (1977) Rate Dependency of the Behavioral Effects of Amphetamine, in *Advances in Behavioral Pharmacology* vol. 1, (Thompson T. and Dews P. B., eds.), Academic, New York.

Eckerman D. A. and Edwards J. D. (1978) Schedule-dependent effect of *d*-amphetamine on pausing by pigeons. *Pharmacol. Biochem. Behav.* **8,** 319–321.

Evans H. L. and Weiss B. (1978) Behavioral Toxicology, in *Contemporary Research in Behavioral Pharmacology* (Blackman D. E. and Sanger D. J., eds.), Plenum, New York.

Falk J. L. (1961) Production of polydipsia in normal rats by an intermittent food schedule. *Science* **133,** 195–196.

Falk J. L. (1971) The nature and determinants of adjunctive behavior.*Physiol. Behav.* **6,** 577–588.

Falk J. L. (1977) The origin and functions of adjunctive behavior. *Anim. Learn. Behav.* **5,** 325–335.

Falk J. L. (1981) The Place of Adjunctive Behavior in Drug Abuse Research, in *Behavioral Pharmacology of Human Drug Dependence* (Thompson T. and Johanson C. E., eds.), NIDA Drug Abuse Research Monograph 37, Dept. of Health and Human Svcs., Washington.

Falk J. L. (1983) Drug dependence: Myth or motive? *Pharmacol. Biochem. Behav.* **19,** 385–391.

Feldon J., Lerner T., Levin D., and Myslobodsky M. (1983) A behavioral examination of convulsant benzodiazepine and GABA antagonist, Ro 5-3663, and benzodiazepine-receptor antagonist Ro 15-1788, *Pharmacol. Biochem. Behav.* **19,** 39–41.

Ferraro D. P. (1976) A Behavioral Model of Marihuana Tolerance, in *The Pharmacology of Marihuana* (Braude M. C. and Szara S., eds.), Raven, New York.

Ferster C. B. and Skinner B. F. (1957) *Schedules of Reinforcement,* Appleton-Century-Crofts, New York.

Ford K. E., Fowler S. C., and Nail G. L. (1979) Effects of clozapine and chlorpromazine upon operant response measures in rats. *Pharmacol. Biochem. Behav.* **11,** 239–241.

Foree D. D., Moretz F. H., and McMillan D. E. (1973) Drugs and punished responding. II. *d*-amphetamine-induced increases in punished responding. *J. Exp. Anal. Behav.* **20,** 291–300.

Fouriezos G. and Wise R. A. (1976) Pimozide-induced extinction of intracranial self-stimulation: Response patterns rule out motor performance deficits. *Brain Res.* **103,** 377–380.

Fowler S. C., Filewich R. J., and Leberer M. R. (1977) Drug effects upon force and duration of response during fixed-ratio performance in rats. *Pharmacol. Biochem. Behav.* **6,** 421–426.

Galbicka G., Lee D. M., and Branch M. N. (1980) Schedule-dependent tolerance to behavioral effects of Δ^9-tetrahydrocannabinol when reinforcement frequencies are matched. *Pharmacol. Biochem. Behav.* **12,** 85–91.

Geller I. and Seifter J. (1960) The effects of meprobamate, barbiturates, *d*-amphetamine and promazine on experimentally induced conflict in the rat. *Psychopharmacologia* **1,** 482–492.

Glick S. D. and Jerussi T. P. (1974) Spatial and paw preferences in rats: Their relationship to rate-dependent effects of *d*-amphetamine. *J. Pharmacol. Exp. Ther.* **188,** 714–725.

Gonzalez F. A. and Byrd L. D. (1977) Mathematics underlying the rate dependency hypothesis. *Science* **195,** 546–550.

Goudie A. J. and Demellweek C. (1986) Conditioning Factors in Drug Tolerance, in *Behavioral Analysis of Drug Dependence* (Goldberg S. R. and Stolerman I. P., eds.), Academic, New York.

Greenshaw A. J., Sanger D. J., and Blackman D. E. (1983) Effects of chlordiazepoxide on the self-regulated duration of lateral hypothalamic stimulation in rat. *Psychopharmacology* **81,** 236–238.

Griffiths R. R., Bigelow G. E., and Henningfield J. E. (1980) Similarities in Animal and Human Drug-Taking Behavior, in *Advances in Substance Abuse* vol. 1, (Mello N. K., ed.), JAI, Connecticut.

Grilly D. M. (1977) Rate-dependent effects of amphetamine resulting from behavioral competition. *Biobehav. Rev.* **1,** 87–93.

Hanson H. M. (1974) Psychophysical evaluation of toxic effects on sensory systems. *Fed. Proc.* **34,** 1852–1857.

Hanson H. M., Witoslawski J. J., and Campbell E. H. (1967) Drug effects in squirrel monkeys trained on a multiple schedule with a punishment contingency. *J. Exp. Anal. Behav.* **10,** 565–569.

Harris R. A., Snell D., and Loh H. H. (1978) Effects of *d*-amphetamine, monomethoxyamphetamines and hallucinogens on schedule-controlled behavior. *J. Pharmacol. Exp. Ther.* **204,** 103–117.

Hayashi T., Tadokoro S., Hashimoto H., and Nakashimo M. (1982) Enhancement of avoidance-suppressing effect after repeated administration of haloperidol and serum haloperidol in rats. *Pharmacol. Biochem. Behav.* **17**, 131–136.

Hearst E. (1961) Effects of *d*-amphetamine on behavior reinforced by food and water. *Psychol. Rep.* **8**, 301–309.

Heffner T. G., Drawbaugh R. B., and Zigmond M. J. (1974) Amphetamine and operant behavior in rats: Relationship between drug effect and control response rate. *J. Comp. Physiol. Psychol.* **86**, 1031–1043.

Houser V. P. (1978) The Effects of Drugs on Behavior Controlled by Aversive Stimuli, in *Contemporary Research in Behavioral Pharmacology* (Blackman D. E. and Sanger D. J., eds.), Plenum, New York.

Huppert F. A. and Iversen S. D. (1975) Response suppression in rats: A comparison of response contingent and noncontingent punishment, and the effects of a minor tranquilliser, chlordiazepoxide. *Psychopharmacologia* **44**, 67–75.

Hymowitz N. and Abramson M. (1983) Effects of diazepam on responding suppressed by response-dependent and independent electric shock delivery. *Pharmacol. Biochem. Behav.* **18**, 769–776.

Johanson C. E. (1978) Drugs as Reinforcers, in *Contemporary Research in Behavioral Pharmacology* (Blackman D. E. and Sanger D. J., eds.), Plenum, New York.

Katz J. L. and Barrett J. E. (1978) Ethanol, pentobarbital and chlordiazepoxide effects in squirrel monkeys responding under fixed-ratio food presentation and stimulus shock termination. *Psychopharmacology* **56**, 153–155.

Katz J. L. and McLeod D. R. (1979) Mathematics relevant to rate-dependent drug effects. *Neurosci. Biobehav. Rev.* **3**, 11–13.

Kelleher R. T. and Morse W. H. (1964) Escape behavior and punished behavior. *Fed. Proc.* **23**, 808–817.

Kelleher R. T. and Morse W. H. (1968a) Determinants of the specificity of behavioral effects of drugs. *Ergeb. der Physiol.* **60**, 1–56.

Kelleher R. T. and Morse W. H. (1968b) Schedules using noxious stimuli. III. Responding maintained by response-produced electric shocks. *J. Exp. Anal. Behav.* **11**, 819–838.

Kida M., Greenshaw A. J., Sanger D. J., and Blackman D. E. (1981) The effects of *d*-amphetamine and chlordiazepoxide on responding maintained by a multiple schedule of food and electrical brain stimulation in rats. *Psychol. Rec.* **31**, 349–356.

Ksir C. (1981) Rate-Convergent Effects of Drugs, in *Advances in Behavioral Pharmacology* vol. 3, (Thompson T., Dews P. B., and McKim W. A., eds.), Academic, New York.

Kumar R. (1974) Editorial: Animal models for evaluating psychotropic drugs. *Psychol. Med.* **4**, 353–359.

Kuribara H. and Tadokoro S. (1981) Correlation between antiavoidance activities of antipsychotic drugs in rats and daily clinical doses. *Pharmacol. Biochem. Behav.* **14**, 181–192.

Laties V. G. (1972) The modification of drug effects on behavior by external discriminative stimuli. *J. Pharmacol. Exp. Ther.* **183**, 1–13.

Laties V. G. (1978) How operant conditioning can contribute to behavioral toxicology. *Environ. Health Perspect.* **26**, 29–35.

Laties V. G. (1979) I. V. Zavadskii and the beginnings of behavioral pharmacology: An historical note and translation. *J. Exp. Anal. Behav.* **32**, 463–472.

Laties V. G. and Weiss B. (1966) Influence of drugs on behavior controlled by internal and external stimuli. *J. Pharmacol. Exp. Ther.* **152**, 388–396.

Leander J. D. (1975) Rate-dependent effects of drugs. II. Effects of some major tranquilizers on multiple fixed-ratio, fixed-interval schedule performance. *J. Pharmacol. Exp. Ther.* **193**, 689–700.

Leander J. D. and McMillan D. E. (1974) Rate-dependent effects of drugs. I. Comparisons of *d*-amphetamine, pentobarbital and chlorpromazine on multiple and mixed schedules. *J. Pharmacol. Exp. Ther.* **188**, 726–739.

Lucki I. (1983) Rate-dependent effects of amphetamine on responding under random-interval schedules of reinforcement in the rat. *Pharmacol. Biochem. Behav.* **18**, 195–201.

Lucki I. and DeLong R. E. (1983) Control rate of response or reinforcement and amphetamine's effect on behavior. *J. Exp. Anal. Behav.* **40**, 123–132.

Lyon M. and Robbins T. (1975) The Action of Central Nervous System Stimulant Drugs: A General Theory Concerning Amphetamine Effects, in *Current Developments in Psychopharmacology* vol. 2, (Essman W. B. and Valzelli L., eds.), Spectrum, New York.

Macht D. I. (1924) A pharmacodynamic analysis of the cerebral effects of atropine, homatropine, scopolamine and related drugs. *J. Pharmacol. Exp. Ther.* **22**, 117–122.

Mackintosh N. J. (1974) *The Psychology of Animal Learning,* Academic, London.

MacPhail R. C. and Gollub L. R. (1975) Separating the effects of response rate and reinforcement frequency in the rate-dependent effects of amphetamine and scopolamine on the schedule-controlled performance of rats and pigeons. *J. Pharmacol. Exp. Ther.* **194,** 332–342.

Masserman J. H. and Yum K. S. (1946) Analysis of the influence of alcohol on experimental neurosis in cats. *Psychosom. Med.* **8,** 36–52.

McKearney J. W. (1974) Effects of *d*-amphetamine, morphine and chlorpromazine on responding under fixed-interval schedules of food presentation or electric shock presentation. *J. Pharmacol. Exp. Ther.* **190,** 141–153.

McKearney J. W. (1980) Fixed ratio schedules of food presentation and stimulus shock termination: Effects of *d*-amphetamine, morphine and clozapine. *Psychopharmacology* **70,** 35–39.

McKearney J. W. (1981) Rate-dependency: Scope and Limitations in the Explanation and Analysis of the Behavioral Effects of Drugs, in *Advances in Behavioral Pharmacology* vol. 3, (Thompson T., Dews P. B., and McKim W. A., eds.), Academic, New York.

McKearney J. W. and Barrett J. E. (1975) Punished behavior: Increases in responding after *d*-amphetamine. *Psychopharmacologia* **41,** 23–26.

McKearney J. W. and Barrett J. E. (1978) Schedule-Controlled Behavior and the Effects of Drugs, in *Contemporary Research in Behavioral Pharmacology* (Blackman D. E. and Sanger D. J., eds.), Plenum, New York.

McKim W. A. (1981) Rate-Dependency: A Nonspecific Behavioral Effect of Drugs, in *Advances in Behavioral Pharmacology* vol. 3, (Thompson T., Dews P. B., and McKim W. A., eds.), Academic, New York.

McMillan D. E. (1968) The effects of sympathomimetic amines on schedule-controlled behavior in the pigeon. *J. Pharmacol. Exp. Ther.* **160,** 315–325.

McMillan D. E. (1975) The determinants of drug effects on punished responding. *Fed. Proc.* **34,** 1870–1879.

McMillan D. E. and Leander J. D. (1975) Drugs and punished responding. V. Effects of drugs on responding suppressed by response-dependent and response-independent electric shock. *Arch. Int. Pharmacodyne. Ther.* **213,** 22–27.

Miczek K. A. (1973) Effects of scopolamine, amphetamine, and chlordiazepoxide on punishment. *Psychopharmacologia* **28,** 373–389.

Miller N. E. (1956) Effects of drugs on motivation: the value of using a variety of measures. *Ann. NY Acad. Sci.* **65,** 318–333.

Moerschbaecher J. M., Thompson D. M., and Thomas J. R. (1979) Effects of methamphetamine and scopolamine on variability of response location. *J. Exp. Anal. Behav.* **32,** 255–263.

Morpurgo C. (1965) Drug-induced modifications of discriminated avoidance behavior in rats. *Psychopharmacologia* **8,** 91–99.

O'Donnell J. M. and Seiden L. S. (1983) Differential-reinforcement-of-low-rate 72-second schedule: Selective effects of antidepressant drugs. *J. Pharmacol. Exp. Ther.* **224,** 80–88.

Pavlov I. P. (1927) *Conditioned Reflexes,* Dover, New York.

Pellow S. and File S. E. (1984) Multiple sites of action for anxiogenic drugs: Behavioural, electrophysiological and biochemical correlations. *Psychopharmacology* **83,** 304–315.

Poling A., Krafft K., and Chapman L. (1980) *d*-Amphetamine, operant history, and variable-interval performance. *Pharmacol. Biochem. Behav.* **12,** 559–562.

Prado de Carvalho L., Grecksch G., Chapouthier G., and Rossier J. (1983) Anxiogenic and non-anxiogenic benzodiazepine antagonists. *Nature* **301,** 64–66.

Pryor G. T., Uyeno E. T., Tilson H. A., and Mitchell C. L. (1983) Assessment of chemicals using a battery of neurobehavioral tests: A comparative study. *Neurobehav. Toxicol. Teratol.* **5,** 91–117.

Rachlin H. (1976) *Behavior and Learning,* W. H. Freeman, San Francisco.

Rawlins J. N. P., Feldon J., Salmon P., Gray J. A., and Garrud P. (1980) The effects of chlordiazepoxide HCl administration upon punishment and conditioned suppression in the rat. *Psychopharmacology* **70,** 317–322.

Ray O. S. and Bivens L. W. (1967) Phenothiazine depression of approach and avoidance behavior. *Psychopharmacologia* **10,** 196–203.

Robbins T. W. (1981) Behavioral Determinants of Drug Action: Rate-Dependency Revisited, in *Theory in Psychopharmacology* vol. 1, (Cooper S. J., ed.), Academic, New York.

Robbins T. W. and Sahakian B. J. (1979) "Paradoxical" effects of psychomotor stimulant drugs in hyperactive children from the standpoint of behavioural pharmacology. *Neuropharmacology* **18,** 931–950.

Robbins T. W. and Watson B. A. (1981) Effects of *d*-Amphetamine on Response Repetition and "Win-Stay" Behaviour in Rat, in *Quantification of Steady-State Operant Behavior* (Bradshaw C. M., Szabadi E., and Lowe C. F., eds.), Elsevier/North Holland Biomedical, Amsterdam.

Roper T. J. (1981) What is meant by the term "schedule-induced," and how general is schedule induction. *Anim. Learn. Behav.* **9,** 433–440.

Rushton R., Steinberg, H., and Tinson C. (1963) Effects of a single experience on subsequent reactions to drugs. *Br. J. Pharmacol.* **20,** 99–105.

Sanger D. J. (1978) Effects of *d*-amphetamine on temporal and spatial discrimination in rats. *Psychopharmacology* **58,** 185–188.

Sanger D. J. (1981) Endorphinergic mechanisms in the control of food and water intake. *Appetite: J. Intake Research* **2,** 193–208.

Sanger D. J. (1985) The effects of clozapine on shuttle-box avoidance responding in rats: Comparisons with haloperidol and chlordiazepoxide. *Pharmacol. Biochem. Behav.* **23,** 231–236.

Sanger D. J. (1986) Drug Taking as Adjunctive Behavior, in *Behavioral Analysis of Drug Dependence* (Goldberg S. R. and Stolerman I. P., eds.), Academic, New York.

Sanger D. J. and Blackman D. E. (1975a) Rate-dependent effects of drugs on the variable-interval behavior of rats. *J. Pharmacol. Exp. Ther.* **194,** 343–350.

Sanger D. J. and Blackman D. E. (1975b) The effects of tranquillizing drugs on timing behavior in rats. *Psychopharmacologia* **44,** 153–156.

Sanger D. J. and Blackman D. E. (1976) Rate-dependent effects of drugs: A review of the literature. *Pharmacol. Biochem. Behav.* **4,** 73–83.

Sanger D. J. and Blackman D. E. (1978) The Effects of Drugs on Adjunctive Behavior, in *Contemporary Research in Behavioral Pharmacology* (Blackman D. E. and Sanger D. J., eds.), Plenum, New York.

Sanger D. J. and Blackman D. E. (1981) Rate-Dependence and the Effects of Benzodiazepines, in *Advances in Behavioral Pharmacology* vol. 3, (Thompson T., Dews P. B., and McKim W. A., eds.), Academic, New York.

Sanger D. J. and Corfield-Sumner P. K. (1979) Schedule-induced drinking and thirst: A pharmacological analysis. *Pharmacol. Biochem. Behav.* **10,** 471–474.

Sanger D. J., Key M., and Blackman D. E. (1974) Differential effects of chlordiazepoxide and *d*-amphetamine on responding maintained by a DRL schedule of reinforcement. *Psychopharmacologia* **38,** 159–171.

Sanger D. J., Leclere J. F., and Lloyd K. G. (1983) Hazard Detection in Behavioral Toxicology, in *Present Problems and Future Trends in Drug Toxicology* (Zbinden G., ed.), John Libby, London.

Schuster C. R. and Zimmerman J. (1961) Timing behavior during prolonged treatment with *d,l*-amphetamine. *J. Exp. Anal. Behav.* **4,** 327–330.

Schuster C. R., Dockens W. S., and Woods J. H. (1966) Behavioral variables affecting the development of amphetamine tolerance. *Psychopharmacologia* **9,** 170–182.

Seiden L. S., MacPhail R. C., and Oglesby M. W. (1975) Catecholamines and drug-behavior interactions. *Fed. Proc.* **34,** 1823–1831.

Sidman M. (1955) Technique for assessing the effects of drugs on timing behavior. *Science* **122,** 925.

Skinner B. F. (1938) *The Behavior of Organisms,* Appleton-Century-Crofts, New York.

Skinner B. F. and Heron W. T. (1937) Effects of caffeine and benzedrine upon conditioning and extinction. *Psychol. Rec.* **1,** 340–346.

Skinner B. F. and Morse W. H. (1975) Concurrent activity under fixed-interval reinforcement. *J. Comp. Physiol. Psychol.* **50,** 279–281.

Smith J. B. and Clark F. C. (1975) Effects of *d*-amphetamine, chlorpromazine, and chlordiazepoxide on intercurrent behavior during spaced-responding schedules. *J. Exp. Anal. Behav.* **24,** 241–248.

Spealman R. D. (1979) Comparison of drug effects on responding punished by pressurized air or electric shock delivery in squirrel monkeys: Pentobarbital, chlordiazepoxide, *d*-amphetamine and cocaine. *J. Pharmacol. Exp. Ther.* **209,** 309–315.

Steinberg H., Rushton R., and Tinson C. (1961) Modification of the effects of an amphetamine-barbiturate mixture by the past experience of rats. *Nature* **192,** 533–535.

Stitzer M. and McKearney J. W. (1977) Drug effects on fixed-interval responding with pause requirements for food presentation. *J. Exp. Anal. Behav.* **27,** 51–59.

Terrace H. S. (1963) Errorless discrimination learning in the pigeon: Effects of chlorpromazine and imipramine. *Science* **140,** 318–319.

Thompson D. M. (1974) Repeated acquisition of behavioral chains under chronic drug conditions. *J. Pharmacol. Exp. Ther.* **188,** 700–713.

Thompson D. M. (1978) Stimulus Control and Drug Effects, in *Contemporary Research in Behavioral Pharmacology* (Blackman D. E. and Sanger D. J., eds.), Plenum, New York.

Thorndike E. L. (1911) *Animal Intelligence,* Macmillan, New York.

Tye N. C., Iversen S. D., and Green A. R. (1979) The effects of benzodiazepines and serotonergic manipulations on punished responding. *Neuropharmacology* **18,** 689–695.

Urbain C., Poling A., Millam J., and Thompson T. (1978) *d*-Amphetamine and fixed-interval performance: Effects of operant history. *J. Exp. Anal. Behav.* **7,** 333–335.

Walker C. H., Faustman W. O., Fowler S. C., and Kazar D. B. (1981) A multivariate analysis of some operant variables used in behavioral pharmacology. *Psychopharmacology* **74,** 182–186.

Weiss B. and Gott C. T. (1972) A microanalysis of drug effects on fixed-ratio performances in pigeons. *J. Pharmacol. Exp. Ther.* **180,** 189–202.

Wenger G. R. and Dews P. B. (1979) The effects of phencyclidine, ketamine, *d*-amphetamine and pentobarbital on schedule-controlled behavior in the mouse. *J. Pharmacol. Exp. Ther.* **196,** 616–624.

Wentink E. A. (1938) The effects of certain drugs and hormones upon conditioning. *J. Exp. Psychol.* **22,** 150–163.

Wetherington C. L. (1982) Is adjunctive behavior a third class of behavior? *Neurosci. Biobehav. Rev.* **6,** 329–350.

Wilder J. (1967) *Stimulus and Response: The Law of Initial Values,* John Wright, Bristol.

Williams J. L. and White J. M. (1984) The effects of amphetamine and scopolamine on adjunctive drinking and wheel-running in rats. *Psychopharmacology* **82,** 360–367.

Wise R. A. (1982) Neuroleptics and operant behavior: The anhedonia hypothesis. *Behav. Brain Sci.* **5,** 39–87.

Wise R. A., Spindler J., and LeGault L. (1978) Major attenuation of food reward with performance-sparing doses of pimozide in the rat. *Can. J. Psychol.* **32,** 77–85.

Wuttke W. and Kelleher R. T. (1970) Effects of some benzodiazepines on punished and unpunished behavior in the pigeon. *J. Pharmacol. Exp. Ther.* **172,** 397–405.

Behavioral Analysis of Anxiolytic Drug Action

Robert Dantzer

1. Introduction

Among the drugs used clinically for their antianxiety (anxiolytic) properties are to be found a wide variety of chemically heterogeneous compounds, which include, as most prominent classes, benzodiazepines, barbiturates, alcohol, and propanediol derivatives. They are among the most widely used (and sometimes abused) drugs, and within less than 20 yr, they have generated an impressive number of papers and symposia dealing with their chemistry, pharmacology, metabolism, structure–activity relationships, and clinical properties. Because benzodiazepine derivatives are the most commonly prescribed anxiolytics, this chapter will focus principally on their behavioral effects.

The study of mechanisms of action of anxiolytics can be conducted at several levels of analysis. Views on their molecular and cellular mechanisms of action have been profoundly modified by the discovery, in 1977, of brain benzodiazepine receptors and their functional coupling with a GABA-activated chloride channel (Mohler and Okada, 1977; Squires and Braestrup, 1977). Behavioral analyses of anxiolytic effects have been, for the most part, independent of these considerations. They aim at describing the behavioral mechanisms by which drugs alter behavior. The psychopharmacology of antianxiety drugs has mainly been dominated by the attempts to develop animal models for the prediction of anxiolytic drug effects and by the use of behavioral tests to investigate neurochemical mechanisms of drug action. However, their specificity of action on punished responding and the deviation of this effect from the law of rate dependency, have been food for thought for experimental psychologists from very early in the story of these compounds. All the questions concerning their possible mechanisms of action were already expressed in the late sixties (e.g., Margules and Stein, 1967), and more recent work has only resulted in more complexity, by demonstrating that, besides their antipunishment properties, anxiolytics exert a wide range of behavioral effects that cannot always be easily accounted for in terms of reduced anxiety or frustration.

The aim of this chapter is first to describe the main behavioral effects of antianxiety drugs, then to attempt to find out what basic behavioral processes they alter, and, finally, to evaluate the prospects for future studies of antianxiety drugs. The emphasis is mainly methodological, and therefore, no attempt has been made to comprehensively review the literature concerning this subject.

2. Behavioral Effects of Antianxiety Drugs

2.1. Effects of Anxiolytics on Behavior Suppressed by Punishment

The most frequently investigated behavioral action of anxiolytics is their ability to increase response rates suppressed by delivery of response-dependent shocks (punishment). In a typical experiment, rats are trained to press a lever for food according to a variable-interval (VI) schedule, i.e., with a food reward available after variable time intervals since the last reward (*see* chapter by Sanger in this volume for discussion of reinforcement schedules). After stabilization of the response rate under this schedule, a signal tone is presented every 15 min with a 3-min duration. During the tone presentation, the reinforcement schedule is modified in such a way that every response produces a food reward, but also a low-intensity electric shock to the feet of the rat. After a few sessions under this multiple schedule, rats generally respond at a high rate during the VI schedule and stop responding when the tone is turned on. They usually emit only a few responses during the punishment segment of the multiple schedule of food reinforcement and resume responding at their previous rate as soon as the tone is turned off. Pretreatment with anxiolytics reinstates responding suppressed by contingent punishment at doses that have little or no effect on food-reinforced responding, although high doses depress this last class of behavior (Fig. 1).

Since their demonstration by Geller, Seifter, and colleagues (1960; Geller et al., 1962), the antipunishment effects of anxiolytic agents have been observed in a number of species and in a variety of behavioral procedures generating conflict between simultaneous presentation of shock and reward. Similar effects have been described in human volunteers, when monetary loss rather than shock was used to suppress operant behavior (Carlton et al., 1981). Although most studies have used as punishers aversive events that have direct effects on response rates, it has been shown that conditioned punishers, i.e., stimuli previously paired with aversive events, are also able to suppress operant responding. In pigeons working for food under a VI schedule, introduction of a conditioned-punishment contingency, by introducing after each key-peck a visual stimulus, occasionally paired with shock, resulted in response suppression that was released by chlordiazepoxide (Valentine and Barrett, 1981).

Several variations to the original technique have been suggested in order to either decrease time required for training the animals or reduce day-to-day variability in individual performance. The most popular version of the approach–avoidance conflict for fast screening of anxiolytics involves punishment of a consummatory response, licking a drinking tube by water-deprived rats or mice (Vogel et al., 1971). This technique offers the advantage of using naive subjects in a one session test. However, it is much less specific than punishment of lever-pressing since suppressed drinking is reinstated by such drugs as anticholinergic agents or phosphodiesterase

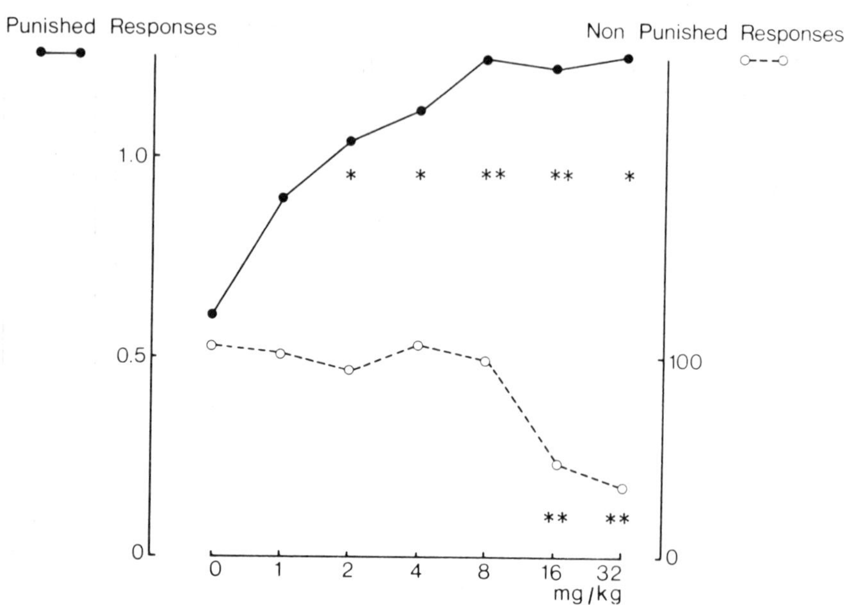

Fig. 1. Effects of benzodiazapine—clorazepate—on punished and unpunished behavior in a multiple schedule of food reinforcement. Rats ($n = 6$) were conditioned to respond on a variable-interval schedule (VI 30 sec), interrupted by two 2-min periods signaled by a light above the lever, during which every third response was simultaneously reinforced by a food pellet and punished by a weak electric shock. Clorazepate was injected intraperitoneally at various doses 30 min before the session in well-trained animals, each subject serving as its own control. Solid line indicates effects on punished responses (after logarithmic transformation), broken line indicates effects on nonpunished responses (expressed as ratio of response rate after this treatment to preceding control response rate). Note that clorazepate at doses as low as 2 mg/kg increased significantly ($* p < 0.05$, $** p < 0.01$) the number of punished responses without altering nonpunished responding, whereas higher doses disrupted nonpunished responding.

inhibitors (Bignami, 1976; Beer et al., 1972). The reasons for this difference are unclear, and there has been little systematic attempt to study the influence of procedural parameters on the effect of anxiolytics on shock-induced suppression of drinking. It must be noted, however, that a chronic version of the technique has been developed (Kilts et al., 1981), and that it compares favorably to the Geller-Seifter technique in terms of sensitivity and specificity.

Large inter-individual differences in the response of animals to anxiolytics in the Geller-Seifter conflict test have been found by several authors, but have not been given systematic attention. In a recent study, Babbini et al., (1982) observed that 20% of rats were insensitive to the anticonflict effects of the benzodiazepine derivative oxazepam. In the other rats, the responsiveness to oxazepam was inversely related to the shock intensities given during training and positively related to the day-to-day spontaneous variation in the absence of drug. It therefore appears that sensitivity of punished responding to anxiolytics covaries with its sensitivity to nonpharmacological factors. This intrinsic variability is not always looked for by pharmacologists who would prefer stabilized performance under standard conditions. As a matter of fact, a major problem with the use of the Geller-Seifter technique is the calibration of the electric shock used for punishment: High intensities of shock produce a total suppression during the conflict portion of the multiple schedule, and this dramatic change in responding is not altered by pretreatment with anxiolytics. In contrast, low intensities of shock can be the source of large day-to-day fluctuations in punished response rate. The usual way to circumvent this problem is to increase the number of responses during the conflict segment of the multiple schedule by using a fixed-ratio schedule (FR) (Cook and Davidson, 1973) or an incremental shock (Pollard and Howard, 1979). Another possibility for increasing the sensitivity of the techhnique is to omit shock during the drug test, although the drug treatment may become a cue for the absence of shock.

The exact factors that are responsible for the sensitivity of punished responding to anxiolytics are not known. Negative evidence is better established than positive evidence. It has been demonstrated that the release of punished responding cannot be accounted for by a deficit in learning and memory, an increase in food motivation, a reduced sensitivity to electric shocks, or general stimulant effects (McMillan, 1975; Miczek, 1973). The reliability of the effects of benzodiazepines on behavior suppressed by contingent punishment contrasts with the inconsistency of their effects on behavior suppressed by response-independent shocks. In the conditioned emotional response procedure, rats trained to press a lever for food are presented with a warning signal followed by an inescapable electric shock. This procedure leads to suppression of responding during the presentation of the signal. Direct comparison of both paradigms is difficult since response-dependent shock is usually more effective in suppressing behavior than response-independent shock. The higher sensitivity of conflict techniques to anxiolytics may therefore simply be a result of rate-dependent effects. According to this interpretation, anxiolytics are more effective on behavioral suppression induced by contingent shock than on behavioral suppression induced by noncontingent shock, just because response rates are lower in the former case (Sanger and Blackman, 1981). In a recent study, Rawlins et al. (1980) varied shock intensity between groups of rats exposed either to response-dependent or response-independent shock in order to ensure a similar degree of suppression for each mode of shock presentation. Chlordiazepoxide increased response rates in both groups to the same extent. In contrast, when shock intensity was held constant, resulting in a more marked behavioral suppression in rats receiving response-dependent shock, chlordiazepoxide was more effective in this latter group. Such data would dismiss the intervention of punishment contingency as a critical variable in the effect of anxiolytics and support a rate-dependency interpretation.

This possibility was reexamined by Hymowitz and Abramson (1983), using a within-subject rather than a between-subject design. Rats trained on a VI schedule of food reinforcement were exposed alternately to FI (response-dependent) or fixed time (response-independent) schedules of shock delivery, with various intensities of shock. Diazepam reliably increased responding suppressed by response-dependent shock and did so in a rate-dependent manner. In contrast, the effects of diazepam on rates of responding during response-independent shock delivery were inconsistent, since only half the animals responded positively to the drug treatment, in spite of a similar degree of behavioral suppression for response-dependent and response-independent shock in all animals.

Although contradictory, the results of these studies suggest that contingency and rate dependency are not critical in the effects of anxiolytics on behaviors suppressed by events. Experiments comparing the effectiveness of various procedural factors (shock intensity and food deprivation levels) with the effects of diazepam on behavior suppressed by signaled and unsignaled shock (Hymowitz, 1981) may give some clue to this issue. Behavioral suppression induced by either procedure was found to be more susceptible to experimental manipulations and diazepam treatment than behavioral suppression during the signal preceding the shock (conditioned suppression). This is another example of the relative insensitivity of behavior under strong stimulus control to the disruptive effects of anxiolytics.

2.2. *Effects of Anxiolytics on Behavior Suppressed by Nonreward*

Withdrawal or omission of an expected reward is another effective way of suppressing previously rewarded behavior. When reward presentations are discontinued in rats conditioned to respond for food, the animals usually stop responding within a few minutes (extinction). Antianxiety agents increase resistance to extinction (Dantzer, 1977a; Gray, 1977), suggesting that the omission of an expected reward is aversive, and that frustration reactions elicited by this event share properties in common with reactions elicited by other aversive agents, such as punishment. On this basis, antianxiety agents have been claimed to have antifrustration effects, in addition to their antipunishment effects. There are some cases, however, in which behavior suppressed by extinction is not reinstated by anxiolytics. For example, when reinforcement was withdrawn during a short period of time, signaled by an appropriate exteroceptive stimulus (timeout procedure), diazepam increased the number of nonreinforced responses during the first presentations of the signal when extinction was not yet well acquired. However, when animals stopped responding during the timeout signal, diazepam was no longer effective (Dantzer, 1977a). This maybe another example of the importance of stimulus control in the effects of anxiolytics on suppressed behavior.

Disruption of behavior by nonreward is less marked in animals that have experienced partial reinforcement during acquisition than in animals that have been reinforced after each response (partial-reinforcement effect). According to the frustration theory (Amsel, 1962), animals that have been exposed to partial reinforcement during acquisition have already experienced conditioned frustration reactions. They should, therefore, be more tolerant to frustration induced by extinction. As a matter of fact, antianxiety agents given during acquisition disrupt the development of tolerance to extinction because of partial reward (Gray, 1977; Wilner and Crowe, 1977).

Shifts from a large to a small reward may also depress performance, in comparison to animals that have experienced only the small reward (negative-contrast effects). Antianxiety agents block this phenomenon, although this effect is more complex than was originally thought. Chlordiazepoxide was able to reduce negative-contrast effects of a shift from 32 to 4% sucrose on speed of running in a runway or on licking rates (Rosen and Tessel, 1970; Vogel and Principi, 1971). But, when chlordiazepoxide was administered during both preshift experience with 32% sucrose and postshift experience with 4% sucrose, it was not effective (Flaherty et al., 1980). In addition, chlordiazepoxide administered during postshift experience was effective in eliminating contrast only if it was given on the second session of presentation of 4% sucrose, but not on the first session. This was not a state-dependent effect since chlordiazepoxide was not effective when injected during the preshift period. Flaherty et al. proposed that in these experiments chlordiazepoxide was effective because it produced disinhibition, in the Pavlovian sense. That is, presentation of a novel stimulus (a tone or, in this case, the internal sensations resulting from the drug treatment) may attenuate response suppression caused by negative contrast (for a fuller definition of disinhibition, *see* Mackintosh, 1974, pp. 15–16).

2.3. *Other Behavioral Effects of Anxiolytics*

Anxiolytics tend to increase overall response rates in schedules that maintain low rates of responding because of a negative contingency, in the form of a decrease in the number of reinforcements if response rates exceed a given value (differential reinforcement of low rates: DRL) (Sanger and Blackman, 1981). The same effect has been observed when responses emitted toward the stimulus preceding a food reward prevents the delivery of food (negative automaintenance) (Poling and Appel, 1979).

Another characteristic effect of anxiolytics is their ability to reduce the inhibitory effects of novelty on locomotor activity or consummatory behavior (Poschel, 1971; Soubrié et al., 1976). In the same manner, these compounds increase the number of transitions between a darkened compartment and an illuminated compartment in a two-compartment cage (Crawley, 1981), as well as the amount of social interaction occurring between two rats when placed in a novel and brightly lit arena (File, 1980).

Acquisition of a conditioned avoidance response can be facilitated by acute or chronic treatment with low doses of benzodiazepines in poor learners, whereas avoidance behavior tends to be depressed by high doses of benzodiazepines in well-trained animals (Dantzer, 1977b).

Anxiolytics have characteristic discriminative-stimulus properties that can be best demonstrated in a free operant procedure, in which animals have the choice between two levers, one of which is reinforced in the presence of the drug, the other being reinforced in the presence of the vehicle or another drug. With this procedure, it can be shown that anxiolytics produce an internal stimulus state that can be perceived and discriminated from the normal physiological state (Fig. 2). This technique offers the advantage of being very specific since animals trained with an anxiolytic generalize only to other anxiolytics (Colpaert et al., 1976). Animals can

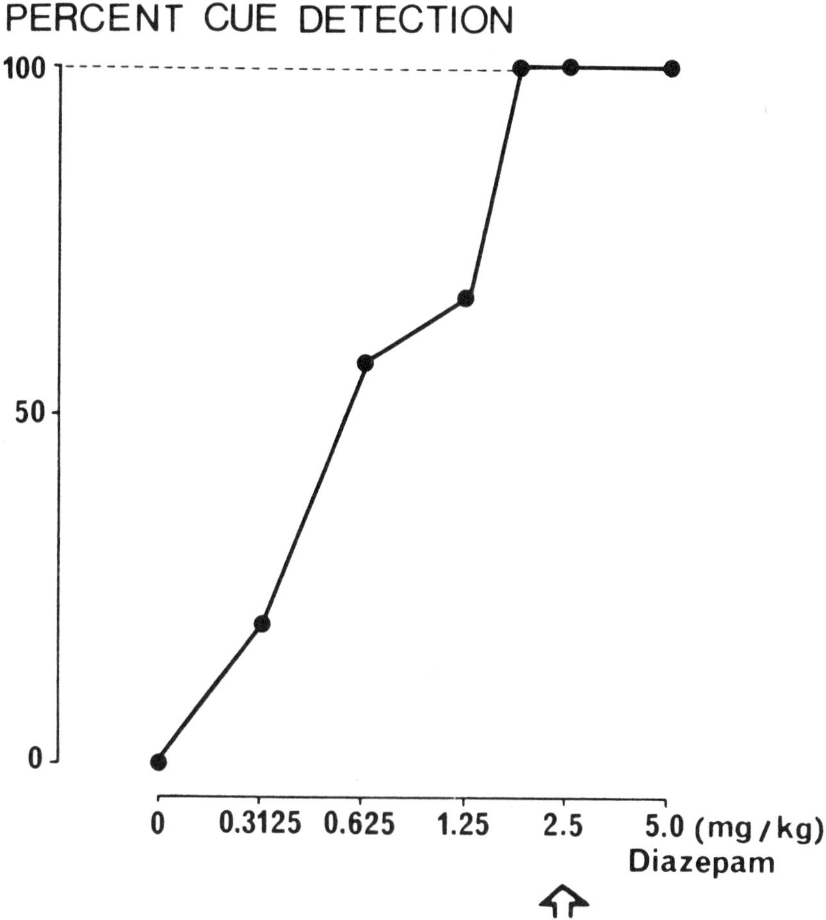

Fig. 2. Diazepam dose–response relationship for rats ($n = 6$) trained to discriminate between saline and 2.5 mg/kg diazepam. The ordinate represents the number of rats (expressed as percent) that selected the diazepam lever in a generalization test during which both levers were reinforced.

even be trained to discriminate between two anxiolytics, such as pentobarbital and chlordiazepoxide (Barry and Krimmer, 1978). In addition, anxiolytics are able to block, in a dose-dependent manner, the discriminative stimulus properties of such stimulants as bemegride and pentylenetetrazol (Shearman and Lal, 1979; also *see* chapter by Järbe in this volume for further discussion of drug discrimination learning).

2.4. Conclusion

In summary, antianxiety drugs reduce behavior-suppressing effects of punishment, nonreward, and novelty; these effects are pharmacologically specific in the sense that they are not induced by other classes of psychotropic drugs. Although not explicitly mentioned in the previously reported data, it must be noted that doses and number of administrations are important variables in the effects of anxiolytics on behavior. In general, sedative and myorelaxant effects are more pronounced at high doses and on acute treatment, so that they may interfere critically with motor performance. Chronic dosage results in a reduction of these effects and a potentiation of the disinhibiting effects on suppressed responding.

From a practical point of view, an important aspect of anxiolytic activity is its pharmacological specificity, since behavioral tests are often used to predict the anxiolytic profile of new compounds. For example, after the discovery of benzodiazepine receptors, a search was initiated for possible endogenous ligands. This search resulted in the isolation of purine derivatives among other putative ligands, one of which was inosine. This compound was described as a benzodiazepine agonist in anticonvulsant tests, but as a benzodiazepine antagonist in an exploration test (Crawley, 1981). However, none of these tests is very specific. Therefore, the effect of inosine in the approach–avoidance conflict test and in animals trained to discriminate a benzodiazepine derivative–clorazepate–from saline, was investigated. In all these tests, inosine displayed little intrinsic activity and neither potentiated nor antagonized the effects of clorazepate (Fig. 3), suggesting that the results described above were related to side

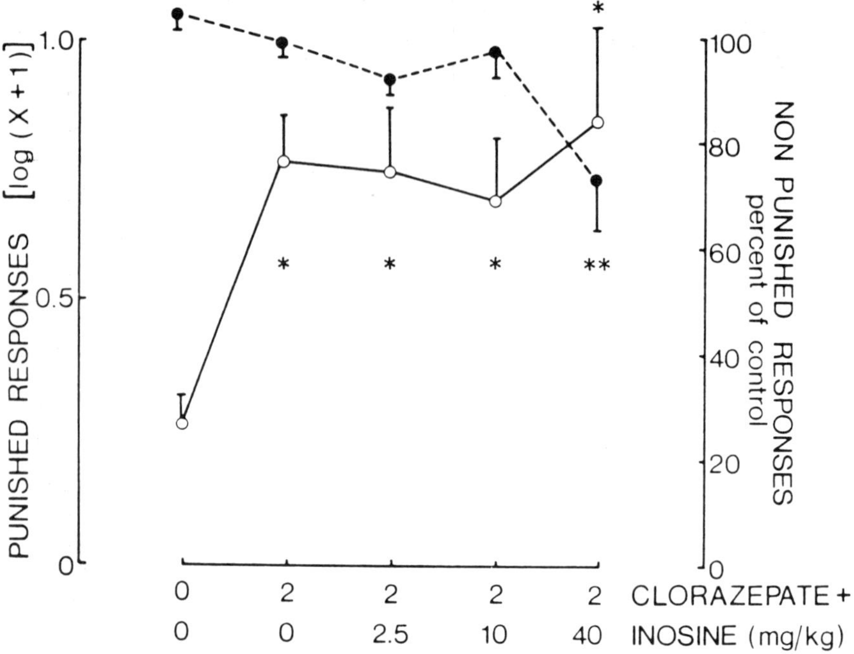

Fig. 3. Absence of interaction between inosine and clorazepate on punished responding. Ten rats, well trained in an approach–avoidance conflict similar to the one described in Fig. 1., were given various combinations of clorazepate (30 min before test) and inosine (10 min before test). Inosine did not modify the effects of clorazepate, except at the higher dose, at which a significant decrease in the number of nonpunished responses was noted.

effects of this compound (Perio, 1983). In the same manner, Ro 15-1788, a compound claimed to have specific antagonist properties, was found to behave like an agonist in the clorazepate-discrimination test (Dantzer and Perio, 1982). This is a very important issue since most of the speculations on new anxiolytic compounds or possible endogenous ligands to the benzodiazepine receptors rely only on crude behavioral tests.

3. Interpretation of the Behavioral Effects of Anxiolytics

3.1. Correlational Approach

During the last two decades, there have been many attempts to construct theoretical models of the behavioral effects of anxiolytics. The interest of pharmacologists for the study of drug effects on conflict behavior grew from the observation that the drug-induced release of behavior suppressed by punishment was not only most prominent with antianxiety drugs, but also positively correlated with their clinical potency. There is a positive correlation amounting to 0.7–0.8 between the minimum effective doses in a rat conflict test and the average daily dose for humans (Cook and Davidson, 1973). The close relationship between the effects of anxiolytics and their clinical activity was further substantiated by the results of chronic treatment. With repeated treatment, the releasing effect of benzodiazepines on behavior suppressed by contingent punishment increased and their depressant effect on nonpunished responding decreased, in a similar way to the development of anxiolytic activity and the attenuation of sedation under chronic treatment in humans (Cook and Sepinwall, 1975; Margules and Stein, 1968). On the basis of such empirical correlations, the approach–avoidance conflict procedure readily became the prototype animal model for the study of anxiety, and there was only a small step to the inference that anxiolytic drugs are effective in this procedure because they make the animals less anxious. The implicit assumption is that aversive stimuli control behavior by generating a state of fear and anxiety, and that this motivational state is altered by anxiolytics. The same analysis has been applied to nonreward, which has been equated to punishment, and also to novelty and uncertainty (Fig. 4).

The problem with this way of reasoning is that it is circular. At the origin, anxiolytics have been defined as such because of their clinical activity, not because of their behavioral effects in animals. As pointed out by Carlton (1978), if we accept that the drugs in question can be meaningfully called anxiolytics, then we are likely to accept the idea that the behavior they modify has some relevance to anxiety.

A recent logical extension of this attitude has been the inference of anxiogenic properties from the observation of increased suppressed behavior in animal tests sensitive to anxiolytics. For example, β-carbolines with a strong affinity for benzodiazepine receptors have been claimed to trigger anxiety when injected into humans. These compounds enhanced shock-induced suppressed drinking (Corda et al., 1983) and lever-pressing (De Carvalho et al., 1983; Rommelspacher et al., 1982), and this effect was antagonized by diazepam and a benzodiazepine antagonist Ro 15-1788.

The weakness of these logical constructions become apparent when effects of benzodiazepines that bear little or no relation to anxiety are considered. In the case of the effects of benzodiazepines on feeding behavior, for example, there is evidence that emotionality is not a necessary condition for the facilitation of the feeding response observed in benzodiazepine-treated rats (Cooper, 1980). As a matter of fact, low doses of chlordiazepoxide increase consumption of familiar food, and this effect is not altered by handling the subjects prior to the experiment or by administering electric shocks. Benzodiazepines may therefore enhance appetite for food by relatively direct means, and specific screening for this pharmacological activity has led to the development of highly effective food-intake stimulants (Baile and McLaughlin, 1979; also *see* chapter by Cooper and Turkish in this volume for further discussion).

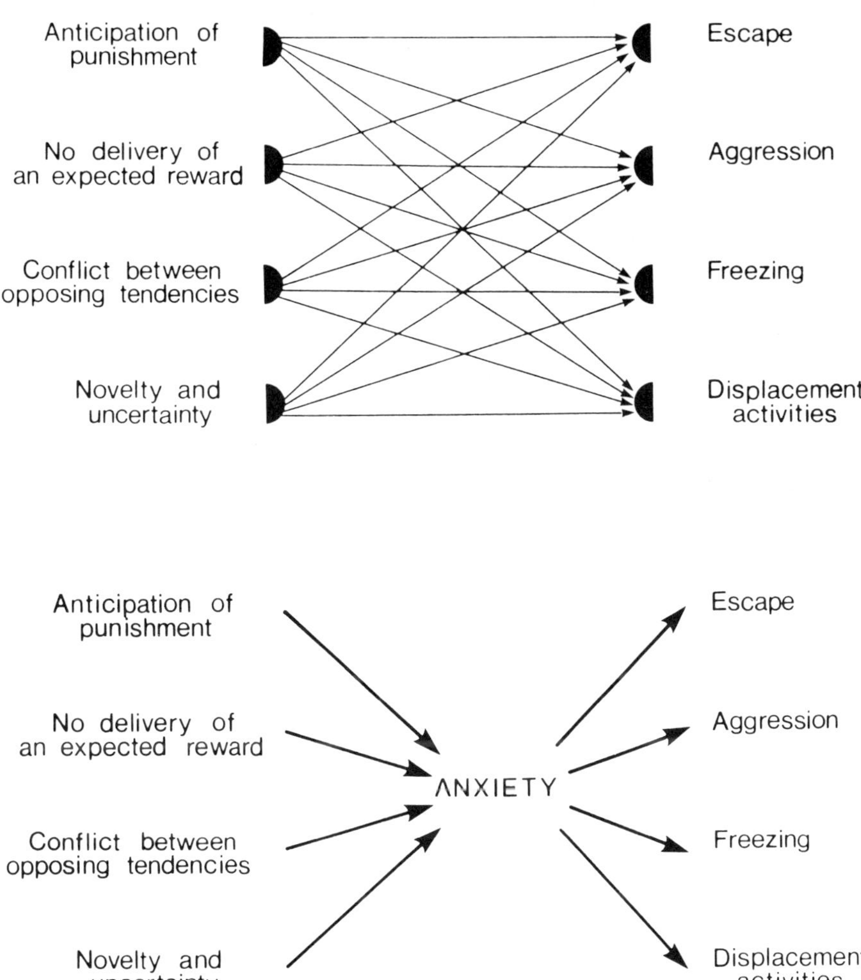

Fig. 4. Motivational analysis of the behavioral effects of antianxiety drugs. Anxiety is conceived of as a common central state, elicited by several situations and giving rise to several responses. The postulation of this motivational state offers the advantage of simplifying the analysis of the relationships between eliciting stimuli and the variety of behavioral reactions that they induce.

3.2. Dissociation Between Effects of Anxiolytics on Behavior Suppressed by, and Behavior Facilitated by, Presentation of Aversive Stimuli

To understand the effects of antianxiety agents on behavior, it may be useful to temporarily forget about their possible anxiolytic activities (which is not the same as denying them) and to attempt to determine the critical factors underlying their activity. Evidence supporting interference of benzodiazepines with responding suppressed by presentation of aversive stimuli has already been considered. However, under certain conditions, aversive stimuli may energize, rather than suppress, behavior. Typical examples are the increase in response force during extinction or facilitation of avoidance produced by presentation of a fear signal, i.e., a signal previously paired with unavoidable electric shocks (conditioned acceleration). If antianxiety agents act at the motivational level, they should decrease both response suppression and response facilitation induced by aversive stimuli. This is not the case. Antianxiety agents do not disrupt conditioned acceleration (Chisholm and Moore, 1970; Dantzer and Mormède, 1976; Dantzer et al., 1976; Morris et al., 1980). Moreover, when diazepam was administered, both before the pairing of the fear signal with unavoidable electric shock and before the test session to control for possible state-dependent effects, this treatment tended to increase conditioned acceleration (Dantzer et al., 1976) (Fig. 5). In the same way, the increase in response force observed during initial exposure to extinction in animals trained to press a lever for a food reward was not reduced by chlordiazepoxide (Fowler, 1974). In another series of experiments, diazepam was administered to pigs trained to get food by pushing a panel with their snout and submitted to extinction by pairs under two conditions, either with access to the response panel and the food trough or without access because of a solid partition. When confronted with another animal during extinction, pigs displayed instances of agonistic behavior interspersed with attempts to reach the panel and the food bowl when these objects were still attainable. In this last case, diazepam-

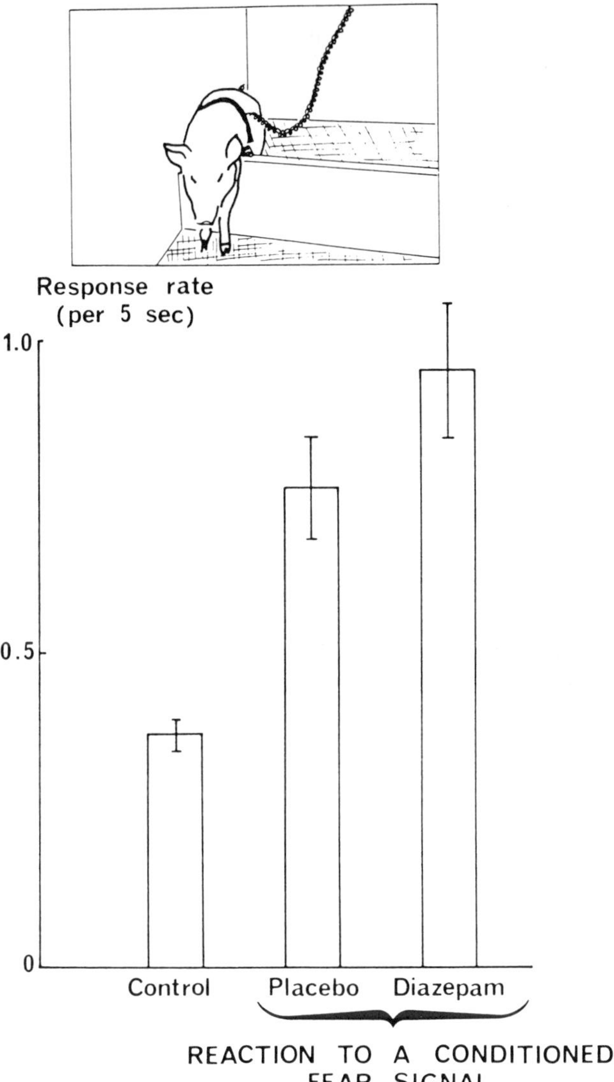

Fig. 5. Effects of diazepam on conditional acceleration of responding produced by presentation of a fear signal. Pigs trained on a continuous avoidance procedure in a shuttle box were submitted to a fear-conditioning procedure during which a neutral tone was repeatedly paired with inescapable electric shock. The next day, they were put back in the shuttle box, and the fear signal was presented without shock 10 times for 5 s. Presentation of the fear signal induced a facilitation of avoidance responding that was increased by diazepam. Each result is the mean performance of 4 pigs.

treated animals spent more time trying to push the panel and reach the trough and fought less than placebo-treated animals. When the cues associated with food were no longer available, fighting was more intense in diazepam-treated animals than in placebo-treated pigs (Arnone and Dantzer, 1980) (Fig. 6). These results show that diazepam decreases or enhances agonistic behavior according to environmental conditions, and that the drug has no generalized antiaggressive or antifrustrative properties.

On the basis of these findings, it has been suggested that most of the behavioral changes induced by antianxiety agents may be regarded as manifestations of a response-persistence effect (Dantzer, 1977b, 1978). A typical example of this response-persistence effect can be found in the changes in response rate observed after a scheduled shock in animals responding on a Sidman avoidance schedule (Dantzer, 1977c). Although normal animals temporarily increase their response rate and return rapidly to their baseline levels, this reaction is amplified and lasts much longer in diazepam-treated animals.

3.3. Respective Role of Response-Independent and Response-Dependent Cues in the Behavioral Effect of Anxiolytics

Response persistence may be produced by several different means. To drive through a red light is a good example. Besides not noticing the red light, one may do so either because one is unable to associate the way of behaving with its possible consequences (e.g., a road accident or a heavy fine) or because one no longer understands the significance of a red light. Antianxiety agents disrupt successive-discrimination learning and performance, but not simultaneous discrimination. However, many of the studies on successive discrimination have used go/no-go procedures that are learned by avoiding particular stimuli so that they can be disrupted if the passive avoidance tendency is altered by the drug treatment. This is the case with anxiolytics that selectively disinhibit no-go responses. The importance of this effect may be decreased by using a successive-conditional discrimi-

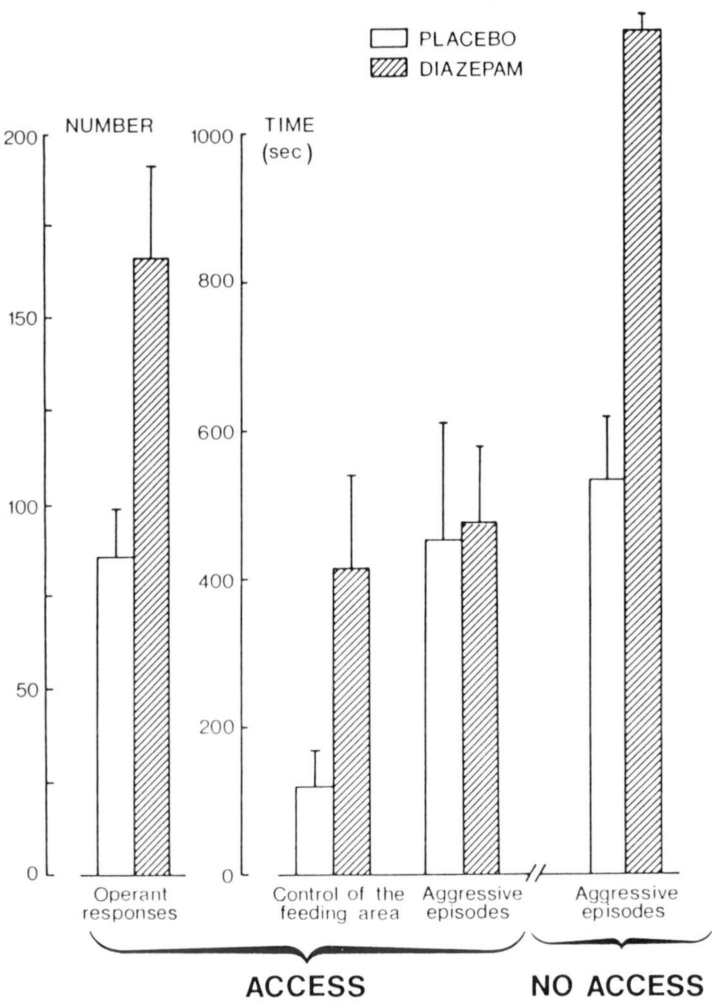

Fig. 6. Effects of diazepam on extinction-induced aggression. Pigs were trained to press a panel with their snout to get food in an operant conditioning chamber. They were then submitted by pairs to extinction with or without access to the response panel and feeding area. When access was permitted, diazepam (1–2 mg/kg) increased the number of operant responses emitted by both animals and the time spent controlling the feeding area, but did not modify aggression (controls = 6 pairs, diazepam = 10 pairs). When access was not permitted, diazepam increased the severity of aggression observed between the animals (controls = 4 pairs, diazepam = 4 pairs).

nation task in which animals have to respond on the appropriate panel among two panels available when presented with one of two discriminative stimuli. Diazepam did not disrupt performance in a successive-conditional discrimination task (Fig. 7), suggesting that anxiolytics do not directly affect discriminative abilities.

Tye et al. (1977) used another type of conditional discrimination task contingent upon the completion of an FI schedule of responding to investigate the respective role of response and sensory factors in the effects of benzodiazepines on discrimination. Briefly, pigeons were trained to peck a center key illuminated with white light on an FI schedule in order to produce a colored light on this key. They had to then shift responding to one of two lateral keys according to the color projected on the center key. Pretreatment with low doses of chlordiazepoxide or flurazepam did not affect discrimination, i.e., pigeons still selected the correct key. However, center key perseveration increased in a monotonic manner with increasing doses of both drugs.

The absence of critical effects of anxiolytics on recognition memory (i.e., decision based on the past perception of a stimulus) has been assessed more directly, using a delayed-matching-to-sample test in which a sample stimulus is presented, followed by a delay interval, followed in turn by the presentation of a number of stimuli, one of which is the same as the one already presented; this last stimulus has to be selected by the subject in order to be rewarded. Chlordiazepoxide did not disrupt performance of monkeys in this test, even at high doses (Sahgal and Iversen, 1980). In addition, studies in humans have shown that diazepam impairs memory by interfering with acquisition of new information, but leaves retrieval processes intact (Ghoneim et al., 1981).

The idea that antianxiety drugs preferentially impair the processing of response-associated cues suggests a reinterpretation of the already described dissociation between effects of these drugs on contingent and noncontingent shock. When shock is delivered following responding, the subject has to rely more on response consequences to modify ongoing

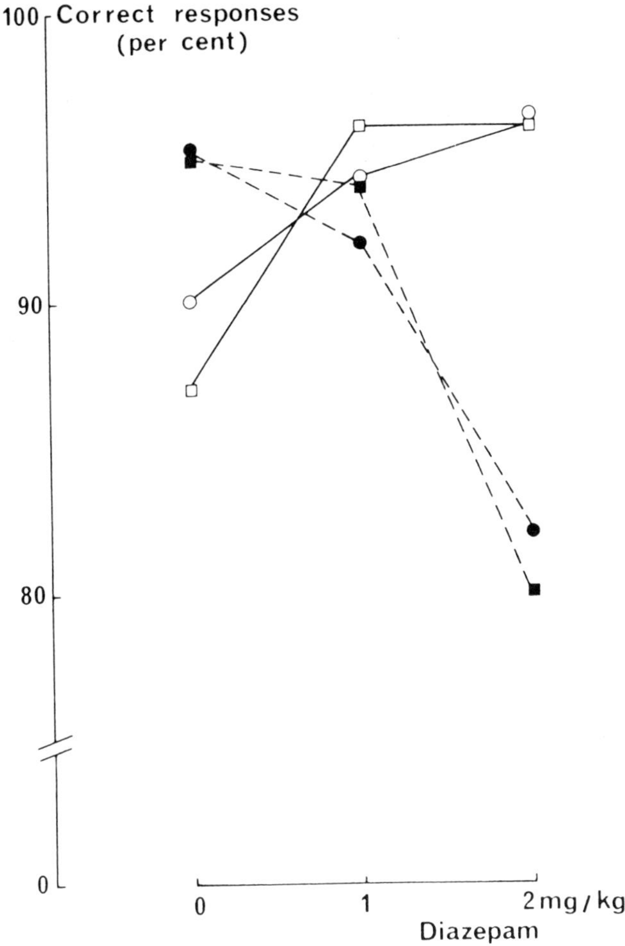

Fig. 7. Effects of diazepam on successive conditional discrimination. Four pigs were trained to get food by pushing a panel with their snout. When presented with one of two auditory discriminative stimuli, they had to push the appropriate panel among two panels available to obtain food. An incorrect response was followed by a timeout period. Once stabilized in this procedure, they were injected with 1 or 2 mg/kg diazepam. Each curve represents the performance of one animal after placebo or diazepam. Diazepam improved performance of two pigs that had reached less than 90% correct discrimination level (solid lines), but decreased at the higher dose the number of correct responses emitted by good performers.

behavior than when shock is scheduled independently of responding. In the latter case, the subject tends to rely mainly on exteroceptive cues provided by the environment (including the time interval since the last shock). According to this interpretation, the effects of anxiolytics should decrease in cases in which stimulus control is important. We have already described evidence favoring this view. However, more direct investigation of the hypothesis is still needed, and could, for example, involve the incorporation of additional exteroceptive cues during punishment or nonreward when investigating the behavioral action of anxiolytics.

Several variants of this interpretation have been proposed recently. In a very elegant synthesis of the psychopharmacology of anxiolytics, neurobiology of the septohippocampal system and clinically defined anxiety disorders, Gray (1982) proposed that anxiolytics disrupt the normal functioning of the septohippocampal system. The primary task of this system is to compare actual with expected stimuli and, in case of mismatch, to activate a whole sequence of behavioral changes enabling analysis of the relevant stimuli over many dimensions. Within this theoretical framework, anxiolytics act on the subcomponents of the system that have for their role the identification of certain stimuli that are particularly important, i.e., requiring careful checking. However, as pointed out by Morris and Gebhart (1981), who used an information processing model to analyze the behavioral effects of anxiolytics, these drugs have some effects on processes involved in recognition of stimuli, but they exert much more potent effects on processes involved in response suppression. More specifically, the response-suppression system is viewed as a neural system that maintains the representation of the correlations between behavior and aversive events. Moreover, by operation of this system, the behavior itself, under appropriate stimulus conditions, becomes the retrieval cue for the memory of past events to which it is correlated. Anxiolytics induce response disinhibition by interfering with this process, and this is apparently the predominant way by which they reduce clinical anxiety (Dantzer, 1978; Morris and Gebhart, 1981) (Fig. 8).

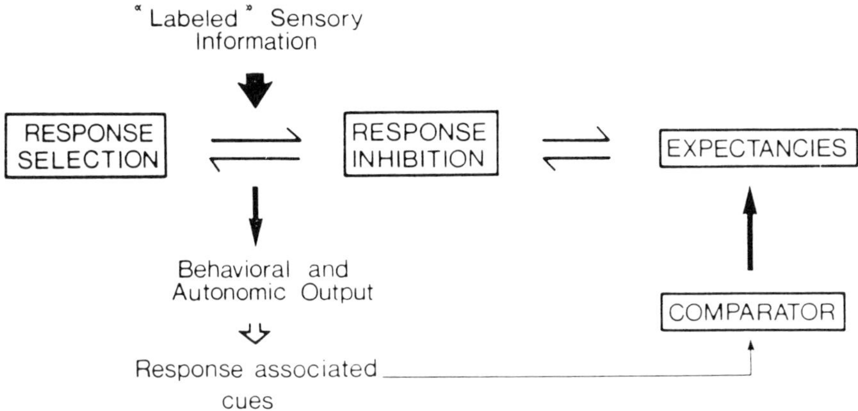

Fig. 8. Schematic representation of processes affected by antianxiety agents. Inferred processes are written into boxes, and words in lower case refer to real world phenomena. Antianxiety agents can impair the acquisition of associations between environmental stimuli and aversive events and therefore alter the affective meaning attributed later to such stimuli. However, in the presence of sensory information already familiar, predominant effects are exercised at the level of response modulatory processes: Antianxiety agents facilitate selection of the prepotent response because of environmental stimuli and the subject's history, and interfere with processes allowing comparison of predictions with the actual result of responding. This results in dissociation of ongoing behavior from its external consequences or its motivational value normally associated with its execution.

4. Prospects for Improving the Behavioral Study of Antianxiety Drugs

4.1. Multiplicity of Behavioral Responses

Much of the literature described in this chapter has been generated by methodological strategies adapted from experimental psychology: Arbitrary responses are selected in the repertoire of animals and associated with arbitrary external consequences in a strictly controlled environment. Behavioral analysis focuses on the factors assumed to be most relevant to behavior change. By doing so, investigators not only neglect other classes of behavior occurring in the situation and having no observable consequences, but they also lose the possibility of extrapolating the results to more natural situations. Understanding of behavioral effects of anxiolytics may be improved by recourse to methodological strategies, putting more emphasis on the multiplicity of response alternatives produced by a given situation, and/or adopting a more natural approach to behavior.

Even in a very simplified situation, such as a Skinner box, many activities are occurring besides the operant selected for reinforcement. In time-interval schedules, for example, terminal activities occurring before the end of the interval and directed toward cues associated with food delivery are reliably preceded by adjunctive behavior (e.g., in pigeons, wing flapping, orienting toward the opposite wall to the food hopper) occurring earlier in the interval, the nature of which varies from subject to subject (Staddon and Simmelhag, 1971). Since adjunctive behavior is generally incompatible with the terminal response, drug effects on the former class of behavior may indirectly alter responding.

Adjunctive behavior can be monitored if, as a result of the arrangement of the environment, there is an opportunity for this behavior to be directed. An example of such adjunctive behavior is schedule-induced polydipsia, which typically develops when water is freely available while rats are lever-pressing for food on an interval schedule. Administration of benzodiazepines tends to facilitate the development of schedule-induced polydipsia, and this effect is more readily apparent when volumes of water intake, rather than rates of licking, are considered (Sanger and Blackman, 1976). The study of schedule-induced behavior represents, however, a rather narrow approach to the issue of the alternation between multiple activities in natural or seminatural environments (*see* chapter by Sanger in this volume for further discussion of drug effects on schedule-induced behavior).

4.2. Seminatural or Natural Environments

Selection of the response to be punished or reinforced has proceeded quite arbitrarily, on the basis of convenience and available equipment. By studying the occurrence of different activities in hamsters put in a relatively large enclosure, Shettleworth (1978) was able to show that all activities are not susceptible to the same extent to punishment and food reward. Scrabbling, i.e., scraping against the wall with forepaws, was readily susceptible to reinforcement and punishment. However, open rearing could be successfully reinforced with food, but was less suppressed by electric shock. Face-washing displayed the opposite pattern of susceptibility. The implicit idea is that some associations are more easily formed than others or, more generally, that there are constraints on learning that differ from species to species (Hinde and Stevenson-Hinde, 1973). Besides the already noted distinction in sensitivity of consummatory responses and leverpressing to the suppressing effects of punishment and release by anxiolytics, this issue has received little attention in the study of behavioral effects of these compounds, in spite of the fact that it is well known that fear is more easily aroused by certain stimuli than by others.

In an attempt to use more natural situations to assess antianxiety effects of drugs, Treit et al. (1981) suggested that the conditioned defensive-burying paradigm is a better model to study behavior of rats toward objects associated with aversive stimuli than more traditional aversive learning tasks. They found that rats shocked once through a prod mounted on the wall of the test chamber returned to the prod and buried it with bedding material from the floor of the chamber. Rats injected with diazepam displayed less defensive burying, but this effect disappeared when strong intensities of shock were delivered through the prod. This contrasted with neuroleptics that were still active even at high intensities of shock.

Another important characteristic of natural behavior is its sequencing. Feeding behavior, for instance, involves several components, including searching, identifying, procuring, and handling of food before consumption. In the laboratory, only the last element of the chain, consumption, is usually taken into account, in spite of the fact that a consideration of the sequencing of behavioral activities may help to understand how drugs modify behavior. For example, in a study of the effects of diazepam on agonistic behavior of pairs of pigs brought together in a neutral pen, it was found that drug-treated animals fought more. This was related to the fact that they were persevering in the mutual pattern of attack from one animal and submission of the other animal, as if the signals of submissiveness displayed by the subordinate were less effective to alter the behavior of the dominant animal (Arnone, 1979).

In a natural environment, animals rarely live alone, but interact actively with conspecifics. An interesting result of the studies on interactions between members of a group is that drug effects depend on the social status of the treated animal. In a monkey colony, treating the dominant animal with chlordiazepoxide increased agonistic interactions before a period of competitive feeding as a result of challenging by subdominant subjects. In contrast, administration of chlordiazepoxide to the lowest-ranking monkey had no noticeable effect (Apfelbach and Delgado, 1974; Lovell et al., 1980). Agonistic behavior may be divided into defense and offense according to the topography of agonistic acts and postures and the targets for bites (*see* chapter by Miczek and Winslow in this volume). In general, anxiolytics appear to increase attack and threat by the dominant at low doses, whereas high doses disrupt these patterns (Miczek and Krsiak, 1979). Antianxiety agents also decrease reactions of defense and flight, and it is possible that effects on attack and defense combine together to account for the enhanced aggression in the paired encounter test noted above. In a recent study, using the colony intruder paradigm in which an animal introduced into a colony is normally the object of intense physical attack from resident males, chronic treatment with chlordiazepoxide of an animal before its introduction into the colony resulted in diminished aggression from the resident, despite the fact that the intruder submitted less and initiated more interactions with residents (File, 1982). These effects may be a result of a decreased tendency of the intruder to display submissive behavior, but they may also be indirect because of altered stimulus properties of the treated animal. For example, Dixon (1983) observed that diazepam increased aggression toward a treated animal placed into the cage of a male resident mouse. However, this effect was the result of changes in the odor of treated animals, since applying urine from drugged animals on the fur of nondrugged animals placed into the cage of a resident resulted in enhanced attack by the resident. Further work is clearly needed in this area to find out at what level antianxiety drugs are acting (*see* also chapter by Miczek and Winslow in this volume).

4.3. Subjective Experiences of Animals

Another potential approach to the study of antianxiety drugs relies on the assessment of subjective experiences in animals. Among others, an experiment by Beninger et al. (1974) shows that appropriate techniques may be devised to investigate subjective experiences in animals. These authors trained rats to press one of four levers in a multiple-response environment, depending on which behavior they were engaged in at the time when a buzzer sounded. If the rat were rearing up on its hind feet when the buzzer was sounded, it had to press one lever, which can be referred to as the "rearing" lever, in order to get a food pellet. None of the other levers yielded food under these circumstances. Rats learned to press different levers depending on whether they were locomoting, rearing up, face-washing, or remaining still. Although it might be argued that it would be difficult to train rats to press a particular lever when they are anxious, this technique is potentially a very powerful tool for assessing internal representations of behavior.

Animals can also be trained to press a lever according to the presence or absence of a drug, and this technique offers a way of investigating the subjective sensations produced by a drug. However, drug-discrimination techniques have mainly served pharmacological purposes, e.g., delimiting classes of drugs giving rise to the same cues and elucidating their cellular and molecular mechanisms of action (*see* chapter by Järbe in this volume). In can be speculated that animals made anxious or fearful by appropriate means should be more able to discriminate antianxiety agents and, more importantly, that discrimination should not necessarily be based on the same qualitative cues as those used by normal animals. A possible way of dealing with this issue would be the use of animals genetically selected for emotionality (e.g., the Maudsley reactive rat strain) and of animals made anxious by early separation from their mother or peers or by introduction to strangers (Suomi et al., 1981).

5. Conclusion

Within recent years, the discovery of brain benzodiazepine receptors has generated an intense search for endogenous ligands and compounds able to bind differentially to subclasses of benzodiazepine receptors, with the hope of finding new and original tranquilizers. The concomitant search for quick and simple techniques for assessing anxiety in animals has resulted in the resurgence of pseudobehavioral studies deducing anxiety or fear from agitated behavior of restrained animals under the influence of brain stimulation or drug injection. As a typical example, monkeys restrained in chairs were implanted with electrodes aimed at the locus ceruleus or the dorsal ascending noradrenergic bundle. Low-intensity stimulation of these electrodes produced alerting and, with increasing intensity of stimulation, mouth chewing and tongue movements, teeth grinding, grasping of the chair, scratching, self-mouthing, yawning, hair-pulling, hand-wringing, escape struggling, and spasmodic body jerks (Redmond and Huang, 1979). These behaviors were claimed to represent fear, since they were similar to those following direct threatening confrontations by humans or those associated with situations of conflict and uncertainty in open field studies, and that they were enhanced by presentation of signaled, unavoidable electric shocks. In the same manner, the "anxiogenic" properties of the methyl ester of β-carboline were deduced from the agitated behavior and the concomitant increases in plasma stress hormones produced by this compound in rhesus monkeys (Ninan et al., 1982).

Although apparently more elaborate, these ways of assessing anxiety are basically similar to the vicious monkey model that was used to demonstrate the tranquilizing properties of benzodiazepines at the beginning of their story (Heise and Boff, 1961). Hopefully, this paper has been able to show that a behavioral approach has much more to offer to the neurobiology of anxiety than behavioral test tubes.

References

Amsel A. (1962) Frustrative nonreward in partial reinforcement and discrimination learning. *Psychol. Rev.* **69,** 306–328.

Apfelbach R. and Delgado J. M. R. (1974) Social hierarchy in monkeys (*Macaca mulatta*) modified by chlordiazepoxide hydrochloride. *Neuropharmacology* **13,** 11–20.

Arnone M., ed. (1979) *Etude Comportementale et Pharmacologique des Conduites Agressives Chez le Porc. Thése 3e cycle,* Université Paul Sabatier, Toulouse.

Arnone M. and Dantzer R. (1980) Effect of diazepam on extinction-induced aggression in pigs. *Pharmacol. Biochem. Behav.* **13,** 27–31.

Babbini M., Gaiardi M., and Bartoletti M. (1982) Benzodiazepine effects upon Geller-Seifter conflict test in rats: Analysis of individual variability. *Pharmacol. Biochem. Behav.* **17,** 43–48.

Baile C. A. and McLaughlin C. L. (1979) A review of the behavioral and physiological response to elfazepam, a chemical feed intake stimulant. *J. Anim. Sci.* **49,** 1371–1395.

Barry H., III and Krimmer E. C. (1978) Similarities and Differences in Discriminative Stimulus Effects of Chlordiazepoxide, Pentobarbital, Ethanol and Other Sedatives, in *Stimulus Properties of Drugs: Ten Years of Progress* (Colpaert F. C. and Rosecrans J. A., eds.), Elsevier, Amsterdam.

Beer B., Chasin M., Clody D. E., Vogel J. R., and Horovitz Z. P. (1972) Cyclic adenosine monophosphodiesterase in brain: Effects on anxiety. *Science* **176,** 428–430.

Beninger R. J., Kendall S. B., and Vanderwolf S. C. (1974) The ability of rats to discriminate their own behaviours. *Can. J. Psychol.* **28,** 79–93.

Bignami G. (1976) Behavioral pharmacology and toxicology. *Ann. Rev. Pharmacol. Toxicol.* **16,** 329–366.

Carlton P. L. (1978) Theories and Models in Psychopharmacology, in *Psychopharmacology: A Generation of Progress* (Lipton M. A., DiMascio, A., and Killman K. F., eds.), Raven, New York.

Carlton P. L., Siegel J. L., Murphree H. B., and Cook L. (1981) Effects of diazepam on operant behavior in man. *Psychopharmacology* **73,** 314–317.

Chisholm D. C. and Moore J. W. (1970) Effects of chlordiazepoxide on discriminative fear conditioning and shuttle avoidance performance in the rabbit. *Psychopharmacologia* **18,** 162–171.

Colpaert F. C., Desmedt L. K. C., and Janssen P. A. J. (1976) Discriminative stimulus properties of benzodiazepines, barbiturates and pharmacologically related drugs: Relation to some intrinsic and anticonvulsant effects. *Eur. J. Pharmacol.* **37,** 113–123.

Cook L. and Davidson A. B. (1973) Effects of Behaviorally Active Drugs in a Conflict–Punishment Procedure in Rats, in *The Benzodiazepines* (Garattini S., Mussini E., and Randall L. O., eds.), Raven, New York.

Cook L. and Sepinwall J. (1975) Behavioral analysis of the effects and mechanisms of action of benzodiazepines. *Adv. Biochem. Psychopharmacol.* **14,** 1–28.

Cooper S. J. (1980) Benzodiazepines as appetite-enhancing compounds. *Appetite* **1,** 7–19.

Corda M. G., Blaker W. D., Mendelson W. B., Guidotti A., and Costa E. (1983) β-carbolines enhance shock-induced suppression of drinking in rats. *Proc. Natl. Acad. Sci. USA* **80,** 2072–2076.

Crawley J. N. (1981) Neuropharmacological specificity of a simple animal model for the behavioral actions of benzodiazepines. *Pharmacol. Biochem. Behav.* **15,** 696–699.

Dantzer R. (1977a) Effects of diazepam on behavior suppressed by extinction in pigs. *Pharmacol. Biochem. Behav.* **6,** 157–161.

Dantzer R. (1977b) Behavioral effects of benzodiazepines: A review. *Biobehav. Rev.* **1,** 71–86.

Dantzer R. (1977c) Etude des effets du diazépam sur le comportement d'évitement continu chez le Porc. *J. Pharmacol.* **8,** 415–426.

Dantzer R. (1978) Dissociation between suppressive and facilitating effects of aversive stimuli on behavior by benzodiazepines. A review and reinterpretation. *Prog. Neuropsychopharmacol* **2,** 33–40.

Dantzer R. and Mormède P. (1976) Fear-dependent variations in continuous avoidance behavior of pigs. I. Lack of effect of diazepam on performance of discriminative fear conditioning. *Psychopharmacology* **49,** 69–73.

Dantzer R. and Perio A. (1982) Behavioural evidence for partial agonist properties of Ro 15-1788, a benzodiazepine receptor antagonist. *Eur. J. Pharmacol.* **81,** 655–658.

Dantzer R., Mormède P., and Favre B. (1976) Fear-dependent variations in continuous avoidance behavior of pigs. II. Effects of diazepam on acquisition and performance of Pavlovian fear conditioning and plasma corticosteroid levels. *Psychopharmacology* **49,** 75–78.

De Carvalho L. P., Grecksch G., Chapouthier G., and Rossier J. (1983) Anxiogenic and nonanxiogenic benzodiazepine antagonists. *Nature* **301,** 64–66.

Dixon A. K. (October, 1983) Indirect drug effects on behavior. *2nd Symposium of the European Society for Research on Aggression Zeist.*

File S. E. (1980) The use of social interaction as a method for detecting anxiolytic activity of chlordiazepoxide-like drugs. *J. Neurosci. Methods* **2,** 219–238.

File S. E. (1982) Colony aggression: Effects of benzodiazepines on intruder behavior. *Physiol. Psychol.* **10,** 413–416.

Flaherty C. F., Lombardi B. R., Wrightson J., and Deptula D. (1980) Conditions under which chlordiazepoxide influences gustatory contrast. *Psychopharmacology* **67,** 269–277.

Fowler S. C. (1974) Some effects of chlordiazepoxide and chlorpromazine on response force in extinction. *Pharmacol. Biochem. Behav.* **2,** 155–160.

Geller I. and Seifter J. (1960) The effects of meprobamate, barbiturates, *d*-amphetamine and promazine on experimentally induced conflict in the rat. *Psychopharmacologia* **1,** 482–492.

Geller I., Kulak J. T., Jr., and Seifter J. (1962) The effects of chlordiazepoxide and chlorpromazine on punishment discrimination. *Psychopharmacologia* **3,** 374–385.

Ghoneim M. M., Mewaldt S. P., Berie J. L., and Hinrichs J. V. (1981) Memory and performance effects of single and 3-week administration of diazepam. *Psychopharmacology* **73**, 147–151.

Gray J. (1977) Drug Effects on Fear and Frustration: Possible Limbic Site of Action of Minor Tranquilizers, in *Handbook of Psychopharmacology* Vol. 8, *Drugs, Neurotransmitters and Behaviour* (Iversen L., Iversen S. D., and Snyder S. H., eds.), Plenum, New York.

Gray J. (1982) *The Neuropsychology of Anxiety: An Enquiry Into the Functions of the Septo-Hippocampal System.* Oxford University, Oxford.

Heise G. A. and Boff E. (1961) Taming action of chlordiazepoxide. *Fed. Proc.* **20**, 393–397.

Hinde R. and Stevenson-Hinde J., eds. (1973) *Constraints on learning.* Academic, New York.

Hymowitz N. (1981) Effects of diazepam on schedule-controlled and schedule-induced behavior under signaled and unsignaled shock. *J. Exp. Anal. Behav.* **36**, 119–132.

Hymowitz N. and Abramson M. (1983) Effects of diazepam on responding suppressed by response-dependent and independent electric shock delivery. *Pharmacol. Biochem. Behav.* **18**, 769–776.

Kilts C. D., Commissaris R. L., and Rech R. H. (1981) Comparison of anti-conflict drug effects in three experimental animal models of anxiety. *Psychopharmacology* **74**, 290–296.

Lovell D. K., Bedford J. A., Grove L., and Wilson M. C. (1980) Effects of *d*-amphetamine and diazepam on paired and grouped primate food competition. *Pharmacol. Biochem. Behav.* **13**, 177–181.

Mackintosh N. J. (1974) *The Psychology of Animal Learning.* Academic, London.

Margules D. L. and Stein L. (1967) Neuroleptics vs. Tranquilizers: Evidence From Animal Behavior Studies on Mode and Site of Action, in *Neuropsychopharmacology* (Brill H., Cole J. O., Deniker P., Hippius H., and Bradley P. B., eds.), Excerpta Medica Foundation, Amsterdam.

Margules D. L. and Stein L. (1968) Increase of "antianxiety" activity and tolerance of behavioral depression during chronic administration of oxazepam. *Psychopharmacologia* **13**, 74–80.

McMillan D. E. (1975) Determinants of drug effects on punished responding. *Fed. Proc.* **34,** 1870–1879.

Miczek K. A. (1973) Effects of scopolamine, amphetamine and benzodiazepines on conditioned suppression. *Pharmacol. Biochem. Behav.* **1,** 401–411.

Miczek K. A. and Krsiak M. (1979) Drug effects on agonistic behavior. *Adv. Behav. Pharmacol.* **2,** 87–162.

Mohler H. and Okada T. (1977) Benzodiazepine receptors: Demonstration in the central nervous system. *Science* **198,** 849–851.

Morris M. D. and Gebhart G. F. (1981) Anti-anxiety agents and emotional behavior: An information processing analysis. *Prog. Neuropsychopharmacol.* **5,** 219–240.

Morris M. D., Berger A. B., and Gebhart G. F. (1980) Effect of chlordiazepoxide on conditioned and unconditioned fear in rats. *Prog. Neuropyschopharmacol.* **4,** 153–160.

Ninan P. T., Insel T. M., Cohen R. M., Cook J. M., Skolnick P., and Paul S. M. (1982) Benzodiazepine receptor-mediated experimental "anxiety" in primates. *Science* **218,** 1332–1333.

Perio A. (1983) *Contribution à l'Etude Psychopharmacologique des Benzodiazépines.* Thèse Doctorat 3e cycle, Université de Bordeaux II.

Poling A. and Appel J. B. (1979) Drug effects on the performance of pigeons under a negative automaintenance schedule. *Psychopharmacology* **60,** 207–210.

Pollard G. T. and Howard J. L. (1979) The Geller-Seifter conflict with incremental shock. *Psychopharmacology* **62,** 117–121.

Poschel B. P. H. (1971) A simple and specific screen for benzodiazepine-like drugs. *Psychopharmacologia* **19,** 193–198.

Rawlins J. N. P., Feldon J., Salmon P., Gray J. A., and Garrud P. (1980) The effects of chlordiazepoxide HCl administration upon punishment and conditioned suppression in the rat. *Psychopharmacology* **70,** 317–322.

Redmond D. E., Jr. and Huang Y. H. (1979) New evidence for a locus coeruleus norepinephrine connection with anxiety. *Life Sci.* **25,** 2149–2162.

Rommelspacher H., Bruning G., Schulze G., and Hill R. (1982) The *in Vivo* Occurring β-Carbolines Induce a Conflict-Augmenting Effect Which is Antagonized by Diazepam:

Correlation to Receptor Binding Studies, in *Neuroreceptors* (Hucho F., ed.), Walter de Gruyter & Co, Berlin.

Rosen A. J. and Tessel R. E. (1970) Chlorpromazine, chlordiazepoxide and incentive shift performance in the rat. *J. Comp. Physiol. Psychol.* **72**, 257–262.

Sahgal A. and Iversen S. D. (1980) Recognition memory, chlordiazepoxide and rhesus monkeys: Some problems and results. *Behav. Brain Res.* **1**, 227–243.

Sanger D. J. and Blackman D. E. (1976) Effects of diazepam and ripazepam on two measures of adjunctive drinking in rats. *Pharmacol. Biochem. Behav.* **4**, 73–83.

Sanger D. J. and Blackman D. E. (1981) Rate-dependence and the effects of benzodiazepines. *Adv. Behav. Pharmacol.* **3**, 1–20.

Shearman G. and Lal H. (1979) Discriminative stimulus properties of pentylenetetrazol and bemegride: Some generalization and antagonism tests. *Psychopharmacology* **63**, 315–321.

Shettleworth S. J. (1978) Reinforcement and the organization of behavior in golden hamsters: Punishment of three action patterns. *Learn. Motiv.* **9**, 99–123.

Soubrié, P., De Angelis L., Simon P., and Boissier J. R. (1976) Effets des anxiolytiques sur la prise de boisson en situation nouvelle et familière. *Psychopharmacologia* **50**, 41–45.

Squires R. F. and Braestrup C. (1977) Benzodiazepine receptors in rat brain. *Nature* **266**, 732–734.

Staddon J. E. R. and Simmelhag V. L. (1971) The "superstition" experiment: A re-examination of its implication for the principle of adaptive behavior. *Psychol. Rev.* **78**, 3–43.

Suomi S. J., Kraemer G. W., Baysinger C. M., and DeLizio R. D. (1981) Inherited and Experiential Factors Associated With Individual Differences in Anxious Behavior Displayed by Rhesus Monkeys, in *Anxiety: New Research and Changing Concepts* (Klein D. F. and Rabkin J., eds.), Raven, New York.

Treit D., Pinel J. P. J., and Fibiger H. C. (1981) Conditioned defensive burying: A new paradigm for the study of anxiolytic agents. *Pharmacol. Biochem. Behav.* **15**, 619–626.

Tye N. C., Sahgal A., and Iversen S. D. (1977) Benzodiazepines and discrimination behaviour: Dissociation of response and sensory factors. *Psychopharmacology* **52**, 191–194.

Valentine J. O. and Barrett J. E. (1981) Effects of chlordiazepoxide and *d*-amphetamine on responding suppressed by conditioned punishment. *J. Exp. Anal. Behav.* **35**, 209–216.

Vogel J. R. and Principi K. (1971) Effects of chlordiazepoxide on depressed performance after reward reduction. *Psychopharmacologia* **21**, 8–12.

Vogel J. R., Beer B. and Clody D. E. (1971) A simple and reliable conflict procedure for testing anti-anxiety agents. *Psychopharmacologia* **21**, 1–7.

Wilner P. J. and Crowe R. (1977) Effect of chlordiazepoxide on the partial reinforcement extinction effect. *Pharmacol. Biochem. Behav.* **7**, 479–482.

Effects of Drugs on Reward Processes

Andrew J. Greenshaw and Thomas B. Wishart

1. Introduction

The study of effects of drugs on reward or reinforcement (*see* Wise, 1978a, for a definition of the terms reward and reinforcement as they are used in this chapter) represents a vast area of research that ranges from the level of experimental studies with laboratory animals to that of drug trials and bioclinical assays with human psychiatric populations. The present chapter focuses on attempts to analyze effects of drugs on reward processes in laboratory animals, typically rodents. This is not intended to be a review of the literature; studies that have been cited are examples of particular experimental approaches in this research area. The main emphasis is on studies of intracranial self-stimulation. Other experimental areas, including drug self-administration and the conditioned place-preference paradigm, are also discussed, but in much less detail. The present treatment is intended to provide a useful introduction to major issues in this research area.

2. Self-Stimulation Studies

The observation that electrical stimulation of local brain areas may act as a positive reinforcer or reward (Olds and Milner, 1954) marked the beginning of an era in behavioral brain research. It was rapidly established that the rewarding properties of electrical brain stimulation were so great at certain stimulation sites that, under selective conditions, animals would forego the opportunity to eat and drink or engage in sexual activities in order to continue performing responses that served to deliver brain stimulation. The self-stimulation paradigm was quickly recognized as a methodology for the analysis of possible mechanisms underlying drug addiction (Olds et al., 1956) and from the early 1960s became established as a paradigm for the investigation of neural substrates of reinforcement (Stein, 1964).

2.1. Response Rate as a Measure of Reward

Much of the early behavioral work involved mapping out which brain areas would yield self-stimulation, using operant procedures involving lever-pressing on a simple continuous-reinforcement schedule (Olds and Olds, 1963). Rate of lever-pressing under these conditions is a good correlate of the intensity of the stimulating current. Rate was, therefore, generally adopted as a measure of self-stimulation (Olds, 1977). Response rate is, however, not necessarily related to reward: This statement may at first seem to be at odds with the functional analysis of reinforcement, but it is apparent that a measure of reinforcement under limited conditions may not be equivalent to a general measure of reinforcement. An early experiment provides a clear illustration of the problem.

Hodos and Valenstein (1962) conducted an elegant study in which effects of current intensity were assessed in relation to response rate and a measure of preference. Rats implanted with stimulating electrodes in both the septal and hypothalamic areas of the brain were trained to self-stimulate in a two-lever behavioral test chamber. The levers were separated by a partition that prevented the animals from operating both levers simultaneously. In the same subjects, stimulation of the septal site generally maintained lower rates of responding than hypothalamic stimulation over a range of current intensities. The rate measure, therefore, indicated that septal stimulation was less reinforcing that hypothalamic stimulation. The animals were then allowed to self-stimulate at either electrode site, depending on their lever choice, with the relationship between site and lever kept constant. Hodos and Valenstein observed a general preference in terms of the relative number of responses for septal stimulation when current intensities were equal for both electrodes. Hypothalamic stimulation was preferred to septal stimulation only when the latter was at a relatively low intensity. Thus, hypothalamic sites in this study maintained the highest response rates, but septal stimulation was generally preferred. In a parametric analysis of choice behavior in the same study, choice was a good correlate of current intensity when different intensities were available for the stimulation of one site. Hodos and Valenstein (1962) have also pointed out that the measure of response rate may not be sufficient for an analysis of reward in view of the tendency of electrical brain stimulation to elicit sequences of motor behavior that may interfere with response performance.

In the study of pharmacology, it is evident that the influences of drugs on rates of behavior may be attributed to a wide range of effects: sedative or stimulant effects, changes in the animal's motivational state, or changes in attentional or memory processes, to name a few of the possibilities (Iversen, 1977). In order to conclude that the effects of a drug are related to reward, it is necessary to rule out other possibilities. Despite apparent inadequacies of response-rate measures (Valenstein, 1964), some researchers have attempted to circumvent this problem by comparing effects of drugs on self-stimulation with those on parallel measures of motor function (Rolls et al., 1974a,b).

The use of rate as a measure of self-stimulation behavior may in some cases be justified on the grounds that some researchers are attempting to use the self-stimulation phenomenon to provide a sensitive procedure with which to analyze drug interactions, without discussing possible effects of drugs on reward (e.g., Wishart and Herberg, 1979). However, despite the early development of procedures for the analysis of drug effects on brain stimulation reward (Stein and Ray, 1960; Stein and Seifter, 1961), significant progress in this area of research has until relatively recently been impeded by the almost standard use of response rate as a behavioral measure. This point is clearly indicated by the fact that out of a total of some 95 papers dealing specifically with the effects of drugs on self-stimulation that were cited in a review in 1976, only 15 studies involved the measure of aspects of behavior other than rates of self-stimulation (Wauquier, 1976). Nevertheless, there have been a few elegant attempts to use a simple response-rate measure to assess the specificity of possible drug effects on reward.

One early study by Stein and Seifter (1961) provided a technique for assessing possible drug effects on reward by measuring response rate. In this experiment, rats were trained to self-stimulate on a continuous-reinforcement schedule. By testing the animals for self-stimulation at different current intensities, the reinforcement threshold for this parameter was established. The animals were then tested with the continuous-reinforcement schedule in operation, but with the stimulation current set just below the reinforcement threshold. Under these conditions the subjects engaged in very little lever pressing. Administration of amphetamine, however, resulted in high rates of self-stimulation that gradually declined to the very low levels of responding seen in the control condition. Amphetamines are known to induce a facilitation of response rates in a wide variety of situations and it is, therefore, possible that this effect of amphetamine may be a nonspecific facilitation of behavior. To control for this possibility, Stein and Seifter compared the effects of amphetamine on lever-pressing under conditions in which subthreshold stimulation was available and in which no stimulation was available. Administration of doses of amphetamine that were without effect in the no-stimulation condition were effective in engendering high response rates when the subthreshold stimulation was available contingent on lever-pressing. The dependence of this drug effect on the availability of subthreshold brain stimulation provides strong evidence that the effects of amphetamines on rates of self-stimulation may be attributed to reward-enhancing effects. Nevertheless, it is apparent that effects of amphetamine on self-stimulation may be at least partly attributable to less specific effects. *d*-Amphetamine has been reported to enhance continuously reinforced rates of lever-pressing maintained by electrical brain stimulation at doses of up to approximately 2 mg/kg and to depress this behavior at higher doses (Stein and Wise, 1973; Domino and Olds, 1972). Stein and Wise (1973) have suggested that the rewarding value of brain stimulation is decreased after administration of high doses, e.g., 5 mg/kg of amphetamine, resulting in the depression of responding. At these doses, however, administration of amphetamine typically results in the onset of perseverative responding, or stereotypy (Randrup and Munkvad, 1967). Thus a decrease in rates of self-stimulation after administration of high doses of amphetamine may be attributed to nonspecific effects on performance. Indeed, recent evidence suggests that this is the case. Carey (1979), on the basis of studies by Yehuda and Wurtman (1972) demonstrating the dependence of amphetamine stereotypy on thermoregulatory factors, investigated the effects of amphetamine on self-stimulation rates when hyperthermia is prevented. In this study, Carey reported that by precooling the subjects and subsequently testing for self-stimulation in a cold room, the facilitatory effects of 5 mg/kg of *d*-amphetamine could be observed. Administration of this dose under normal temperature conditions resulted in a complete cessation of self-stimulation. The involvement of motor impairment in the depression of self-stimulation rates after high doses of *d*-amphetamine has also been suggested by Zacharko and Wishart (1979). In their experiment, the effects of a range of doses of amphetamine were assessed under conditions in which rats were trained to self-stimulate by interrupting a photobeam. A dose-dependent facilitation of responding was observed after administration of the drug. These authors have suggested that, under the conditions of their experiment, administration of the highest dose of *d*-amphetamine (5 mg/kg) did not result in decreased response rates because the operant requirement, i.e., interruption of the photobeam, was compatible with the changes in response topography elicited by the drug (Lyon and Randrup, 1972; Randrup and Munkvad, 1967). Similar results have been reported for effects of up to 4 mg/kg of *d*-amphetamine on lever-pressing under a fixed-interval schedule of reinforcing hypothalamic stimulation (Greenshaw et al., 1985).

2.2. The Spatial Distribution of Responses at a Set Intensity of Stimulation

A novel and potentially useful approach to the analysis of effects of drugs on relative self-stimulation rates in terms of reward has been described by Glick et al. (1980, 1981). Glick and his colleagues reported that the two sides of the rat brain are differentially sensitive to brain stimulation. In these studies, rats tested for self-stimulation with bilateral hypothalamic electrodes displayed asymmetries in reinforcement thresholds and induced movements (circling). Regardless of the side of the brain that was stimulated, rotational behavior almost always occurred in the same direction and the direction of circling induced by stimulation was equivalent to that for circling behavior induced by a 1-mg/kg dose of *d*-amphetamine. Interestingly, reward thresholds were lower on the side contralateral to the direction of rotation, and the rate–intensity functions (i.e., curves depicting response rate as a function of current intensity) were displaced to the left for the electrode placement on that side of the brain. On the basis of these results, Glick and his colleagues (1981) conducted an experiment in which rats with bilateral hypothalamic electrodes that supported self-stimulation were tested in a choice procedure providing concurrent access rewarding stimulation on either side of the brain. Stimulation current intensity was titrated so that, under control conditions, rats displayed fairly equal rates of self-stimulation at each lever, with each lever being allocated to a different site. Amphetamine at 0.25–2.0 mg/kg induced a clear preference for stimulation to the more sensitive side of the brain. The possibility that this effect of *d*-amphetamine was simply related to the drug-induced preferences for a particular lever was ruled out by reversing the relationship between the stimulation sites and the levers. This is an interesting technique with which to analyze possible drug effects on reward. However, it remains to be demonstrated whether this procedure will be sensitive to the effects of other compounds.

2.3. The Temporal Distribution of Responses at a Set Intensity of Stimulation

An interesting approach to the dissociation of reward and performance effects, in terms of the local distribution of response rates (i.e., interresponse times), has been described by Huston and Mills (1971). This procedure provides a measure of reinforcement thresholds in terms of the emergence of relatively long interresponse times. Huston and Mills reported that it was possible to measure reinforcement thresholds using a procedure involving a concurrent schedule. Rats responding on a fixed-ratio schedule typically display a relatively long pause after the delivery of reinforcement until the next response (the postreinforcement pause). By training rats on a concurrent fixed-ratio, continuous-reinforcement schedule, Huston and Mills showed that the emergence of postreinforcement pauses was dependent upon the relative intensities of stimulation delivered on each component schedule. Thus, when the intensity of stimulation on the fixed-ratio was held at a constant suprathreshold level, the emergence of typical fixed-ratio patterning (i.e., a postreinforcement pause followed by a sustained high response rate until the delivery of the next reinforcer) was dependent on whether the stimulation delivered on the concurrent continuous-reinforcement schedule was above or below the reinforcement threshold intensity. This procedure has been used to assess the effects of various drugs on reward. Cassens and Mills (1973) have compared the effects of the administration of lithium and *d*-amphetamine using this procedure, and have reported that the administration of lithium increases reward thresholds measured in this way, whereas administration of *d*-amphetamine was reported to have the opposite effect. Withdrawal of *d*-amphetamine after chronic administration has also been reported to result in increased reward threshold (Cassens et al., 1981).

In these experiments, the threshold of reinforcement was defined in terms of the relative frequency of postreinforcement pauses, with a postreinforcement pause being defined as an interresponse interval of three or more standard deviations above the mean interresponse interval at a given current level in the continuous-reinforcement condition. Unfortunately, this procedure does not provide an adequate assessment of the reinforcement threshold that is independent of other effects of drugs. It has been demonstrated that the administration of *d*-amphetamine may result in a decrease in postreinforcement pause durations (Sanger, 1978), and a shift in the distribution of interresponse times toward shorter interresponse intervals (Ando, 1975). It is well established that a wide range of drugs may effect the distribution of interreponse times (Ando, 1975). Thus, with the concurrent fixed-ratio, continuous-reinforcement procedure, it may not be possible to dissociate drug-induced changes in pausing or interresponse times that are caused by a change in reinforcement threshold and other less specific effects of drugs on this measure.

The Hodos and Valenstein (1962) experiment described earlier clearly indicates that measures of choice may have advantages over response rate *per se*. Choice or preference is usually expressed in terms of relative rates of responding, as in the Hodos and Valenstein study and the recent studies by Glick et al. (1980, 1981) described above.

2.4. Autotitration of Current Intensity

A procedure for measuring reinforcement thresholds in terms of a choice measure was first described by Stein and Ray (1960). These investigators trained animals to regulate the intensity of brain stimulation that maintained their behavior. In this experiment, animals were trained to self-stimulate and then exposed to a situation in which each animal was given access to two widely spaced levers set into one wall of a behavioral test chamber. The intensity of the reinforcing brain stimulation was initially set at a high level.

The apparatus was programmed so that each response on one lever served to deliver brain stimulation and also reduce the intensity of the next available reinforcer by a predetermined amount. At any time the operation of the second lever reset the intensity of the brain stimulation to its initial high value. Under these conditions, animals reliably reset the intensity of brain stimulation when it was reduced below a certain level. Thus, by measuring current intensity at the time of the reset response, Stein and Ray were able to measure each animal's reward threshold. This effect yields reliable threshold estimates because animals typically press the reset lever at the same intensity of brain stimulation regardless of the initial intensity of the reinforcement (Schaefer and Holtzman, 1979). In most experiments, a fixed ratio is operative for decreasing current, e.g., every fifth lever press (FR5) may serve to decrease available current by a preset amount.

In early research, the effects of the administration of amphetamine and of the neuroleptic drug chlorpromazine were investigated using this procedure (Stein and Ray, 1960; Stein, 1964). Relatively large doses of amphetamine (1 mg/kg and above) were reported to have distinct "threshold-lowering" effects, since resetting occurred at lower current intensities after administration of these drugs (Stein and Ray, 1960; Stein, 1964). Administration of chlorpromazine resulted in resetting at higher intensities when doses of up to 2 mg/kg were used. Higher doses (2–3 mg/kg) resulted in a complete cessation of responding (Stein, 1964). These data were interpreted in terms of effects on reinforcement threshold, and were thus proposed as evidence for the effects of these compounds on reward (Stein, 1964). However, this interpretation must be dependent on a dissociation of the effects of the drug on perseveration of responding.

Administration of psychomotor stimulants such as *d*-amphetamine may result in the display of repetitive motor patterns or stereotypy (Randrup and Munkvad, 1967). Furthermore, spatial preferences on operant schedules may be markedly affected by these drugs (Glick and Jerussi, 1974; Sanger, 1978). Thus, with the procedure developed by Stein and Ray (1960), it is unclear whether the effects of amphetamine, and perhaps certain other drugs, are determined by relative rates of responding on either lever under control conditions. Notably, chlorpromazine and other neuroleptics also affect motor output, and these drugs are known to interact with neural systems mediating behavioral effects of drugs such as amphetamine (Iversen, 1977). The recent observation that injections of amphetamine into the nucleus accumbens increase reward thresholds with this procedure suggests a specific effect of this drug on reward (Neill and Justice, 1981). Nevertheless, without an analysis of effects of intraaccumbens amphetamine on spatial aspects of performance, this remains a controversial issue.

Threshold alterations have been reported after administration of a number of drugs using this procedure. Amphetamines (Stein and Ray, 1960; Schaefer and Holtzman, 1979; Zarevics and Setler, 1979), the GABA antagonist picrotoxin (Nazzaro and Gardner, 1980), and morphine (Nazzaro et al., 1981) are reported to decrease reward thresholds. Interestingly, the morphine effect was dependent on the site of stimulation (ventral-tegmental area). Rats self-stimulating at the substantia nigra pars compacta displayed an increase in the reward threshold after administration of morphine (Nazzaro et al., 1981). Various neuroleptics (Schaefer and Holtzman, 1979; Schaefer and Michael, 1980; Zarevics and Setler, 1979) are also reported to increase thresholds with this procedure.

It is interesting to note that a comparison of the effects of *d*- and *l*-amphetamine, haloperidol, and α-methyl-*p*-tyrosine on continuously reinforced rates of self-stimulation and on autotitration thresholds in the same animals revealed that drug-induced changes in reinforcement threshold were not consistently related to drug-induced changes in response rates with either procedure (Schaefer and Holtzman, 1979). It is apparent that although these studies represent impressive evidence for drug-induced alterations in the rewarding properties of brain stimulation, this interpretation of their data remains equivocal in the absence of appropriate controls for effects of drugs on spatial aspects of performance.

2.5. Method of Limits

A threshold determination procedure based on response frequency has been advocated by Esposito and Kornetsky (1977). This approach involves the determination of the reinforcement threshold in a discrete trial procedure. Animals are initially trained to self-stimulate by turning a wheel manipulandum. Following this training, each trial typically begins with the delivery of a noncontingent 0.5-s train of stimulation. A response within 7.5 s of this stimulus results in a delivery of a train of stimulation identical in all parameters to the noncontingent stimulus, thus terminating the trial. Failure to respond has no scheduled consequences and the trial terminates after 7.5 s in the absence of responding. Intervals between trials are varied, with an average of 15 s. Responses during the intertrial interval result in a 15-s delay before the start of the next trial. Thus, under these conditions, the initial noncontingent stimulation may serve as a discriminative stimulus indicting the availability of response-contingent stimulation, and as a comparative stimulus in the sense that it is a predictor of the parameters of the contingent stimulus.

By varying current intensity according to the method of limits (using a block of ten trials at each tested value), the reinforcement threshold is measured for each animal. This measure is determined by calculating the mean current for the midpoint between the intervals in which an animal made more than five and less than five responses. The latency to respond (i.e., time between noncontingent stimulation and wheel-turning and total intertrial responses) may provide measures of behavioral impairment or disrupted responding in this procedure.

Esposito and colleagues have reported various drug effects on self-stimulation using this procedure, including threshold-lowering after morphine (Esposito and Kornetsky, 1977) and amphetamine (Esposito et al., 1980), and threshold-increasing after haloperidol (Esposito et al., 1979). These effects are reported to be specifically related to drug-induced changes in reward because they were not accompanied by increases in response latencies or by consistent effects on error responding.

This procedure is interesting in that it provides a simultaneous assessment of measures related to reinforcement and to response performance. However, the presence of a punishment contingency (i.e., intertrial delays contingent on error responses) may be a variable that has a significant influence on drug effects. The significance of this factor under these conditions has not been assessed so far.

2.6. *Self-Regulated Duration of Brain Stimulation*

The discovery that animals will readily acquire responses that terminate prolonged trains of self-administered electrical brain stimulation (Bower and Miller, 1958; Roberts, 1958) has provided another self-regulation procedure with which it may be possible to assess drug effects on reinforcement. There has, however, been a certain amount of controversy over the mechanism of reinforcement underlying this phenomenon. The relevant issues are, therefore, briefly dealt with below.

There have been two main proposals for the explanation of this self-regulated duration phenomenon. One hypothesis is that an initially rewarding brain stimulation becomes aversive if prolonged (Bower and Miller, 1958). Bower and Miller further suggest that although animals could learn to respond in order to escape from such a stimulus, they could not learn to avoid it. However, Stein (1962) proposed that the neural response to brain stimulation undergoes adaptation and therefore the animal must interrupt the stimulus in order to feel the next onset and further reward.

Many experiments have been conducted in an attempt to resolve these two proposals. The evidence up to 1973 was reviewed by Deutsch, who concluded at that time that there was good evidence in favor of adaptation, but suggested, "whether this aversive factor is actually present remains for further work to determine" (Deutsch, 1973, p. 311). Recently, Sutherland and Nakajima (1980) have provided clear evidence for the existence of an aversive component with prolonged rewarding brain stimulation.

Their experiment was based on the work of Ettenberg and White (1978), who demonstrated that rats may develop a preference for flavors previously associated with rewarding hypothalamic stimulation. In another report, Ettenberg (1979) demonstrated that the degree of preference induced by pairing a flavor with brain stimulation was dependent upon the intensity of stimulation. Sutherland and Nakajima (1980) proposed that if there was an aversive component to prolonged rewarding brain stimulation, then this should be reflected by the relationship between the duration of stimulation and the degree of preference for the flavor with which it is paired. They hypothesized that if prolonged stimulation became nonrewarding through adaptation, then there should be a maximum preference displayed in response to all pairings with stimulation at or above the optimally rewarding duration. Alternatively, the presence of an aversive component may act to attentuate a taste preference induced with stimulation longer than the optimal duration. Sutherland and Nakajima (1980) reported an inverted U-shaped function relating the duration of rewarding hypothalamic stimulation to flavor preference (measured as a percentage of total fluid intake). In view of this result, it is clear that there can be an aversive component to prolonged rewarding hypothalamic stimulation.

It is apparent that the aversive effects of stimulation, measured in terms of escape responses, are dependent upon the site of stimulation (Hoebel, 1976). Therefore, the effects of experimental manipulations on self-regulated duration of stimulation may be caused by influences on reward or adaptation to reward (or aversion, depending upon the self-stimulation site), making the interpretation of such data difficult. The complexity of this issue has been discussed at length in a recent report (Atrens et al., 1983).

The problem of analyzing the effects of experimental manipulations on behavioral measures of the self-regulated duration of electrical brain stimulation has been the concern of a number of papers by Atrens and his colleagues (e.g., Atrens, 1973; Atrens et al., 1974, 1976). The approach adopted in these studies has been to use a shuttle-box procedure (similar to that originally described by Margules in

1966). Typically, in these experiments animals are exposed to a schedule in which movement to within 15 cm of one end of a shuttle box interrupts a photobeam, resulting in the initiation of a continuous train of brain stimulation that may be terminated only by interrupting another photobeam transecting the chamber 15 cm from the opposite end. Both the latency to initiate and to escape brain stimulation are measured under these conditions. These measures have been shown to be sensitive to changes in both frequency (Edwards et al., 1979) and intensity (Atrens et al., 1974) of rewarding brain stimulation.

With this procedure, the latency to initiate stimulation is generally regarded as a measure of the rewarding component of stimulation. The escape latency is usually taken as an index of the aversive component of the stimulation (Atrens, 1973). Atrens originally proposed that selective changes in these two response latencies permit the evaluation of specificity of any pharmacologically induced change in self-stimulation. If administration of a drug resulted in an increase or decrease of both latencies, it would not be possible to rule out an interpretation of this effect in terms of a nonspecific facilitatory or depressant effect of the drug on shuttling behaviors. However a change in only one latency, or opposite changes in both latencies, could not reasonably be attributed to nonspecific motor effects.

Using this procedure, Atrens et al. (1974) investigated the effects of *d,l*-amphetamine on hypothalamic stimulation. The results demonstrated that amphetamine (0.5–2 mg/kg) specifically enhanced reward (i.e., decreased latency to initiate stimulation) at sites in the medial, lateral, and periventricular hypothalamus at several intensities of rewarding stimulation. Administration of amphetamine was also reported to increase the latency to terminate stimulation at these sites in a number of animals. In contrast to these results, Atrens et al. (1974) reported that administration of this drug generally produced a current- and dose-dependent decrease in reward when behavior was maintained by stimulation of thalamic sites (i.e., latency to initiate stimulation was increased).

In a series of further studies, Atrens and his colleagues have demonstrated reward-decreasing effects of the a_2-noradrenergic agonist clonidine (Hunt et al., 1976, 1981) and the tetracyclic antidepressant mianserin (Hunt et al., 1981). Hunt et al. (1976) have also demonstrated reward-reducing effects of the catecholamine synthesis inhibitor a-methyl-p-tyrosine. A reduction in reward has also been demonstrated after administration of clozapine (Atrens et al., 1976), but in the same study, administration of another neuroleptic drug—haloperidol—increased latencies to both initiate and terminate stimulation. Thus, with this procedure the effects of haloperidol could have been the result of a nonspecific decrement in performance. Specific reductions in the latency to terminate stimulation have been reported after administration of etorphine (Baltzer et al., 1977) and morphine (Levitt et al., 1977). An earlier study using a similar technique demonstrated that this procedure is also sensitive to the effects of benzodiazepines. Margules and Stein (1967) tested rats at high current levels that induced short latencies of initiation and termination. In this study they reported that administration of oxazapam resulted in a marked decrease in latency to terminate stimulation.

Another early study utilized a combination of rate and latency measures in an attempt to elucidate the possible influences of another benzodiazepine, chlordiazepoxide, on the reinforcing poperties of brain stimulation. In this experiment, Panksepp et al. (1970) compared the effects of chlordiazepoxide on self-stimulation rates with rats that displayed differential latencies to escape from rewarding hypothalamic stimulation. They reported that administration of chlordiazepoxide (15 mg/kg) resulted in increased rates of self-stimulation (10–15 μA above reward threshold) at sites that yielded reliable escape behavior. However, drug administration resulted in decreased rates of self-stimulation that did not consistently yield escape behavior. These authors suggested that this differential drug effect was the result of a specific change in the aversive component of stimulation after administration of chlordiazepoxide. However, the observation that administration of chlordiazepoxide does not appear to affect escape behavior elicited by tegmental stimulation (Olds, 1966) limits the generality of this interpretation (*see* also, Caudarella et al., 1982, for similar site-dependent effects).

Edwards et al. (1979) investigated the effects of various drugs when the duration of brain stimulation was controlled in a shuttle box, as in the experiments by Atrens and his associates, or in an operant test chamber by a combination of lever-pressing at one side of the test chamber (to initiate stimulation) and shuttling to the other side (to terminate stimulation). The effects of administration of haloperidol, phentolamine, scopolamine, propranolol, and FLA-63 were investigated in relation to stimulation at different frequencies of electrical brain stimulation. The behavioral measures used in this study were on-time, the mean duration of brain stimulation; off-time, the mean interval between the offset of stimulation and the initiation of the next stimulation; and time-on, as a percentage of the total session durations. Haloperidol consistently decreased percentage time-on by elevating off-times (without consistent effects on on-times); these effects of haloperidol were greater at lower frequencies. Phentolamine, an α-adrenergic antagonist, also differentially decreased off-times with consistently greater effects at lower frequencies; other drugs were without consistent effects on behavior. Various drugs have been recently tested with this procedure in a series of studies by Liebman and colleagues (*see* Liebman, 1983, for an extensive review that includes these studies). This researcher has suggested that the present approach is relatively sensitive and easy to employ in terms of time required to train animals.

The differential effect of haloperidol in a study by Edwards et al. (1979) is inconsistent with the effect described earlier in the study reported by Atrens et al. (1976). There is no explanation for this discrepancy at the present time, although it may possibly be attributed to subtle differences in procedure between the two studies.

The Edwards study is particularly interesting in terms of the use of a number of behavioral measures (*vide supra*). Wauquier et al. (1983) have pointed out that multiple measures with this procedure are necessary for a satisfactory appraisal of drug effects, particularly when comparing effects of drugs with effects of changes in current intensity.

From these reports it is apparent that this approach has provided a useful and sensitive technique for the evaluation of the influences of drugs on reward and what is generally assumed to be aversion in self-stimulation. However, it has been suggested that this approach does not provide a clear measure of reward. Fibiger (1978) has proposed that a decrease in reward (i.e., an increased latency to initiate stimulation) may possibly be attributed to a drug-induced deficit in the animal's ability to initiate operant responses. This is a valid criticism, particularly considering the effects of neuroleptic drugs, a class of compounds that decrease operant responding maintained by a variety of schedules at doses that do not appear to affect unconditioned responses (Margules and Stein, 1967). Another limitation of the procedure is illustrated by a report of effects of haloperidol in a study by Atrens et al. (1976). As described earlier, this drug increased both latency to initiate and terminate stimulation in this experiment. It is clear that a nonspecific performance decrement may not be ruled out as an interpretation of this effect. However, it is possible that administration of haloperidol resulted in a general reinforcement decrement (i.e., decreased both reward and aversion) in this study. The available data do not allow an assessment of this possibility. Clearly, the only way to demonstrate the absence of a general performance decrement under these conditions would be to show that the effect of the drug on a response that controlled the duration of reinforcement is different from its effect on an equivalent behavior.

A recent study by De Witte (1981) has provided such an analysis. In this study, De Witte investigated the effects of naloxone on self-regulated duration of hypothalamic stimulation under different procedural conditions. De Witte observed that administration of naloxone resulted in an increase in the duration of stimulation with rats that had previously received foot-shock in the presence of stimulation. No such effect was apparent with animals that had not been exposed to the stimulation-foot-shock pairing conditions. Thus the effects of naloxone could not have been caused by a nonspecific performance decrement.

In relation to the use of a unitary "stimulation-duration" measure in the self-stimulation paradigm (Redgrave, 1978; Olds, 1975; De Witte, 1981), it is apparent that in the absence of other measures, it is difficult to assess the specificity of possible drug effects in terms of reinforcement. This is particularly evident in view of recent reports that administration of drugs may result in changes of the duration of responses that are unrelated to reinforcement duration on schedules of food and water delivery (*see* Fowler, 1974; Faustman et al., 1981).

A recent approach has used intermittent delivery of brain stimulation on fixed-interval schedules to address this problem. Under these conditions, effects of drugs on the self-regulated duration of brain stimulation and on the duration of nonreinforced responses (i.e., responses in the absence of brain stimulation) may be compared. With this procedure, chlordiazepoxide is reported to increase the duration of stimulation, the duration of nonreinforced responses, and overall response rate. Notably, the effect of chlordiazepoxide on the duration of nonreinforced responses was greater in magnitude than the effect on the duration of stimulation (Greenshaw et al., 1983). With d-amphetamine and β-phenylethylamine over a wide range of doses, effects on rate and nonreinforced response duration have been observed in the absence of changes in the duration of stimulation (Greenshaw et al., 1985). The latter result is interesting in view of previous reports of amphetamine-induced increases (Zacharko and Wishart, 1979; Zacharko and Kokkinidis, 1982) and decreases (Atrens et al., 1974) in the duration of brain stimulation. Since the duration of stimulation on a fixed-interval schedule is a good correlate of the intensity of stimulation, whereas response rate and the duration of non-reinforced responses are not, these results have been interpreted in terms of schedule-dependent effects of drugs on measures of reinforcement (Greenshaw et al., 1985). The implications of these data, together with clear demonstrations of response-dependent effects of drugs on self-stimulation (Ettenberg et al., 1981; Wauquier and Niemegeers, 1979; White et al., 1978), are particularly important when considering the results of self-stimulation experiments in relation to theories of the "neural basis of reward" (*see* Ettenberg et al., 1981, for an interesting example of the problem).

2.7. The Reward-Summation Function

In an attempt to circumvent the difficulties associated with determining the specificity of drug effects on reward in the self-stimulation paradigm, Edmonds and Gallistel have devised a method that provides a measure of reward that is relatively unaffected by changes in the animal's level of arousal or motor abilities (Edmonds and Gallistel, 1974).

Under this procedure an animal is run between a start box, in which it receives "priming" stimulation (i.e., independent of responding), and a goal box at the other end of an alley, where it has access to rewarding brain stimulation contingent on lever-pressing. By independently varying the parameters of the priming and reinforcing stimulation, it is possible to determine the functions that relate changes in performance to the parameters of brain stimulation. With the parameters of priming stimulation held constant, the function relating running speed to the number of electrical pulses the rat receives as a reward (the reward-summation function) has a distinctive shape. With short pulse trains, the running speed is low, but as train length is increased, the running speed suddenly increases to an asymptote. The location (on the pulse train axis) of the sharp rise in the reward-summation function is a measure of the reward value of the stimulation that appears to be unaffected by factors that alter general performance levels (Edmonds and Gallistel, 1974).

Edmonds and Gallistel (1977) have used this technique to investigate the effects of the catecholamine-synthesis inhibitor α-methyl-*p*-tyrosine on self-stimulation behaviors. These authors reported that administration of this compound resulted in a decrease in reward (i.e., the locus of the rise in the reward-summation function was shifted toward an increased number of pulses per reward). However, this effect was dependent on the site of brain stimulation.

In a subsequent study, Franklin (1978) used this procedure to investigate the effects of pimozide, clonidine, and piperoxane on brain-stimulation reward. Administration of the neuroleptic drug pimozide at 0.1 and 0.2 mg/kg resulted in a shift in the reward-summation function in the direction indicating a decrease of reward, but did not proportionately depress the maximum running speed; higher doses of this drug (up to 0.9 mg/kg) abolished responding in this experiment. Clonidine (0.03 and 0.15 mg/kg) similarly reduced the rewarding value of stimulation and also depressed running speed. Piperoxane (5 mg/kg) had no effects on either running speed or the reward-summation function when administered alone. However, when administered in combination with clonidine, piperoxane abolished the effect of clonidine on the reward-summation function and potentiated the clonidine-induced depression of running speed. These data are particularly interesting in that they demonstrate that it is possible to dissociate reward and performance effects of drugs with the reward-summation function technique. Furthermore, the results of Franklin's 1978 study indicate that this is a sensitive procedure for the study of drug interactions.

Gallistel and Karras (1984) have used an adaptation of this technique using rates of lever-pressing alone to demonstrate facilitation of reward in response to administration of amphetamine and attenuation of reward in response to administration of pimozide. This effect of amphetamine was blocked by pimozide treatment.

Recent studies have demonstrated that this technique may be useful for assessing emergent changes in reward sensitivity, as induced by chronic antidepressant treatment (O'Regan et al., 1985).

A limitation of using this method is that it does not allow a distinction to be made between possible effects of drugs on reward and aversion. Atrens' work, described earlier, indicates that this is an important issue in the analysis of the effects of drugs on reward. Nevertheless, this is a very powerful approach that provides a measure of reinforcement sensitivity truly independent of (maximal) response rates. There are to date no severe criticisms of this approach. It is noteworthy, however, that this technique will only work when response rate is sensitive to changing current intensity. Although other approaches (i.e., choice) may be effective even with drug treatments that induce stereotyped responding, this approach may not (Franklin, personal communication).

2.8. Studies of "Functional Equivalence"

As described earlier in this chapter, a study conducted by Stein and Seifter (1961) compared the effects of the administration of amphetamine with the availability of brain stimulation using response rate as a measure of reinforcement. The rationale for this analysis was that rewarding electrical stimulation of the brain and amphetamine had equivalent effects on a brain-reward system. Thus, this experiment was designed to demonstrate that brain stimulation and administration of amphetamine resulted in functionally equivalent changes in response rate.

Other experiments that have so far been described in this chapter have not entailed the assumption that effects of administration of drugs are simply equivalent to changes in brain stimulation. The approach that has been adopted in these studies is a more sophisticated one, accepting that the behavioral effects of the drugs may be multiple and complex and, therefore, attempting to dissociate between different components of drug action.

In relation to the hypothesis that catecholamine activity is the principle neuropharmacological basis of reward (Stein and Wise, 1973), it has been proposed that manipulations of catecholamine activity within the central nervous system induces changes in behavior that are directly equivalent to behavioral changes induced by altering the availability of reinforcement (Wise, 1978a,b). This simple hypothesis is now no longer tenable, since it is established that a number of neurotransmitters may be involved in the expression, establishment, and maintenance of reinforcement; nevertheless, these studies that have primarily assessed the possible involvement of dopamine are particularly important because they illustrate the general approach.

2.9. Analyses of Within-Session Response Patterning

Wise suggested that the blockade of dopamine systems in the central nervous system, induced by administration of dopamine receptor blockers, such as the neuroleptic drugs (particularly pimozide), results in a state of drug-induced nonreward or "anhedonia" (Wise, 1978a,b). Wise has attempted to demonstrate the equivalence of administration of pimozide and of withholding reinforcement by comparing the effects of the two treatments on within-session changes in rates of lever-pressing normally maintained by hypothalamic stimulation (Fouriezos and Wise, 1976; Fouriezos et al., 1978).

In these studies, administration of graded doses of pimozide (0.125–0.5 mg/kg) resulted in patterns of self-stimulation on a continuous-reinforcement schedule that were observed to be equivalent to those caused by a graded reduction of current intensity (Fouriezos and Wise, 1976; Fouriezos et al., 1978). With the lowest doses of pimozide and small reductions in current intensity, rates of responding were observed to be similar to control rates for the first 5–10 min, after which rates of responding dropped to between 10 and 15% of control rates. With larger doses of pimozide and greater decreases in current intensity, the responding was observed to decelerate more rapidly; however, the initial rates of responding again were reported to be equivalent in the two conditions. The presence of an initial period of responding that was similar to control rates in both conditions was interpreted as evidence against any nonspecific performance decrements resulting from administration of pimozide.

Similar evidence of graded decreases in response measures after pretreatment with pimozide were reported with a straight-alley runway task (Fouriezos et al., 1978). In this study, animals were trained to run a 5-ft alley for access to rewarding brain stimulation. On each trial, latency to leave the start box, running speed in the alley, and lever-pressing rates for the delivery of 15 reinforcers (on a continuous-reinforcement schedule) in the goal box were recorded. After 15 reinforced responses in the goal box, a new trial was initiated, the lever was retracted, and the animal was required to run back to the other end of the alley for another 15 responses with the lever now available at that side.

After administration of 0.5 mg/kg of pimozide, animals exhibited response latencies, running times, and lever-pressing rates for about the first six trials that were equivalent to control measures. After this initial period of normal responding, performance deteriorated. This pattern of response decrement observed after drug administration was reported to be equivalent to the effects of nonreward. Wise (1978a,b) suggested that these results are in favor of the drug-induced blockade of reward with pimozide. However, although this approach of establishing functional equivalence between drug effects and the effects of nonreward through an analysis of in-session response patterning is an elegant one, it remains a possibility that this apparent equivalence of treatment effects may be artifactual.

In a recent study, Ettenberg and his colleagues (Ettenberg et al., 1979) examined this possibility by investigating the effects of pimozide on responding in extinction. Ettenberg et al. proposed that if administration of pimozide resulted in behavioral changes that are caused by a blockade of reward, then the effects of combinations of pretreatment with pimozide and exposure to nonreward should be equivalent to the effects of exposure to either condition. In this experiment, rats were trained to self-stimulate on a continuous-reinforcement schedule. Response rates were recorded for every 5-min period of each 30-min session. Ettenberg et al. (1979) reported that administration of pimozide under conditions of nonreward led to a greater decrease in response rates over the session than nonreward alone. Thus, they suggested that administration of pimozide resulted in a motor decrement that may parallel the effects of nonreward. Essentially similar discrepancies between effects of pimozide and nonreward have been reported by Fibiger et al. (1976), Phillips and Fibiger (1979), and Greenshaw et al. (1981).

Clearly, the results of the above studies are inconsistent with the initial proposal of Wise (1978a). However, despite this result, further evidence for an interpretation of this equivalence of changes in response patterning in terms of reward blockade has been provided by Franklin and McCoy (1979). These authors hypothesized that if administration of pimozide results in a progressive decrement in the animal's ability to respond, self-stimulation, once blocked, should not recommence until the animal recovers either from the drug or from the previous bout of activity (*see* Franklin and McCoy, 1979). Alternatively, if the pimozide-induced suppression of responding is caused by a blockade of reward, then it should be possible to reinstate responding with a discriminative stimulus that has previously signaled the availability of reward. An experiment was conducted in which two groups of animals were exposed to a multiple-variable interval, 15-s, fixed-ratio 4 schedule of hypothalamic stimulation. Each group was then exposed to a different schedule under which each 3-min period of variable interval, 15 s or fixed-ratio 4, was separated by 3-min periods in which no stimulation was delivered. With one group, onset of a flashing light was correlated with commencement of the fixed-ratio component. The light remained on through the nonreward component and was switched off on the commencement of the variable-interval component. Thus, with this group both onset and offset of the light correlated with the availability of reward. The second (unsignaled) group exerienced the onset and offset of the light for an equal proportion of time; the light onset and offset were random in relation to the availability of reward. The effects of reduced brain-stimulation current under pimozide on responding were assessed in separate sessions. In each case the effects of the treatment were first assessed with the schedule in operation, but with the light off for the first 40 min. The effects of reinstating the light were compared in each treatment condition. With pimozide treatment and reduced brain-stimulation intensity, the gradual reduction in responding was observed over the first 40 min of the session. When the light was reinstated, the group for which the light had been a signal for availability of reward displayed a marked increase in response rates, both under conditions of reduced brain stimulation and after administration of pimozide. These effects were not observed with the group for which the light had not signaled availability of reward. This increase in responding induced by the light-signaled group extinguished after approximately 10 min. Franklin and McCoy ruled out an interpretation of nonspecific arousal effects of the light by the use of an unsignaled group and their failure to reinstate responding by manually shaking the subjects in the pimozide condition. In some respects this experiment may, in a sense, represent the "tip of the iceberg," since it bridges the gap between the simple "reinforcement hypothesis" and experiments designed to assess the relative contribution of "learning processes." Indeed, this has proved to be a fruitful avenue of research (e.g., *see* Beninger, 1983).

3. Drug Self-Administration

Drugs such as alcohol, marijuana, morphine, heroin, amphetamine, and cocaine, to name a few, have the potential for human drug abuse. When used chronically, physical dependence may occur that subsequently may play a role in the maintenance of drug intake. Nevertheless, drug-taking seems to be related to feelings of pleasure and euphoria elicited by many psychoactive drugs. For this reason, research directed toward an understanding of basic reward-reinforcement mechanisms has employed drug self-administration techniques. Using operant conditioning and procedures for chronic intravenous infusions, it was shown that animals will perform responses to obtain infusions of these same drugs, and a vast literature now exists on these "animal models" of human drug abuse (Griffiths et al., 1979). These studies have included a range of procedures for drug administration, including intravenous, intramuscular, and oral injection routes. In relation to the latter route, problems of drug palatability (e.g., with ethanol) and conditioned taste-aversion learning (Goudie, 1986) have proved to be problematic (*see* Grant and Samson, 1985, for an interesting approach to the induction of oral ethanol consumption in the rat). Much of the earlier literature was directed toward an understanding of the various parameters that determined the self-administration of drugs, and the interested reader is referred to Johanson (1978) for an overview of this field. Some important features of drug self-administration merit discussion here.

For a drug to have rewarding properties in the self-administration paradigm, it must be established that behavior will be maintained only when drug delivery is response-contingent. The use of yoked-control procedures has been invaluable in this respect (Pickens and Thompson, 1971). Furthermore, the demonstration of schedule control with intermittent drug reinforcement has also provided useful evidence concerning the relative reinforcing properties of different drugs. For example, Shannon and Thompson (1985) have demonstrated second-order schedule maintenance with β-phenylethylamine, but not with the structurally similar compound phenylethanolamine, indicating that the former compound is a more powerful reinforcer.

In terms of varying reward magnitude (either in terms of varying the dose of the reinforcing drug per delivery or administering various pharmacological agents to alter the efficacy of the reinforcing drug stimulus), it is evident that the drug self-administration paradigm may have some advantages over electrical self-stimulation of the brain. These advantages have been clearly outlined by Wise (1978a) with numerous examples, but will be described briefly here.

3.1. Response Rate and Reinforcement: An Inverse Relationship

In studies of intravenous drug self-administration using schedules of continuous reinforcement, a reduction of reward magnitude (i.e., dose per delivery) will, within the range of doses that maintain sustained responding, increase rates of responding. Thus, animals will apparently respond to maintain optimal levels of drug-stimulation. Conversely, increased doses per delivery will (within limits: *vide supra*) decrease rates of responding. Consequently (and in contrast to electrical brain self-stimulation studies), pharmacological and physiological manipulations that result in reward attenuation will increase response rates and those that facilitate reward will decrease responding (Yokel and Wise, 1975, 1976). Many drugs that are reported to decrease reward in the self-stimulation paradigm (such as pimozide) also decrease operant responding; an increase in rates of drug self-administration after such treatment, therefore, represents rather strong evidence for effects on the reinforcing value of drug stimuli (*see* Wise, 1978a, pp. 233–237, for a most useful discussion on this subject). Nevertheless, it is clear that this form of analysis is less readily applied to schedules of drug self-administration whereby reinforcement density is relatively independent of response rate (i.e., fixed- and variable-interval schedules). More recent work is concerned with the use of the technique of self-administration to better understand the neuronal and neurochemical basis of reward and reinforcement. A brief summary of some of these studies, and their findings, follows.

3.2. *Central Aspects of Drug Self-Administration*

The early drug self-administration studies required the subject—most frequently a rat or monkey—to perform a response, usually pressing a lever, to produce a small infusion of drug directly into a vein, while, at the same time, the experimenter attempted some manipulation of brain structure (or some aspect of brain chemistry) thought to be involved in the mediation of reward. Thus, for example, Glick et al. (1975) reported that lesions of the caudate nucleus alter the self-administration of, and physical dependence upon, morphine in rats. Lesions in the hypothalamus have similar effects (Amit et al., 1973).

Current research efforts also involve the direct self-administration of drugs into specific brain regions. If it can be shown that animals will self-administer a psychoactive agent into one brain region but not another, it is highly likely that the former contains, or is part of, a neural system subserving reward or reinforcement. The results of a number of studies show that rats willingly learn to press a lever that results in the delivery of a small quantity of morphine directly into the lateral hypothalamus (Olds, 1979), septum (Stein and Olds, 1977), nucleus accumbens (Olds, 1982), and ventral tegmental area (Bozarth and Wise, 1981). There are, however, some conflicting findings; for example, Britt and Wise (1981) suggest on the basis of lesion studies that the self-administration of morphine into the lateral hypothalamus is actually mediated by the ventral tegmental area, probably as a result of drug diffusion from the former to the latter site.

The areas of the brain that support morphine self-administration contain high concentrations of opioid receptors, and are also part of the mesolimbic-mesocortical dopamine system that is believed to play a critical role in reward. Olds and Williams (1980) have shown that the areas that most strongly support brain self-stimulation also support opiate self-administration, further demonstrating the relationship between these two phenomena.

Using a newly developed microinjection technique permitting the delivery of nanoliter quantities of drug, Goeders and Smith (1983) have reported the observation that medial prefrontal cortex (MFC) supports the self-administration of cocaine, whereas the nucleus accumbens and ventral tegmental area do not. Responding for cocaine in the MFC was dose-dependent and maintained by a fixed-ratio schedule of reinforcement. Furthermore, animals learned to effectively distinguish between two levers of which only one resulted in drug delivery when activated. Goeders and Smith conclude, based on their finding that sulpiride, a dopamine D_2 receptor antagonist, reduced the self-administration of cocaine in the MFC, and that the reinforcing effects of cocaine (like those of morphine) are related to activity of the mesolimbic-mesocortical dopamine system. Further studies of this nature may serve to widen and clarify our current understanding of neural systems underlying reward.

4. Place-Conditioning Studies

An additional approach has arisen for the assessment of drug effects on reinforcement: namely, the conditioned place-preference paradigm. Basically, this procedure involves the forced pairing of a distinct environment with drug treatment and the assessment of the subject's subsequent preference for the drug-paired environment. Typically, animals are tested in a three-compartment apparatus consisting of a large cubic compartment at either end, separated by a narrower, middle choice compartment. With this procedure, after the assessment of baseline choice behavior in an initial adaptation phase, each animal receives drug injections in one compartment (A) and vehicle injections in the other compartment (B) on alternate days. After a number of drug-A, vehicle-B pairings, the choice of the animals for A vs B is assessed by placing the animal in the middle compartment and then measuring the relative time spent in A and B. This particular approach probably stems mainly from the work of Reicher and Holman (1977), who demonstrated an amphetamine-induced location preference. Nevertheless, there has recently been a great surge of interest in this paradigm, presumably because of the apparent simplicity and the apparent ease of data interpretation that it affords. It should be noted that certain basic issues may affect the outcome of place-preference conditioning experiments. The main factors are: (1) the nature of the test apparatus, i.e., salience of the environmental cues, which will determine the relative baseline preference for A or B (as above), and (2) the allocation of preferred or nonpreferred side in relation to drug-side pairing (Mucha and Iversen, 1984). Other considerations, such as, of course, drug dose, are also pertinent to the outcome of such studies.

4.1. Problems of Interpretation

Although this paradigm has mainly yielded results similar to those of self-stimulation and drug self-administration studies, a few cautionary remarks may be appropriate in relation to the spatial-conditioning approach. It seems clear in the light of certain experiments that, for some drugs at least, "place preference" (or its inverse, "place avoidance") may not be attributable to state-dependent learning (Mucha and Iversen, 1984). Furthermore, as preference testing is carried out in the absence of drug treatment, the observed effects are clearly not directly due to drug-induced impairment or facilitation of motor activity. Nevertheless, there is an increasing body of literature that describes conditioned drug effects in terms of altered motor activity. This is well illustrated by a recent demonstration of environment-specific enhancement of motor activity with amphetamine as the unconditioned stimulus. Beninger and Hahn (1983) have reported that animals with a history of amphetamine injections in a specific environment exhibited a specific enhancement of activity in that environment after saline injections. Similar conditioned responses to cocaine have been demonstrated by Barr et al. (1983). In this study, the extinction of conditioned activity changes was assessed. Notably, the conditioned drug effect decayed over 15 d, but little extinction was evident over four daily trials. The implications of these data for confounding the interpretation of place-preference data are self-evident. Unfortunately, extinction data for the place-preference paradigm are sparse. Mucha and Iversen (1984) have reported retention of a conditioned place-preference for at least 1 mo. Similarly, Bardo et al. (1984) have reported that in over four extinction trials, their subjects did not display any change in the total duration of time spent in the drug-paired environment. Nevertheless, these authors did report a significant decrease in time on the preferred side relative to the number of entries (i.e., time spent per entry into the preferred compartment).

An analysis of the extinction of conditioned place preferences or place aversions may possibly prove to be worthwhile, if not necessary, for the clear interpretation of the results of place-preference conditioning.

In relation to the issue of conditioned changes in locomotor activity *per se,* it is rather interesting to note that Swerdlow and Koob (1984) have reported that restrained rats (i.e., rats rendered immobile during conditioning) exhibit conditioned locomotor responses to amphetamine, but do not exhibit an amphetamine-induced place preference. These authors suggest that drug-induced locomotor activity *per se* is necessary for the induction of a place preference. A possible limitation in this study is that the restraint procedure may have had aversive consequences. However, this observation of a dissociation between conditioned activity changes and conditioned place preference is fairly strong evidence in favor of the reinforcement interpretation of the amphetamine-induced place preference. Nevertheless, conditioned activity changes represent a major possible source of interpretative error with this approach.

5. Conclusion

This chapter has dealt mainly with procedures for assessing drug effects on reward in the context of electrical self-stimulation of the brain. The areas of drug self-administration and place-preference conditioning with drugs have also briefly been considered. It is apparent that various approaches to the analysis of reward have been adopted, and that the data from most, if not all, suffer from problems of interpretation. These problems, which have been considered in the preceding sections, clearly indicate the difficulties of establishing the specificity of influences of drugs on reinforcement processes. Despite these complexities, it is evident that certain classes of compounds may facilitate reward or act as reinforcers in their own right. In this respect, the parallel between known drugs of abuse (in human terms) and the results of these laboratory studies is striking (Griffiths et al., 1979). Nevertheless, although theories concerning neural substrates of reinforcement are apparently developing away from the simplistic, single-reward transmitter view (Wise, 1980), we remain far from any clear understanding of this area (*see* Amit and Brown, 1982; Wise and Bozarth, 1982, for recent and somewhat contrasting views).

A number of researchers have recently indicated the need for an attempt to explore the multifaceted nature of the reinforcement process in this context (De Witte and Bruyer, 1980; Wauquier et al., 1983). That such an approach is necessary is indicated by the lack of support for simple "global hypotheses," such as the anhedonia hypothesis (at least in its original form), proposed by Wise (*see* Wise, 1982, for a recent overview). In the view of the present authors, progress may be achieved more readily by reassessing the vast database already accrued, particularly in terms of sensitive behavioral test procedures, and by avoiding the pitfalls of developing theories of neurotransmitter function beyond the limits of available behavioral data. This is particularly important when considering discussions of *drive, motivation,* and *reward* and the underlying neural substrates. In fact, looking back at the early experiments concerning self-stimulation and drugs, it is evident that progress has been rather limited (Greenshaw, 1985). Wauquier and his colleagues (1983) have suggested what we feel is a desirable direction for future research in relation to effects of neuroleptics on self-stimulation. This statement could usefully be applied to the area of "drugs and reinforcement" in general.

Instead of an interpretation of the effects of neuroleptics on brain self-stimulation in terms of the dichotomy reward-performance, it might be worthwhile to discuss these in terms of behavioral elements, their intensity and their sequence in specific situations. Alternatively, the development of paradigms of self-stimulation by which specific stimulus properties can be dissociated from the behavioral components induced by or concomitant with brain-stimulation, are urgently required.

(From Wauquier et al., 1983, p. 163, with permission from authors and publishers.)

References

Amit Z. and Brown Z. W. (1982) Actions of drugs of abuse on brain reward systems: A reconsideration with specific attention to alcohol. *Pharmacol. Biochem. Behav.* **17,** 233–238.

Amit Z., Corcoran M. E., Amir S., and Urca G. (1973) Ventral hypothalamic lesions block the consumption of morphine in rats. *Life Sci.* **13**, 805–816.

Ando D. (1975) Profile of drug effects on temporally spaced responding in rats. *Pharmac. Biochem. Behav.* **3**, 833–841.

Atrens D. M. (1973) A reinforcement analysis of rat hypothalamus. *Am. J. Physiol.* **224**, 62–65.

Atrens D. M., Ljungberg T., and Ungerstedt U. (1976) Modulation of reward and aversion processes in the rat diencephalon by neuroleptics: Differential effects of clozapine and haloperidol. *Psychopharmacology* **49**, 97–100.

Atrens D. M., Sinden J. D., and Hunt G. E. (1983) Dissociating the determinants of self-stimulation. *Physiol. Behav.* **31**, 787–799.

Atrens D. M., Von Vietinghoff-Riesch F., Der Karabetian A., and Masliyah E. (1974) Modulation of reward and aversion processes in the rat diencephalon by amphetamine. *Am. J. Physiol.* **22**, 874–880.

Baltzer J. H., Levitt R. A., and Furby J. E. (1977) Etorphine and shuttle box self-stimulation in the rat. *Pharmacol. Biochem. Behav.* **7**, 413–416.

Bardo M. T., Miller J. S., and Neiswander J. L. (1984) Conditioned place preference with morphine: The effect of extinction training on the CR. *Pharmacol. Biochem. Behav.* **21**, 545–549.

Barr G. A., Sharpless N. S., Cooper S., Schiff S. R., Paredes W., and Bridger W. H. (1983) Classical conditioning, decay and extinction of cocaine-induced hyperactivity and stereotypy. *Life Sci.* **33**, 1341–1351.

Beninger R. J. (1983) The role of dopamine in locomotor activity and learning. *Brain Res. Rev.* **6**, 173–196.

Beninger R. J. and Hahn B. L. (1983) Pimozide blocks establishment but not expression of amphetamine-produced environment-specific conditioning. *Science* **220**, 1304–1306.

Bower G. H. and Miller N. E. (1958) Rewarding and punishing effects from the same place in the rat's brain. *J. Comp. Physiol. Psychol.* **51**, 669–678.

Bozarth M. A. and Wise R. A. (1981) Intracranial self-administration of morphine into the ventral tegmental area in rats. *Life Sci.* **28**, 551–555.

Britt M. D. and Wise R. A. (1981) Opiate rewarding action: Independence of the cells of the lateral hypothalamus. *Brain Res.* **222**, 213–217.

Carey R. J. (1979) Facilitation of responding for rewarding brain stimulation by a high dose of amphetamine when hyperthermia is prevented. *Psychopharmacology* **61**, 267–271.

Cassens G. P. and Mills A. W. (1973) Lithium and amphetamine: Opposite effects on threshold of intracranial reinforcement. *Psychopharmacologia* **30**, 283–290.

Cassens G., Actor C., Kling M., and Schildkraut J. (1981) Amphetamine withdrawal: Effects on threshold of intracranial reinforcement. *Psychopharmacology* **73**, 318–322.

Caudarella M., Campbell K. A., and Milgram N. W. (1982) Differential effects of diazepam (Valium) on brain stimulation reward sites. *Pharmacol. Biochem. Behav.* **16**, 17–21.

Deutsch J. A. (1973) Prolonged rewarding brain-stimulation. *Psych. Learning Motiv.* **7**, 297–311.

De Witte P. (1981) Effect of naloxone on the self-stimulation behaviour of the postero-lateral area of the hypothalamus in rats: Influence of procedural conditions. *Psychopharmacology* **73**, 391–393.

De Witte P. H. and Bruyer R. (1980) Self-stimulation behavior: Methods evaluating intracranial reward and their relations with motivational states. *Physiol. Psychol.* **8**, 386–394.

Domino E. F. and Olds M. E. (1972) Effects of *d*-amphetamine, scopolamine, chlordiazepoxide and diphenylhydantoin on self-stimulation behaviour and brain acetylcholine. *Psychopharmacologia* **23**, 1–16.

Edmonds D. E. and Gallistel C. R. (1974) Parametric analysis of brain-stimulation reward in the rat. III. Effect of performance variables on the reward summation function. *J. Comp. Physiol. Psychol.* **87**, 860–869.

Edmonds D. E. and Gallistel C. R. (1977) Reward versus performance in self-stimulation: Electrode-specific effects of alpha-methyl-*para*-tyrosine on reward in the rat. *J. Comp. Physiol. Psychol.* **91**, 962–974.

Edwards M., Wishik J., and Sinnamon H. M. (1979) Catecholaminergic and cholinergic agents and duration regulation of ICSS in the rat. *Pharmacol. Biochem. Behav.* **10**, 723–731.

Esposito R. and Kornetsky C. (1977) Morphine lowering of self-stimulation thresholds: Lack of tolerance with long-term administration. *Science* **195**, 189–191.

Esposito R. U., Faulkner W., and Kornetsky C. (1979) Specific modulation of brain-stimulation reward by haloperidol. *Pharmac. Biochem. Behav.* **10**, 937–940.

Esposito R. U., Perry W., and Kornetsky C. (1980) Effects of *d*-amphetamine and naloxone on brain-stimulation reward. *Psychopharmacology* **69**, 187–191.

Ettenberg A. (1979) Conditioned taste preferences as a measure of brain stimulation reward in rats. *Physiol. Behav.* **23**, 167–172.

Ettenberg A. and White N. (1978) Conditioned taste preferences in the rat induced by self-stimulation. *Physiol. Behav.* **21**, 363–366.

Ettenberg A., Cinsavich S. A., and White N. (1979) Performance effect with repeated-response measures during pimozide-produced dopamine receptor blockade. *Pharmacol. Biochem. Behav.* **11**, 557–561.

Ettenberg A., Koob G. F., and Bloom F. E. (1981) Response artifact in the measurement of neuroleptic-induced anhedonia. *Science* **213**, 357–359.

Faustman W., Fowler S., and Walker C. (1981) Time-course of chronic haloperidol and clozapine upon operant rate and duration. *Eur. J. Pharmacol.* **70**, 65–70.

Fibiger H. C. (1978) Drugs and reinforcement mechanisms: A critical review of the catecholamine theory. *Ann. Rev. Pharmacol. Toxicol.* **18**, 37–51.

Fibiger H. C., Carter D. A., and Phillips A. G. (1976) Decreased intracranial self-stimulation after neuroleptics or 6-hydroxydopamine: Evidence for mediation by motor-deficits rather than by reduced reward. *Psychopharmacology* **47**, 21–27.

Fouriezos G. and Wise R. A. (1976) Pimozide-induced extinction of intracranial self-stimulation: Response patterns rule out motor or performance deficits. *Brain Res.* **103**, 377–380.

Fouriezos G., Hansson P., and Wise R. A. (1978) Neuroleptic-induced attenuation of brain-stimulation reward. *J. Comp. Physiol. Psychol.* **92**, 659–669.

Fowler S. C. (1974) Some effects of chlordiazepoxide and

chlorpromazine on response force in extinction. *Pharmacol. Biochem. Behav.* **2,** 155–160.

Franklin K. B. J. (1978) Catecholamines and self-stimulation: Reward and performance effects dissociated. *Pharmacol. Biochem. Behav.* **9,** 813–820.

Franklin K. B. J. and McCoy S. N. (1979) Pimozide-induced extinction in rats: Stimulus control rules out motor deficits. *Pharmacol. Biochem. Behav.* **11,** 71–75.

Gallistel C. R. and Karras D. (1984) Pimozide and amphetamine have opposing effects on the reward summation function. *Pharmacol. Biochem. Behav.* **20,** 73–77.

Glick S. D. and Jerussi T. P. (1974) Spatial and paw preferences in rats: Their relationship to rate-dependent effects of *d*-amphetamine. *J. Pharmacol Exp. Ther.* **188,** 714–725.

Glick S. D., Cox R. S., and Crane A. M. (1975) Changes in morphine self-administration and morphine dependence after lesions of the caudate nucleus in rats. *Psychopharmacologia* **41,** 219–224.

Glick S. D., Weaver L. M., and Meibach R. C. (1980) Lateralization of reward in rats: Differences in reinforcing thresholds. *Science* **207,** 1093–1095.

Glick S. D., Weaver L. M., and Meibach R. C. (1981) Amphetamine enhancement of reward asymmetry. *Psychopharmacology* **73,** 323–327.

Goeders N. E. and Smith J. E. (1983) Cortical dopaminergic involvement in cocaine reinforcement. *Science* **221,** 773–775.

Goudie A. J. (1986) Aversive Stimulus Properties of Drugs: The Conditioned Taste Aversion Paradigm, in *Methods in Experimental Psychopharmacology* (Greenshaw A. J. and Dourish C. T., eds.) Humana, New Jersey.

Grant K. A. and Samson H. H. (1985) Induction and maintenance of ethanol self-administration without food deprivation in the rat. *Psychopharmacology,* **86,** 475–479.

Greenshaw A. J. (1985) Commentary—dopamine and reinforcement: Circling or décalage? *Behav. Brain Sci.* **8,** 175–176.

Greenshaw A. J., Sanger D. J., and Blackman D. E. (1981) The effects of pimozide and of reward omission on fixed-interval behaviour of rats maintained by food and electrical brain stimulation. *Pharmacol. Biochem. Behav.* **15,** 227–233.

Greenshaw A. J., Sanger D. J., and Blackman D. E. (1983) The effects of chlordiazepoxide of the self-regulated duration of lateral hypothalamic stimulation in rats. *Psychopharmacology* **81**, 236–238.

Greenshaw A. J., Sanger D. J., and Blackman D. E. (1985) Effects of *d*-amphetamine and *β*-phenylethylamine on fixed-interval responding maintained by self-regulated electrical hypothalamic stimulation in rats. *Pharmacol. Biochem. Behav.* **23**, 519–523.

Griffiths R. R., Brady J. V., and Bradford D. L. (1979) Predicting the Abuse Liability of Drugs With Animal Drug Self-Administration Procedures: Psychomotor Stimulants and Hallucinogens, in *Advances in Behavioural Pharmacology* vol. 2 (Thompson T. and Dews P. B., eds.), Academic, New York.

Hodos W. and Valenstein E. S. (1962) An evaluation of response rate as a measure of rewarding intracranial stimulation. *J. Comp. Physiol. Psychol.* **55**, 80–84.

Hoebel B. G. (1976) Brain Stimulation Reward and Aversion in the Rat Brain, in *Brain Stimulation Reward* (Wauquier A. and Rolls E. T., eds.), Elsevier, New York.

Hunt G. E., Atrens D., Chesher G. B., and Becker F. T. (1976) alpha-Noradrenergic modulation of hypothalamic self-stimulation: Studies employing clonidine, *l*-phenylephrine and alpha-methyl-*para*-tyrosine. *Eur. J. Pharmacol.* **37**, 105–111.

Hunt G. E., Atrens D., and Johnson G. F. S. (1981) The tetracyclic antidepressant mianserin: Evaluation of its blockade of presynaptic alpha-adrenoceptors in a self-stimulation model using clonidine. *Eur. J. Pharmacol.* **70**, 59–63.

Huston J. P. and Mills A. W. (1971) Threshold of reinforcing brain stimulation. *Commun. Behav. Biol.* **5**, 331–340.

Iversen S. D. (1977) Brain Dopamine Systems and Behaviour, in *Handbook of Psychopharmacology* vol. 8 (Iversen L. L., Iversen S. D., and Snyder S. H., eds.), Plenum, New York.

Johanson C. E. (1978) Drugs as Reinforcers in *Contemporary Research in Behavioral Pharmacology* (Blackman D. E. and Sanger D. J., eds.), Plenum, New York.

Levitt R. A., Baltzer J. H., Evers T. M., Stillwell D. J., and Furby J. E. (1977) Morphine and shuttle-box self-stimulation in the rat: A model for euphoria. *Psychopharmacology* **54**, 307–311.

Liebman J. M. (1983) Discriminating between reward and performance: A critical review of intracranial self-stimulation methodology. *Neurosci. Biobehav. Rev.* **7,** 45–72.

Lyon M. and Randrup A. (1972) The dose-response effect of amphetamine upon avoidance behaviour in the rat seen as a function of increasing stereotypy. *Psychopharmacologia* **23,** 334–347.

Margules D. L. (1966) Separation of positive and negative reinforcing systems in the diencephalon of the rat. *Am. J. Physiol.* **79,** 205–211.

Margules D. L. and Stein L. (1967) Neuroleptics vs. Tranquilizers: Evidence From Animal Studies of Mode and Site of Action, in *Neuro-Psychopharmacology* (Brill H., Cole J. O., Deniker P., Hippius H., and Bradley P. B., eds.), Excerpta Medica Foundation, New York.

Mucha R. F. and Iversen S. D. (1984) Reinforcing properties of morphine and naloxone revealed by conditioned place preferences: A procedural examination. *Psychopharmacology* **82,** 241–247.

Nazzaro J. M. and Gardner E. L. (1980) GABA antagonism lowers self-stimulation thresholds in the ventral tegmental area. *Brain Res.* **189,** 279–283.

Nazzaro J. M., Seeger T. F., and Gardner E. L. (1981) Morphine differentially affects ventral tregmental and substantia nigra brain reward thresholds. *Pharmac. Biochem. Behav.* **14,** 325–331.

Neill D. B. and Justice J. B., Jr. (1981) An Hypothesis for a Behavioral Function of Dopaminergic Transmission in the Nucleus Accumbens, in *The Neurobiology of the Nucleus Accumbens* (Chronister R. B. and de France J. F., eds.), Haer Institute, Brunswick, Maine.

Olds J. (1977) *Drives and Reinforcements: Hypothalamic Studies of Behavioral Function.* Raven Press, New York.

Olds J., Killam K. F., and Bach-y-Rita P. (1956) Self-stimulation of the brain used as a screening method for tranquillizing drugs. *Science* **124,** 265–266.

Olds M. E. (1975) Effects of intraventricular 6-hydroxydopamine and replacement therapy with norepinephrine, dopamine and serotonin on self-stimulation in diencephalic and mesencephalic regions in the rat. *Brain Res.* **98,** 327–342.

Olds M. E. (1966) Facilitatory action of diazepam and chlordiazepoxide on hypothalamic reward behaviour. *J. Comp. Physiol. Psych.* **62,** 136–140.

Olds M. E. (1979) Hypothalamic substrate for the positive reinforcing properties of morphine in the rat. *Brain Res.* **168,** 351–360.

Olds M. E. (1982) Reinforcing effects of morphine in the nucleus accumbens. *Brain Res.* **237,** 429–440.

Olds J. and Milner P. (1954) Positive reinforcement produced by electrical stimulation of septal area and other regions of rat brain. *Physiol. Psychol.* **47,** 419–427.

Olds M. E. and Olds J. (1963) Approach-avoidance analysis of rat diencephalon. *J. Comp. Neurol.* **120,** 259–295.

Olds M. E. and Williams K. N. (1980) Self-administration of *d*-ala-met-enkephalinamide at hypothalamic self-stimulation sites. *Brain Res.* **194,** 155–170.

O'Regan D., Kwok R., Bailey B. A., Yu P. H., and Greenshaw A. J. (1985) Chronic effects of clorgyline and of *l*-deprenyl on rewarding hypothalamic stimulation and regional brain monoamine metabolism in rats. (abstract) *J. Neurochem.* **44,** S92A.

Panksepp J., Gandelman R., and Trowill J. (1970) Modulation of hypothalamic self-stimulation and escape behaviour by chlordiazepoxide. *Physiol. Behav.* **5,** 965–969.

Phillips A. G. and Fibiger H. C. (1979) Decreased resistance to extinction after haloperidol: Implications for the role of dopamine in reinforcement. *Pharmacol. Biochem. Behav.* **10,** 751–768.

Pickens R. and Thompson T. (1971) Characteristics of Stimulant Drug Reinforcement, in *Stimulus Properties of Drugs* (Thompson T. and Pickens R., eds.), Appleton Century Crofts, New York.

Randrup A. and Munkvad J. (1967) Stereotyped activities produced by amphetamine in several animal species and man. *Psychopharmacologia* **11,** 300–310.

Redgrave P. (1978) Modulation of intracranial self-stimulation behaviour by local perfusions of dopamine noradrenaline and serotonin within the caudate nucleus and nucleus accumbens. *Brain Res.* **155,** 277–295.

Reicher M. A. and Holman E. W. (1977) Location preference and flavour aversion reinforced by amphetamine in rats. *Anim. Learn. Behav.* **5**, 333–346.

Roberts W. W. (1958) Both rewarding and punishing effects from stimulation of posterior hypothalamus of cat with same intensity. *J. Comp. Physiol. Psychol.* **51**, 400–407.

Rolls E. T., Kelly P. H., and Shaw S. G. (1974a) Noradrenaline, dopamine and brain stimulation reward. *Pharmacol. Biochem. Behav.* **2**, 735–740.

Rolls E. T., Kelly P. H., Shaw S. G., Woods R. J., and Dale R. (1974b) The relative attenuation of self-stimulation, eating and drinking produced by dopamine receptor blockade. *Psychopharmacology* **38**, 219–230.

Sanger D. J. (1978) Effects of *d*-amphetamine on temporal and spatial discrimination in rats. *Psychopharmacology* **58**, 185–188.

Schaefer G. J. and Holtzman S. G. (1979) Free operant and autotitration brain self-stimulation procedures in the rat: A comparison of drug effects. *Pharmacol. Biochem. Behav.* **10**, 127–135.

Schaefer G. J. and Michael R. P. (1980) Acute effects of neuroleptics on brain self-stimulation thresholds in rats. *Psychopharmacology* **67**, 9–15.

Shannon H. E. and Thompson W. A. (1985) Behavior maintained under fixed-interval and second-order schedules by intravenous injections of endogenous noncatecholic phenylethylamines in dogs. *J. Pharmacacol. Exp. Ther.* **228**, 691–695.

Stein E. A. and Olds J. (1977) Direct intracerebral self-administration of opiates in the rat. *Soc. Neurosci. Abst.* **3**, 302.

Stein L. (1962) An analysis of stimulus-duration preference in self-stimulation of the brain. *J. Comp. Physiol. Psychol.* **55**, 405–414.

Stein L. (1964) Self-stimulation of the brain and the central stimulant action of amphetamine. *Fed. Proc.* **23**, 836–841.

Stein L. and Ray O. S. (1960) Brain stimulation reward "thresholds" self-determined in rats. *Psychopharmacologia* **1**, 251–256.

Stein L. and Seifter J. (1961) Possible mode of antidepressive action of imipramine. *Science* **134**, 286–287.

Stein L. and Wise C. D. (1973) Amphetamine and Noradrenergic Reward Pathways, in *Frontiers in Catecholamine Research* (Usdin E. and Snyder S., eds.), Pergamon, New York.

Sutherland R. J. and Nakajima S. (1980) taste-preferences induced by trains of rewarding lateral hypothalamic stimulation of differing durations. *Physiol. Behav.* **24,** 633–636.

Swerdlow N. R. and Koob G. F. (1984) Restrained rats learn amphetamine-induced locomotion, but not place preference. *Psychopharmacology* **84,** 163–166.

Valenstein E. S. (1964) Problems of measurement and interpretation with reinforcing brain stimulation. *Psychol. Rev.* **71,** 415–437.

Wauquier A. (1976) The Influence of Psychoactive Drugs on Brain Self-Stimulation in Rats: A Review, in *Brain Stimulation Reward* (Wauquier A. and Rolls E. T., eds.), American Elsevier, New York.

Wauquier A. and Niemegeers C. J. E. (1979) A comparison between lick- or lever-pressing contingent reward and the effects of neuroleptics thereon. *Arch. Int. Pharmacodyn. Ther.* **239,** 239–240.

Wauquier A., Clincke G. H. C., and Fransen J. F. (1983) Parameter selection in a rate independent test of brain self-stimulation: Towards an alternative interpretation of drug effects. *Behav. Brain Res.* **7,** 155–164.

White N., Brown Z., and Yachnin M. (1978) Effects of catecholamine manipulations on three different self-stimulation behaviours. *Pharmacol. Biochem. Behav.* **9,** 273–278.

Wise R. A. (1980) Action of drugs of abuse on brain reward systems. *Pharmacol. Biochem. Behav.* **13: 1** Suppl, 213–233.

Wise R. A. (1978a) Catecholamine theories of reward: A critical review. *Brain Res.* **152,** 215–247.

Wise R. A. (1978b) Neuroleptic attenuation of intra-cranial self-stimulation, reward or performance deficits? *Life Sci.* **22,** 535–542.

Wise R. A. (1982) Neuroleptics and operant behavior: The anhedonia hypothesis. *Behav. Brain Sci.* **5,** 39–87.

Wise R. A. and Bozarth M. A. (1982) Action of drugs of abuse on brain reward systems: An update with specific attention to opiates. *Pharmacol. Biochem. Behav.* **11,** 625–629.

Wishart T. B. and Herberg L. J. (1979) Central cholinergic mechanisms in electrical self-stimulation and in drug-induced tremor in rats. *Pharmac. Biochem. Behav.* **11,** 625–629.

Yehuda S. and Wurtman R. (1972) Release of brain dopamine as a probable mechanism for the hyperthermic effect of *d*-amphetamine. *Nature* **240,** 477–478.

Yokel R. A. and Wise R. A. (1975) Increased lever-pressing for amphetamine after pimozide in rats: Implications for a dopamine theory of reward. *Science* **187,** 547–549.

Yokel R. A. and Wise R. A. (1976) Attenuation of intravenous amphetamine reinforcement by central dopamine blockade in rats. *Psychopharmacology* **48,** 311–318.

Zacharko R. M. and Kokkinidis L. (1982) Preference for fixed vs self-selected durations of brain stimulation in rats administered *d*-amphetamine sulphate. *Life Sci.* **30,** 1029–1034.

Zacharko R. M. and Wishart T. B. (1979) Facilitation of self-stimulation with high doses of amphetamine in the rat. *Psychopharmacology* **64,** 247–248.

Zarevics P. and Setler P. (1979) Simultaneous rate-independent and rate-dependent assessment of intracranial self-stimulation: Evidence for the direct involvement of dopamine in brain reinforcement mechanisms. *Brain Res.* **169,** 499–512.

Aversive Stimulus Properties of Drugs

The Conditioned Taste Aversion Paradigm

Andrew J. Goudie

1. Conditioned Taste Aversion

1.1. The Basic Phenomenon

The majority of psychoactive drugs induce conditioned taste aversion (CTA). The basic CTA procedure usually involves pairing ingestion of a novel-tasting fluid with drug injection. Following recovery from the drug studied, subjects are again presented with the novel fluid. Acquisition of CTA is assessed in terms of either a reduced intake of the fluid relative to the preconditioning base-line, or a reduced preference for the drug-paired fluid in a choice procedure. Almost universally, reductions in intake of drug-paired substances have been assumed to be a result of the development of an association between some aversive stimulus property of the drug and the taste of the novel fluid—this being the derivation of the term "conditioned taste aversion." However, as argued elsewhere (Goudie, 1979) and discussed below, *some* conditioned taste aversions may be misnamed phenomena, and there may be little justification for assuming that they involve aversive stimulus properties of drugs (*see* also Stolerman and D'Mello, 1981).

CTA *appears* to be a simple form of associative learning, involving association between a taste (usually termed the conditional stimulus, or CS), and some "aversive" treatment (usually termed the unconditioned stimulus or UCS). Such a learning process should have considerable adaptive value, since subjects can avoid ingestion of foods that may be "toxic." The phenomenon has been reported in a wide range of species, including (among others) the slug, cougar, coyote, hawk, cod, bear, sparrow, magpie, hamster, gerbil, quail, mouse, and rat (Gustavson, 1977). CTA has also been described in humans. On the basis of a self-report questionnaire, Garb and Stunkard (1974) concluded that CTA had developed in 38% of their sample of 696 subjects when illness coincided with food intake. Empirical evidence for CTA in humans was provided by Bernstein (1978) in children receiving chemotherapy for cancer. Subjects received chemotherapy after ingestion of a novel ice cream; they subsequently showed a reduced preference for the ice cream in a choice test compared to a control group that received chemotherapy alone (*see* Bernstein and Webster, 1980, for similar data from adult cancer patients).

CTA has clearly been observed in many species, including man. The ubiquity of the phenomenon is further demonstrated by the fact that the ability to acquire CTA is present very early in ontogeny (Rudy and Cheatle, 1977). There is even remarkable evidence that CTA can be acquired *in utero* (Stickrod et al., 1982).

Despite, or perhaps because of, its apparent simplicity, CTA has been the subject of intensive study over three decades, e.g., Riley and Clarke (1977) listed some 632 articles published since 1950 on various aspects of the phenomenon. In *pharmacological* studies, it has been conclusively demonstrated that the majority of psychoactive agents induce CTA (reviews by Gamzu, 1977; Cappell and Le Blanc, 1977; Stolerman and D'Mello, 1981; Goudie, 1979). However, before discussing relevant psychopharmacological studies, some aspects of CTA methodology are outlined, since methodology can affect the conclusions drawn about the nature of drug-induced CTA.

1.2. Methodology

1.2.1. Single-Bottle Procedures

The procedure used most often in the study of drug-induced CTA is a simple one-bottle test in which subjects are adapted to restricted fluid access followed by one or more pairings of a novel-tasting fluid with drug administration. Drug-taste pairings are usually separated by a few days, to allow adipsic or "toxic" effects to dissipate between conditioning trials. Most studies that use this technique are essentially derived from the early report of Cappell et al. (1973). The basic datum in single-bottle studies is amount of fluid consumed. CTA is assessed in terms of reduced intake relative to changes in intake of controls. A fundamental limitation with this approach lies in the "floor" and "ceiling" effects that constrain fluid intake. Because of "floor" effects, it may be possible to demonstrate *apparent* similarities between subjects treated in different ways if all show maximal suppression of intake; in such circumstances it is possible to detect differences between groups in CTA potency by using an extinction procedure (Elkins, 1974), as described below.

A major factor to consider in using one-bottle tests is the tendency of many species to restrict intake of novel-tasting substances, showing "neophobia" (Domjan, 1975). The magnitude of the neophobic response shown by individual subjects is not predictable *a priori*. In our laboratory, we have repeatedly noted marked individual differences in neophobia. Since subjects differ in extent of neophobia in an unpredictable way, significant differences may exist between groups in preconditioning levels of intake because of chance variations in neophobia. Such differences could confound CTA studies, since the amount of solution consumed may affect potency of conditioning (e.g., Bond and Di Giustio, 1975). There are two potential solutions to this problem. One is to eliminate the effect if it develops by the use of data transformations (e.g., suppression ratios, percentage scores) whose validity may be questionable. An alternative approach is to use large groups of subjects in an attempt to prevent the occurrence of significant differences in preconditioning intakes. The latter strategy has been adopted by many researchers in CTA studies.

A potential interpretative problem for CTA studies raised by the neophobic response is that it dissipates as a consequence of ingestion of the novel fluid. If an appetitive taste (e.g., saccharin) is used, fluid intake in controls may increase above preconditioning levels of water intake. The aversive effects of drug treatments are therefore evaluated against an increasing level of intake in controls. It is therefore possible to demonstrate statistically significant drug-induced CTA in subjects whose intake remains constant or even increases over trials (e.g., Goudie et al., 1978). As shown in Fig. 1, a reduction in intake in *absolute* terms is not a necessary prerequisite for demonstration of drug-induced CTA.

1.2.2. Two-Bottle Procedures

Two-bottle preference tests are more sensitive than one-bottle tests. For example, D'Mello et al. (1977) detected a CTA induced in rats by *d*-amphetamine at 0.1 mg/kg with a two-bottle test administered after repeated one-bottle conditioning trials that failed to detect any CTA. The greater sensitivity of the two-bottle test is a result of the fact that subjects do not need to consume *any* of the fluid that is paired with drug administration to satisfy their thirst. The two-bottle test is also of value in that it controls for drug effects on motivation to drink. Figure 2 shows an example of a dose-related CTA induced by nitrous oxide detected with a two-bottle procedure. However, despite its sensitivity, the two-bottle test suffers from the limitation that, since it is an extinction test, it can only be administered once, unless extinction of CTA is itself being studied. During repeated conditioning trials with a two-bottle test, subjects might develop an aversion to *both* choice substances if each trial was followed by an aversive treatment.

1.2.3. Extinction Procedures

Under some conditions, potent CTA will develop after conditioning so that subjects consume little of the novel fluid in either one or two-bottle tests. Because of such "floor"

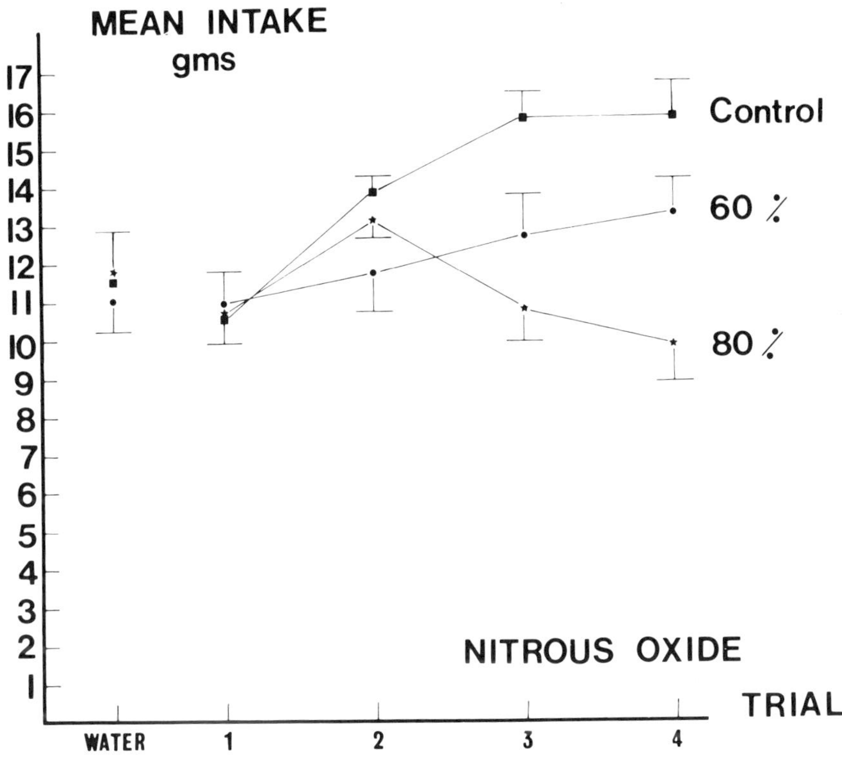

Fig. 1. Nitrous oxide-induced conditioned taste aversion in rats demonstrated with one-bottle tests. Subjects were adapted to a regimen of restricted water access and baseline levels of water intake then recorded (water). Subsequently, subjects in three different experimental groups received repeated conditioning trials in which 0.1% saccharin was paired with concentrations of nitrous oxide between 0 (control), 60, and 80%. Conditioning trials were separated by 2 d of water access. Note the increase in intake seen in controls over trials as a result of the attenuation of neophobia for saccharin, and also the conditioned aversion (relative to controls) seen in subjects treated with 60% nitrous oxide *despite* the fact that these subjects actually increased their fluid intake over trials. Measures of variance shown on the figure are ±SEM (reproduced from Goudie and Dickens, 1978, with permission of the publisher).

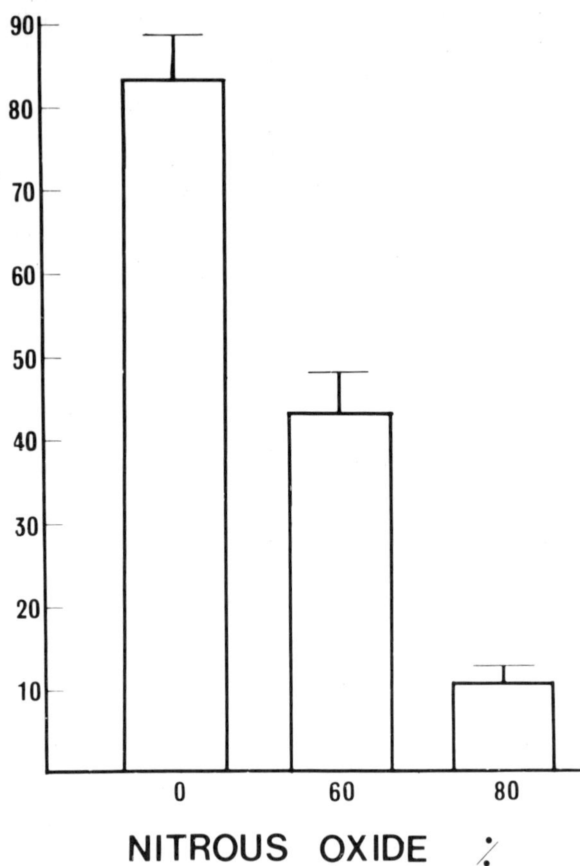

Fig. 2. Nitrous oxide-induced CTA demonstrated with a two-bottle choice test. The mean ±SEM percentage saccharin preference scores are shown for three groups of subjects that had previously received four pairings of the relevant concentration of nitrous oxide gas with 0.1% saccharin prior to a saccharin/water choice test (*see* Fig. 1). Control subjects received 100% oxygen (0% nitrous oxide). A clear dose-related CTA was induced by exposure to nitrous oxide gas (reproduced from Goudie and Dickins, 1978, with permission of the publisher).

effects, it is, by definition, impossible to demonstrate differences between groups showing complete suppression of intake. In these circumstances, an extinction test may well demonstrate differences between groups (Elkins, 1974). A one-bottle test is usually the procedure of choice when studying extinction, because CTA extinction using two-bottle procedures usually develops extremely slowly, since subjects do not have to consume *any* of the averted taste during the extinction tests (Elkins, 1974). Rapid extinction of CTA with a two-bottle test procedure is strong evidence for the existence of very weak CTA (e.g., Greenshaw and Dourish, 1984b) (*see* Fig. 3). However, extinction of CTA with two-bottle test procedures can be facilitated by the use of severe fluid deprivation regimes (Wellman and Boissard, 1981).

1.2.4. Drinkometer Procedures

Drinkometer procedures have been used by relatively few groups in CTA studies (*see* Berger 1972; Coil et al., 1978a; Vogel and Nathan, 1975). The apparent reluctance of researchers to conduct CTA studies with drinkometers may appear surprising, since they allow recording of many aspects of drinking behavior (latency, pattern, number of licks, and so on) allowing more sophisticated behavioral analyses than one- and two-bottle procedures. However, commercially available drinkometers often record licking by passing a current through the animal via the tongue to a metal base on which the animal stands.The passage of current through the tongue, even at very low levels, is a biologically significant event. Rats prefer to lick at a rod associated with current passage than to lick at a nonelectrified rod. This effect ("current licking") can be detected at current intensities as low as 0.5 μA, and rats will lever-press to gain access to an electrified rod (Weijnen, 1972). "Current licking" is probably dependent on taste sensations from the tongue, since lesions of the chorda tympani, which receives afferents from the gustatory receptors of the tongue, abolish the phenomenon (Weijnen, 1972). Thus, drinkometer techniques involving current passage probably modify taste sensations. The possible significance of such effects in CTA studies was demonstrated by Martonyi and Valenstein (1971), who showed that rats were more willing to ingest quinine from a drinkometer when the current was on than when no current flowed. If CTA is mediated by a shift in palatability of the "averted" taste (Garcia et al., 1974; Parker, 1982), *any* effect of current passage on palatability confounds the data to an unknown

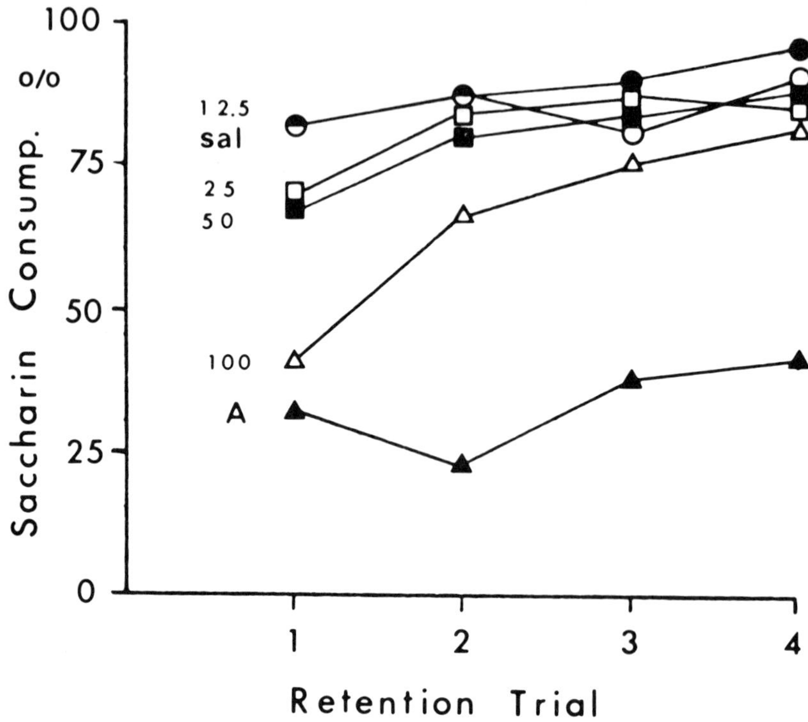

Fig. 3. Extinction of conditioned aversions induced by amphetamine (A) at 2.5 mg/kg and β-phenylethylamine at doses between 12.5 and 100 mg/kg. Also shown are control group data (Sal). The data plotted are saccharin-preference scores (percentages) over four extinction trials after a single pairing of each treatment with saccharin ingestion. Note the complete absence of extinction of amphetamine-induced CTA over the four extinction trials, which contrasts markedly with the very rapid extinction of the aversion induced by a very high (100 mg/kg) dose of phenylethylamine. These data indicate clearly that phenylethylamine is a very weak CTA-inducing agent (reproduced from Greenshaw and Dourish, 1984b, with the permission of authors and publishers).

extent, and may limit the sensitivity of the procedure. Weijnen (1972) even demonstrated that rats injected with cyclophosphamide following water-licking paired with current passage showed an aversion for the water plus current combination in a choice test between water and water plus current. This finding ("current aversion") demonstrates clearly that in CTA studies with many drinkometers, the technique for measuring CTA is inextricably intertwined with the cues utilized in acquiring CTA. A situation that would have delighted Heisenberg! Because of the problems inherent in the use of electrical drinkometers, procedures based upon photobeam interruptions (which do not involve passage of current through the tongue) are the procedures of choice in this area. Such drinkometers are commercially available (Colbourn Instruments, USA).

1.2.5. Operant/Instrumental Procedures

Since most studies of drug-induced CTA have used consummatory licking during CTA acquisition and recall, all such studies have, to some extent, utilized instrumental behaviors (Spiker, 1977). However, we consider here a restricted range of instrumental behaviors—operants such as lever-pressing. There have been relatively few studies of CTA using such techniques. Suppression of lever-pressing by presentation of an "averted" taste following taste/lithium-pairing was reported by Morrison and Collyer (1974). Stolerman and D'Mello (1978a) and D'Mello and Stolerman (1978) reported similar effects with *d*-amphetamine. Subjects maintained on an FR40 or FI60-s schedule of liquid reinforcement showed complete suppression of responding following a single encounter (0.08 mL) with an "averted" flavor when CTA was established on the base-line by pairing response-contingent flavor intake with *d*-amphetamine administration (*see* also Matsuzawa and Hasegawa, 1982). In contrast, Holman (1975) demonstrated that, following training for saccharin on a VI60-s schedule, the establishment of a lithium-induced CTA to saccharin off the base-line failed to affect operant responding in *extinction* tests. These studies might be taken to suggest that "averted" tastes only suppress operant responding when their presentation is contingent on lever-pressing. However, Morrison and Collyer (1974) reported that after VI 3-min training, a *light* stimulus suppressed operant responding for water in *extinction* when the light had previously been paired with a distinctive flavor to which CTA was established on the base-line. The light failed to suppress responding when paired with lithium treatment in the absence of a distinctive flavor cue (i.e., the light associated with the flavor suppressed operant responding provided that the effect of the light was mediated via a taste cue). It is consequently clear that both "averted" flavors and stimuli associated with them can *potentially* suppress operant responding. However, the conditions under which operant responding is suppressed by "averted" tastes remain to be fully delineated. There is evidence (Dickinson et al., 1983) that CTA may have differential effects on behavior maintained by random-interval and random-ratio schedules of reinforcement; the former schedule is resistant to effects of reinforcer "devaluation" by CTA induction off the base-line, an effect seen in both extinction tests and in tests involving response-contingent presentation of the reinforcer. There is also evidence (Hasegawa and Matsuzawa, 1981) that in monkeys, establishing a CTA to a reinforcer off the base-line can induce avoidance of the food in the home cage, but have no effect on key-pressing for the same food on an FR schedule in an operant situation. Thus, CTA may be context specific (*see* Archer et al., 1980, for a context effect in rats). Clearly, the use of operant techniques for assessment of drug-induced CTA should be considered with some caution at present. Inferences drawn about aversive properties of drugs may depend critically on precise experimental parameters.

1.2.6. Conditioned Food Aversions

The majority of studies on drug-induced CTA have involved conditioned fluid as opposed to food aversions. However, there is reliable evidence for the existence of potent conditioned food aversions in rodents (e.g., Bernstein and Goehler, 1983a,b). Bernstein et al. (1983) reported that conditioned food aversions differ from fluid aversions in that they are resistant to interference from novel tastes (presented in *both* foods and fluids) when such tastes are presented during ingestion of the "target" food (i.e., prior to drug treatment). Resistance to associative interference of this type is not seen in *fluid* aversion studies, leading Bernstein et al. (1983) to conclude that:

> *It is possible that foods (and not drinks) are the likely targets that learned taste aversions evolved for ... Whatever the reason, dilute solutions appear to be but a pale imitation of foods ... our results suggest that learning about dilute solutions may reflect only a fraction of the potential potency of taste aversion learning (p. 148).*

If this conclusion is justified, it may be significant for studies of drug-induced CTA that have almost without exception involved fluid intake. The study of drug-induced food aversions may hold considerable promise for the future, particularly for individuals developing sensitive assays for aversive properties of drugs (e.g., behavioral toxicologists).

1.2.7. Conditioned Aversions Acquired Without Ingestion

As noted above, the taste stimulus in CTA studies is typically described as a CS, and the aversion-inducing treatment as a UCS. It is therefore assumed that CTA learning represents an example of classical/Pavlovian conditioning. The CTA procedure certainly does not constitute an operant conditioning procedure (Spiker, 1977), even though operant contingencies are often involved in the measurement of CTA, as described in section 1.2.5. However, studies have demonstrated that CTA can be acquired in the absence of *any* consummatory response, e.g., curarized animals that are, of course, unable to move, have been exposed to forced infusions of a fluid (Domjan and Wilson, 1972). Alternatively, CTA has been acquired when the procedure has involved administering the taste by iv or ip injection in the absence of any drinking behavior (Bradley and Mistretta, 1971; Miceli et al., 1980). Since it is possible to establish CTA in the absence of *any* response, CTA is clearly best classified as a form of Pavlovian conditioning. However, the fact that CTA can be established following injection of the taste CS may be significant for studies of drug-induced CTA, because the drug itself, given as a *putative* UCS, may actually have CS (taste) properties (Miceli et al., 1980; Cunningham, 1978). There is evidence from studies of CTA induced to the taste of orally ingested ethanol that the putative CS (ethanol) can interact pharmacologically with some aversion-inducing UCSs (Zabik and Roache, 1983). The possibility that the aversion-inducing (UCS) treatment may also have CS properties may further complicate interpretation of studies of drug-induced CTA. The putative CS *may* be acting as, or interacting with, the UCS, and vice versa.

1.2.8. *Observational Procedures for Detecting Conditioned Taste Aversions*

Superficially, it may appear rather odd to consider the role of behavioral techniques for detecting CTA, since the obvious way to detect CTA is clearly to measure intake of a fluid or food with a distinctive taste. However, consideration of the nature of CTA learning suggests that observation of behavioral responses to "averted" tastes may not be quite as idiosyncratic as it may, at first sight, appear to be. In conventional classical conditioning paradigms, the acquisition of the conditioned response (CR) is often assessed by measurement of some parameter (size, latency, frequency, and so on) of the CR itself. However, in the CTA paradigm, it is not clear what the UCR and the CR actually are (Goudie, 1979). It has frequently been *assumed* that the CR is conditioned "nausea" or "illness," and the UCS is usually *assumed* to be gastrointestinal "toxicity" or "illness." However, as described below, the conditioned nausea interpretation of CTA is not without its critics. Furthermore, in CTA studies the CR (nausea?) is clearly not measured directly. What *is* measured is some effect of CS/UCS pairings on behavior—usually suppression of drinking. However, there is no strong *a priori* theoretical reason for measuring suppression of drinking rather than any other CR elicited by the taste paired with the drug in question. Thus, insight into the nature of CTA learning might be gained by considering other CRs elicited by tastes paired with putative aversive drug UCSs. For example, Krane (1980) reported that stimuli paired with lithium elicited conditioned defecation in rats. Similarly, Mitchell et al. (1977) argued that, in rats, pica (the consumption of nonnutritive substances) is a species-specific analog of vomiting that provides symptomatic relief from gastric malaise for a species that cannot vomit. They showed that pica is elicited by treatments that induce CTA (including nonpharmacological treatments, such as rotation). Furthermore, Mitchell et al. (1977) showed that if saccharin is paired with lithium or cyclophosphamide, then saccharin presentation alone elicits conditioned pica, an effect attributed to the presence of taste-mediated conditioned illness. Clearly, such examples of noningestive CRs elicited by "averted" CSs support the general notion that CTA is intimately related to gastrointestinal malaise, since the CRs measured (pica and defecation) are linked to the functioning of the gastrointestinal tract. However, recent studies involving other CRs shed doubt on the *universal* validity of this analysis. Berridge et al. (1981) have described distinctive orofacial behavioral responses observed in rats during ingestion of a palatable fluid and rejection of unpalatable quinine solution. The ingestion sequence involves rhythmic movements of the tongue and mouth followed by lateral tongue protrusions. The rejection sequence consists of response components of a gaping mouth, chin-rubbing along the floor, head shaking, and face washing. The ingestion sequence seen after sucrose infusion into the oral cavity was converted into a rejection sequence after sucrose was paired with lithium, *suggesting* that the palatability of sucrose had changed (*see* also Garcia et al., 1974). In a subsequent related study (Pelchat et al., 1983), orofacial CRs to sucrose were studied in rats trained to avoid sucrose either by pairing ingestion with shock (punishment), lithium (CTA), or ingestion of a large quantity of lactose (which causes diarrhea, abdominal cramps, and flatulence in humans). In subjects matched for sucrose avoidance, *only* the group treated with lithium showed the characteristic quinine-like CR of gaping and chin-rubbing following sucrose ingestion. The two other groups showed a typical ingestion response to sucrose. The authors concluded that food rejection can be based on either distaste (as in the lithium-treated subjects who showed quinine-like CRs) or on anticipated danger (as in the two other groups); avoidance based on anticipated danger is not associated with a palatability shift for the taste. The significant finding in the present context is that the CR to lactose was different from that to lithium, despite the fact that both substances caused avoidance of sucrose. In a related independent study, Parker (1982) reported that orofacial CRs elicited by saccharin following pairing with amphetamine and lithium differed markedly. Although both drugs induced equipotent strong CTA, *only* the lithium-paired subjects showed the chin-rub CR previously described as part of the typical orofacial rejection sequence for unpalatable flavors. Parker (1982) concluded that only lithium-induced CTA was mediated by an acquired shift in the palatability of the taste. Thus, reliable evidence has been provided for the existence of *qualitatively* different types of CTA. The existence of such a qualitative distinction between CTA induced by different drugs *has* been hypothesized before (Amit et al., 1977; Riley and Zellner, 1978; Riley et al., 1978; Goudie, 1979). However, these data provide the first empirical evidence in support of the assumed distinction between CTA induced by gross toxins (e.g., lithium) and by other types of drugs. An extension of work in this area should be important from the pharmacological viewpoint, providing a classification of drug-induced CTA into those drugs whose avoidance is based on distaste (e.g., lithium) and those whose avoidance is based on anticipated danger (e.g., amphetamine). These findings provide strong support for the idea that CTA measurement in terms of amounts of solution drunk alone (as has typically been the case in pharmacologically oriented studies) is insensitive to differences that may exist between different types of CTA (Pelchat et al., 1983). A strong case can therefore be made for the use of multiple indices in the measurement of drug-induced CTA. To date, work in this area has neglected this question almost completely.

2. Conditioned Taste Aversion: A Measure of Toxicity?

2.1. Drugs That Induce CTA: Are They All Toxins?

The majority of early studies on CTA involved treatments with known toxic effects in humans, such as radiation and lithium or cyclophosphamide injection. Such studies were initiated in the belief that CTA was induced by "illness" or "malaise" (e.g., Garcia et al., 1967). For example, Nachman and colleagues (1970) reported that pairing saccharin or ethanol intake with *p*-chlorophenylalanine injection resulted in CTA to the relevant fluid. They suggested that:

> *The degree of 'unpleasantness' of a drug may be determined on the basis of whether or not the drug produces a learned aversion. Thus the behaviour of the animal may yield a more sensitive bioassay than other toxicological or pharmacological procedures (p. 1246).*

Berger (1972) subsequently reported that scopolamine, chlorpromazine, and lorazepam also induced potent CTA. However, since *these* drugs were effective at doses that did not elicit overt toxicity, Berger (1972) argued that sickness was not a necessary condition for CTA, a conclusion that contrasted with earlier analyses. To this day, the role of "nausea/sickness/illness" in CTA remains a subject of controversy, as discussed below.

The range of drugs that has subsequently been shown to induce CTA is broad, including virtually all types of drugs. Goudie (1979) noted that among drugs effective in the CTA paradigm were barbiturates and benzodiazepines; cannabis, cannabidiol, and Δ^9 THC; ethanol and acetaldehyde; histamine and antihistamines, amphetamine, methylphenidate, cocaine and related psychostimulants; cholinergics and anticholinergics; caffeine; fenfluramine; morphine, naloxone, and other narcotic agonists and antagonists; nitrous oxide and other anesthetics. CTA had also been reported with drugs that penetrate the blood–brain barrier poorly (e.g., *p*-hydroxyamphetamine, methylscopolamine, and methylatropine), and even with nontoxic nutrients such as glucose (*see* references in

Goudie, 1979). As long ago as 1977, Cappell and Le Blanc argued that further demonstrations of drug-induced CTA with novel drugs were essentially trivial unless directed at analyzing mechanisms involved in CTA, since it was obvious that drugs with very different pharmacological properties induced CTA. However, the number of agents reported to induce CTA continues to grow. Recent reports have extended the range of effective drugs to include phencyclidine and ketamine (Etscorn and Parsons, 1979), cathinone (Foltin and Schuster, 1981), carbamazapine (Smith, 1983), nicotine (Etscorn, 1980), bupropion and amitriptyline (Miller and Miller, 1983), 5-hydroxytryptophan (Zabik and Roache, 1983), phenylpropanolamine (Wellman et al., 1981), and hydralazine and other hypotensive agents (Kresel and Barofsky, 1979).

In recent years there has also been a tendency for the CTA paradigm to be used in behavioral toxicology. Recent studies indicate that the following "toxic" agents induce CTA: chloroform (Landeaur et al., 1982), lead (Dantzer, 1980), tin (Leander and Gau, 1980), the pesticide chlordimeform (Macphail and Leander, 1980), the neurotoxin acrylamide (Anderson et al., 1982), the herbicide 2,4,5-trichlorophenoxyacetic acid (Sjoden et al., 1979), physostigmine (Parker et al., 1982), the carcinogen aflatoxin B_1 (Rappold et al., 1984), and toluene (Miyagawa et al., 1984). Almost without exception, these studies report that CTA is induced by "toxic" agents at low doses with no effect in other tests such as operant behavior, rotarod screening, open field behavior, and so on. However, the interpretation of CTA as a sensitive index of toxicity that appears in the absence of other behavioral signs is essentially irrefutable, since: "It accounts for CTA by means of effects that can be inferred only from the phenomenon they purport to explain" (Stolerman and D'Mello, 1981, p. 164). Although most drugs induce CTA, the interpretation of the effect remains unclear. Some authors (e.g., Dantzer, 1980; Leander and Gau, 1980) suggest that the demonstration of CTA is sufficient evidence of a "toxic" drug effect. In contrast, as noted above, other authors (e.g., Gamzu, 1977; Goudie, 1979) have argued that the phenomenon cannot be attributed simply to "toxicity." Even authors working with "toxic" agents such as chloroform, acrylamide, and toluene have noted that the mechanism by which toxins induce CTA is unclear (Anderson et al., 1982; Landaeur et al., 1982; Miyagawa et al., 1984). This controversy clearly begs the question as to what exactly a "toxic" drug effect is. However, there is no simple answer to this question; *any* drug effect on behavior can be considered to be caused by "toxicity." For example, Klauenberg and Sparber (1983) suggest that the well-known ability of amphetamine to suppress Fixed Ratio responding is a "toxic" effect. In a major review of behavioral toxicology, Evans and Weiss (1978) suggested that a principle feature of behavioral toxicology (which differentiated it from behavioral pharmacology) arose "from the type of compound studied (environmental contaminants versus drugs and neurochemical tools)." These authors also suggested that CTA was a useful way of obtaining evidence of toxicity. Clearly, Evans and Weiss (1978) consider that a demonstration of CTA is sufficient *in itself* to demonstrate a "toxic" effect, despite the fact that it is possible to induce CTA with drug doses that are routinely used in more conventional psychopharmacology and with many drugs that they do not consider to be the *type* of agent usually studied in toxicology. The "toxicity" interpretation of CTA continues therefore to be influential and is increasingly prevalent in behavioral toxicology. However, there are many arguments against the "toxicity" interpretation. Since these have been addressed in detail before (Cappell and LeBlanc, 1975, 1977; Goudie, 1979), they are only briefly outlined in Table 1.

The arguments against the "toxicity" interpretation of CTA clearly have considerable weight. However, it is impossible to refute the hypothesis that "toxicity" mediates CTA since "toxicity" is a vague concept with no general operational definition. Nevertheless, the "toxicity" interpretation of CTA is strengthened by evidence, discussed below, that relates CTA to neural systems that mediate nausea and vomiting, since such actions would probably be universally considered "toxic" effects.

Table 1
Arguments Against the Toxicity Interpretation of
Drug-Induced Conditioned Taste Aversion

Gross behavioral measures of "illness" induced by different agents (e.g., ataxia, seizures, stereotypy, stimulation, sedation, diarrhea) do not predict the potency of conditioned aversions (Nachman and Hartley, 1975; Barker et al., 1977; Greenshaw and Dourish, 1984b).

Some grossly "toxic" agents fail to induce conditioned aversions at high doses (30–50% of the LD_{50}) e.g., gallamine, malonate, cyanide, and strychnine (Nachman and Hartley, 1975; Ionescu and Buresova, 1977).

Many drugs induce conditioned aversions at very low doses that are not usually considered "toxic", e.g., *d*-amphetamine is effective at a dose as low as 0.1 mg/kg in rats (D'Mello et al., 1977; Sanger et al., 1980).

Some drugs (e.g., chlordiazepoxide, ethanol) induce conditioned aversions at doses that increase rates of operant responding and increase food intake (Cappell and Le Blanc, 1975). Such behavioral effects are not usually considered toxic.

Drugs (e.g., amphetamine, morphine) can induce conditioned aversions at doses that are positively reinforcing in other procedures (Wise et al., 1976; Switzman et al., 1978; Sherman et al., 1980; Van der Kooy et al., 1983).

Humans receiving chemotherapy for cancer acquire conditioned aversions in the absence of subjective reports of nausea and vomiting (Bernstein and Webster, 1980).

Qualitatively different types of conditioned aversions may exist. Some of these do not appear to be associated with nausea or a shift in the palatability of the averted taste (Parker, 1982; Pelchat et al., 1983).

2.2. *Conditioned Aversions: An Analog of Nausea and Vomiting?*

Coil et al. (1978b) suggested that, in the rat, the systems mediating CTA are functionally related to those mediating nausea and vomiting in species that, unlike the rat, can vomit.

Sectioning the vagus nerve (which carries afferents from the gut to the medullary "vomiting center") blocks CTA induced by the gastric irritant $CuSO_4$ given ip or intragastrically. However, this effect is not seen when $CuSO_4$ is given iv. Coil et al. (1978b) therefore argued that two separate systems mediate CTA: a vagal afferent system responsive to peripheral irritants and a circulatory system that detects toxins via the area postrema, the medullary chemoreceptive trigger zone for vomiting (Borison and Wang, 1953).The effects of vagotomy that Coil et al. (1978b) observed on CTA in rats are similar to the effects of vagotomy on vomiting in other species, suggesting that CTA and nausea/vomiting are functionally related. In support of this analysis, Coil et al. (1978a) reported that in rats, CTA recall is antagonized by pretreatment with antiemetic drugs that were considered to block CTA because they inhibited *conditioned* nausea. The analysis outlined by Coil et al. (1978a,b) is clearly elegant and strongly supported by their data. However, it has since become clear that this analysis will not account for all examples of CTA. We summarize below evidence in support of and against this analysis.

2.2.1. Supportive Evidence

A number of reports indicate that area postrema lesions antagonize CTA acquisition. Antagonistic effects have been reported (Coil and Norgren, 1981) following treatment with iv, but not intragastric, $CuSO_4$ (as predicted by the two systems analysis); following injection of histamine, lithium, and methylscopolamine (Ritter et al., 1980; McGlone et al., 1980; Rabin et al., 1983), and following radiation treatment (Ossenkopp, 1983a; Rabin et al., 1983). These reports all support the analysis of Coil et al. (1978a,b) by demonstrating that lesions of the area postrema, the chemoreceptive trigger zone for vomiting induced by blood-borne toxins, antagonize the effects of various treatments that induce CTA.

2.2.2. Contrary Evidence

Berger et al. (1973) and Ritter et al. (1980) both reported that area postrema lesions in rats blocked the action of methylscopolamine in the CTA paradigm (presumably by an action on methylscopolamine's effects via the circulatory route on the area postrema, since this drug does not penetrate the blood–brain barrier). However, such lesions did not antagonize amphetamine-induced CTA. Amphetamine-induced CTA is probably predominantly mediated by a direct central effect of the drug (Booth et al., 1977; Roberts and Fibiger, 1975; Lorden et al., 1980; Wagner et al., 1981; Wellman et al., 1981; although, *see* Greenshaw and Buresova, 1982). Therefore, if amphetamine CTA is centrally mediated and unaffected by area postrema lesions, it cannot induce CTA by either of the two pathways to the vomiting center postulated by Coil et al. (1978a,b).

Further evidence against Coil et al.'s (1978a,b) analysis is provided by the finding that radiation-induced CTA in humans develops without subjective reports of nausea (Bernstein and Webster, 1980). Furthermore, two independent extensive studies (Goudie et al., 1982; Rabin and Hunt, 1983) failed to replicate Coil et al.'s (1978a) report that antiemetic drugs block CTA recall. Similarly, Cairnie and Leach (1982) reported that at high doses the antiemetic domperidone did not block the acquisition of radiation-induced CTA. The general link between nausea/vomiting and CTA is therefore tenuous. In support of this conclusion, Kumar et al. (1983) noted that nicotine-induced CTA in rats in antagonized by mecamylamine, but *not* by hexamethonium, the latter being an anticholinergic that acts only peripherally. These data indicate that nicotine-induced CTA is centrally mediated, but that nicotine does not act via mechanisms mediating nausea/vomiting, since hexamethonium antagonizes the emetic effect of nicotine in species that can vomit, presumably by an action at the area postrema (Kumar et al., 1983).

Other reports suggest that the functions of the area postrema may extend beyond that of mediating vomiting. Ossenkopp (1983b) reported that area postrema lesions in rats (which blocked methylscopolamine-induced CTA) actually *potentiated* rotation-induced CTA. Furthermore, Van der Kooy et al. (1983) reported that area postrema lesions (which again blocked methylscopolamine-induced CTA) did not antagonize apomorphine-induced CTA—an effect considered "particularly surprising" by these authors, since apomorphine-induced vomiting in dogs is blocked by area postrema lesions (Borison and Wang, 1953). These two reports are clearly difficult to reconcile with Coil et al.'s (1978a,b) analysis of CTA. The *may* be related to the finding (Edwards and Ritter, 1981) that area postrema lesions cause hyperphagia for palatable, but not for unpalatable, foods, reflecting a possible hypersensitivity to sensory qualities of foods. If some, but not all, examples of CTA are mediated by a shift in the palatability of the taste (Pelchat et al., 1983; Parker, 1982), the effects of area postrema lesions may depend upon the *qualitative* nature of the CTA (i.e., whether or not it is mediated by a palatability shift). Such interactions may account for some of the complexity in the literature on effects of area postrema lesions on CTA acquisition.

Data obtained from studying the effects of vagotomy are equally contentious as they relate to Coil et al.'s (1978a,b) analysis. Thus, Martin et al. (1978) failed to detect any effect of vagotomy on drug-induced CTA. Furthermore, Bernstein and Goehler (1983a) reported that vagotomy *itself* causes conditioned aversion to novel foods. Thus, somewhat ironically, the vagus nerve cannot be the only source of afferent information mediating CTA, since sectioning the vagus itself causes CTA mediated presumably by a nonvagal neural mechanism. At the very least, the overall pattern of data is not sufficiently clear to allow conclusions such as those of Kiefer et al. (1980), who suggested that because vagotomy did not block ethanol-induced CTA, ethanol must be acting in the CTA paradigm via the area postrema as a blood-borne toxin.

2.2.3. Limitations of the Coil et al. (1978a,b) Analysis and Their Implications

Clearly, the analysis put forward by Coil et al. (1978a,b) relating CTA to nausea/vomiting cannot account for *all* the available data. However, much of the data is in accord with predictions from the analysis (e.g., the general pattern of effects of area postrema lesions on CTA acquisition). To attempt to clarify some of the confusion at present prevailing, we suggest that the activation of mechanisms involved in nausea/vomiting is probably a sufficient but *not* necessary condition for a treatment to be effective in inducing CTA (*see* also Bernstein and Webster, 1980). This conclusion is easily reconciled with data suggesting that qualitatively different types of CTA may exist (Parker, 1982), since some, but not all, examples of CTA may be mediated by mechanisms related to nausea/vomiting.

The conclusion that nausea/emesis is a sufficient but not necessary condition for CTA induction has implications for behavioral toxicologists using the CTA paradigm, since it removes much of the face validity of the procedure. If a drug induces CTA, and if this effect is not necessarily related to actions on emetic systems, the significance of the finding is unclear. For example, if constituents of tap water induce CTA at relatively low doses in animals (Landaeur et al., 1982), does this imply that the CTA-inducing "toxin" may cause nausea/vomiting and should be removed from tap water? Since the mechanism involved in the acquired aversion is not known, there can be no simple answer to this question. Effectively, all that a positive finding indicates to the behavioral toxicologist is that the "toxin" induces CTA!

3. The "Paradox" of Conditioned Aversion Induced by Self-Administered Drugs: Attempted Theoretical Solutions

One major finding that promoted interest in CTA was an early report (Cappell and Le Blanc, 1971) that *d*-amphetamine induced CTA in rats at doses that are self-administered in operant procedures. Later studies demonstrated similar "paradoxical" effects with barbiturates and morphine. The clearest way to conceptualize this apparent "paradox" is to suggest that rather than inducing CTA, self-administered drugs should induce conditioned preferences. Such preferences can be conditioned by pairing tastes with alleviation of vitamin deficiency (Zahorik, 1977), or with reinforcing intracranial self-stimulation (Ettenberg et al., 1979). However, although it is possible to condition taste preferences with these procedures, all attempts to induce robust preferences with drugs have failed. In a recent report (Sherman et al., 1983), ethanol at low doses induced a robust conditioned taste preference in food-deprived rats, which was shown to be caused by the caloric properties of ethanol rather than by ethanol-induced intoxication, supporting the conclusion that is is very difficult to obtain *drug*-induced conditioned preferences. There have been occasional reports (e.g., Marfaing-Jallat and Le Magnen, 1979) of very weak (nonsignificant) conditioned preferences induced in subjects undergoing withdrawal when drug injections that alleviated withdrawal are paired with ingestion of a novel-tasting fluid. However, withdrawal from a variety of drugs itself induces CTA (e.g., Pilcher and Stolerman, 1976), and the available data indicate unequivocally that although drug injections given during withdrawal protect against withdrawal-induced CTA, they do not produce conditioned preferences (Crawford and Baker, 1982). Since alleviation of withdrawal does not produce reliable evidence for conditioned taste preferences, it is perhaps not surprising that preferences cannot be conditioned in drug-naive subjects.

The "paradoxical" nature of drug-induced CTA has recently surfaced in a somewhat different form than originally conceptualized. Specifically, it has been reported that drugs can induce CTA and "paradoxical" conditioned place preferences at the same doses (Van der Kooy et al., 1983). If the self-administration paradigm and the place-preference paradigm are functionally equivalent (which at present remains unclear), then the finding that drugs induce CTA and "paradoxical" conditioned place preferences is to be expected on the basis of previous reports of "paradoxical" self-administration of CTA-inducing drugs.

It is clear, therefore, that drugs can possess both reinforcing and aversive properties at the same doses. Attempts to resolve the "paradox" of drug-induced CTA (or the "paradox" of drug self-administration) have been initiated in the belief that it should be possible to isolate variables that determine why drugs have one type of reinforcing effect in one procedure and an *apparently* opposite type of reinforcing effect in other procedures (Stolerman and D'Mello, 1981). If such variables could be isolated, our understanding of factors controlling drug self-administration might be enhanced. We describe below some theoretical analyses of this "paradox."

Vogel and Nathan (1975) suggested that a critical distinction between the self-administration and CTA procedures lay in the subject's control over drug intake in the former procedure, which is absent in the latter. Control over intracranial self-stimulation can determine whether or not such stimulation is reinforcing or aversive (Steiner et al., 1969). Vogel and Nathan (1975) suggested, therefore, that in the CTA procedure, drug effects are aversive because subjects do not control drug intake. However, this analysis is refuted by studies that have shown: (1) that tastes presented prior to sessions in which rats self administer apomorphine become "averted" (Wise et al., 1976); (2) that noncontingent (experimenter-administered) injections both reinforce place preference and induce CTA (Reicher and Holman, 1977); and (3) that non-contingent morphine injections both reinforce maze-running and simultaneously induce CTA to food consumed in the goalbox (White et al., 1977).

A second potential difference between the CTA and the self-administration paradigms lies in the route of drug administration. The self-administration procedure typically (but not always) involves iv drug injections, whereas the CTA procedure typically involves ip injections. Coussens (1974) and Wise et al. (1976) demonstrated that iv amphetamine is less potent in inducing CTA than ip amphetamine. However, iv injections still induced CTA at self-administered doses, so that route of drug administration does not dissociate reinforcing from aversive effects of amphetamine. Large variations in dose also do not dissociate these effects. D'Mello et al. (1977) demonstrated that although *d*-amphetamine induced CTA in rats at doses between 0.1 and 1.0 mg/kg, lower doses did not induce *either* conditioned aversion *or* preference.

The potential role of exteroceptive stimuli acting as secondary reinforcers has also been studied in the CTA paradigm (D'Mello et al., 1977), since stimuli paired with drug administration can themselves be potent reinforcers of operant behavior related to drug self-administration (Goldberg et al., 1975). However, presenting flavors in a distinct spatial location fails to affect CTA acquisition when amphetamine is administered following flavor ingestion, suggesting that the "paradox" cannot be explained in terms of a lack of secondary reinforcing stimuli in the CTA procedure. This hypothesis also seems implausible in the light of evidence that under some circumstances exteroceptive stimuli paired with drug injections acquire marked *aversive* rather than reinforcing properties (Glowa and Barrett, 1983).

A further factor differentiating CTA and self-administration procedures lies in the type of response involved. The former procedure usually involves consummatory licking, whereas the latter typically involves an operant such as lever-pressing. However, as discussed above (section 1.2.5), flavor/drug pairings can suppress operant behavior maintained by flavor presentation in the same way that flavor/drug pairings suppress consummatory licking. Thus, the "paradoxical" nature of CTA cannot be explained in terms of the different types of responses required in the two procedures.

Yet another explanation of the "paradox" is based on the idea that drug-induced CTA may not actually be caused by aversive drug states at all! Reductions in fluid intake observed after taste/drug pairing might be caused by conditioned anorectic or adipsic effects of the drug elicited by food or flavor presentation (Carey, 1978). However, the "conditioned anorexia/adipsia" hypothesis of CTA is clearly inadequate. Studies with amphetamine and related compounds indicate that the hypodipsic potencies of these compounds do *not* correlate with their CTA potency (Stolerman and D'Mello, 1981; Foltin and Schuster, 1981).

An alternative attempt to explain the paradox centers on the idea that pharmacokinetic factors may dissociate aversive and reinforcing effects of drugs (Goudie and Dickins, 1978; Switzman et al., 1981). Cappell and Le Blanc (1977) suggested that short-acting drugs (e.g., cocaine) were relatively ineffective in inducing CTA. Goudie and Dickins (1978) subsequently demonstrated that the efficacy in the CTA procedure of inhalation of the anesthetic nitrous oxide (which is believed to equilibrate with brain tissue within minutes), was proportional to duration of exposure to the gas. Goudie and Dickins (1978) suggested that rapid-onset "state changes" induced by many drugs might be positively reinforcing and selectively associated (Garcia and Koelling, 1966) with short duration operant responses involved in procedures used to assess reinforcing effects of drugs (e.g., lever-pressing or maze-running). In contrast, drug intoxication that is maintained over extended time periods may be aversive and, because of its long duration, should be selectively associated with the long-duration interoceptive stimuli presumed to be involved in food-aversion conditioning (Testa and Ternes, 1977). Unfortunately, the empirical evidence relevant to this analysis is difficult to evaluate conclusively at present. Switzman et al. (1981) reported that although heroin is more potent than morphine in inducing *analgesia,* it is much less potent in the CTA procedure, a finding attributed to heroin's rapid onset of action, in accord with Goudie and Dickins' (1978) analysis. Also in support of this analysis are data that indicate that prolonging the duration of the action of cocaine (Foltin et al., 1981) or lithium (Domjan et al., 1981) by giving divided drug doses separated by some minutes, enhances the aversive action of these drugs compared to that seen when a single large dose is given after fluid intake (although *see* D'Mello et al., 1981). However, other data are not easily reconciled with the analysis proposed by Goudie and Dickins (1978). D'Mello et al. (1981) compared the aversive potencies of apomorphine and cocaine with long-acting derivatives of each parent compound, and reported that prolonging the duration of action of cocaine and apomorphine did not result in increased potency in the CTA procedure that could be attributed to prolonged duration of drug action. Greenshaw and Dourish (1984b) reported that β-phenylethylamine (PEA) only induces a weak CTA at near-lethal doses. Superficially, these data might appear to support the duration-of-action hypothesis, since PEA is very rapidly metabolized by MAO type B and has a half-life of only a few minutes. However, prolonging the duration of action of PEA by either deuterium substitution (Dourish et al., 1983) or inhibition of MAO type B with deprenyl (Greenshaw and Dourish, 1984a) both failed to enhance PEA-induced CTA. Further evidence against the analysis of Goudie and Dickins (1978) is provided by the data of Sherman et al. (1980), who analyzed the effects of altering the injection to conditioning interval in a paradigm involving simultaneous conditioned-place preference and taste-aversion conditioning. Temporal factors failed to dissociate the aversive (CTA) and reinforcing (place-preference) actions of amphetamine, as predicted by Goudie and Dickins' (1978) analysis. However, the relevance of these data to Goudie and Dickins' (1978) analysis depends upon the assumption that the conditioned place-preference and self-administration procedures are functionally equivalent measures of reinforcing effects of drugs. At present this is not established. For example, although it is known that ethanol is self-administered in operant procedures (Smith et al., 1977), the actions of ethanol in the conditioned place-preference paradigm have to date generally proved negative, i.e., the drug induces place aversion (Cunningham, 1979, 1981; Sherman et al., 1983).

Although the jury remains out on the validity of Goudie and Dickins' (1978) explanation of the paradox, sufficient evidence exists that does *not* support their analysis for it to be considered questionable at present (*see* also, Goudie and Newton, 1985).

An alternative approach to the paradox is to try to differentiate neurochemical systems mediating reinforcing and aversive actions of drugs. Many reports implicate catecholaminergic systems in CTA acquisition following treatment with drugs such as ethanol, morphine, and amphetamine (Goudie, 1979). For example, on the basis of studies with icv 6-hydroxydopamine (6-OHDA), Wagner et al. (1981) demonstrated that central dopaminergic systems mediate methamphetamine-induced, but not lithium-induced, CTA. Dopaminergic systems in the brain have frequently been implicated in reinforcement processes (Wise, 1982), and they also appear to play an important role in at least some examples of drug-induced CTA. However, one report (Van der Kooy et al.,

1983) has provided some evidence for a dissociation of the neurochemical systems mediating reward and CTA. Bilateral 6-OHDA lesions of the nucleus accumbens had no effect on apomorphine-induced CTA in rats, but *potentiated* apomorphine-induced place preference (which may be a reliable measure of apomorphine's reinforcing effect). It is *possible* that an extension of this work may dissociate the neuroanatomical systems mediating reward and aversion, and thus at least partially resolve the "paradox" of CTA induced by reinforcing drugs.

However, it is clear that attempts to explain the "paradoxical" nature of drug-induced CTA have not been very successful to date (*see* also, Stolerman and D'Mello, 1981). Studies that demonstrate that drug injections have both reinforcing effects and aversive effects in the same subjects in the same experimental sessions (Wise et al., 1976; White et al., 1977; Switzman et al., 1978; Reicher and Holman, 1977; Sherman et al., 1980) suggest that it may prove difficult, and perhaps impossible, to dissociate the reinforcing and aversive effects of drugs at any level of analysis.

Since the paradox of CTA induced by self-administered drugs has not been resolved, some authors have suggested that demonstrations of CTA with self-administered drugs may not really be paradoxical at all (Gamzu, 1977; Cappell and LeBlanc, 1977). Gamzu (1977) argued that drugs have many different behavioral effects, suggesting that any drug can have different effects on different types of behavior. This argument is not contentious, since an axiom of contemporary psychopharmacology is the idea that drug effects depend upon the type of behavior studied. However, Gamzu's (1977) explanation of the paradox is really no more than a denial of it. He fails to suggest any variable(s) that might determine why drugs have one type of reinforcing effect in one situation and an apparently opposite type of effect in another. Cappell and Le Blanc (1977) have taken a similar position to Gamzu (1977), suggesting that the behavioral effects of reinforcing stimuli depend upon a subject's reinforcement history, the schedule of reinforcement currently operative, and so on. They cite, as an example of this principle, behavior maintained by shock presentation (Morse and Kelleher, 1977).

However, Cappell and Le Blanc (1977) also fail to suggest any critical variable(s) that differentiate the CTA and self-administration procedures. In the case of shock-maintained responding, a past history of shock avoidance is usually necessary for subjects to show the effect (Morse and Kelleher, 1977); consequently, the subject's past history is a variable that partially "explains" shock-maintained responding. In the case of CTA, it is difficult to isolate any similar factor. The suggestion (Gamzu, 1977; Cappell and Le Blanc, 1977) that CTA induced by self-administered drugs is not really paradoxical seems to raise as many questions as it answers. Furthermore, more recent reports from authors working with the place-preference procedure for measuring reinforcing effects of drugs indicate clearly that it *is* still considered paradoxical that a drug induces both place preference and CTA (Van der Kooy et al., 1983). Nevertheless, the possibility that the paradox is more apparent than real merits consideration. The paradox is related to (generally unstated) fundamental *assumptions* about hedonistic factors implicated in reinforcement processes. It is often implicitly assumed that drug self-administration is maintained by euphoric or positive hedonic effects of drugs of abuse. This assumption is questionable, simply because reinforcement is defined operationally in terms of response frequency. It is also generally assumed that CTA learning involves an association between a taste and a dysphoric (negative hedonic) drug effect. This assumption may also be questionable, as highlighted by evidence that there may exist qualitatively different types of CTA (Parker, 1982). It is possible that some examples of CTA learning are misnamed phenomena, and that they do not necessarily involve *aversive* stimulus properties of drugs (*see* also Goudie, 1979). Clearly, if it is suggested that self-administration is not necessarily mediated by euphoriant drug effects, *and* that CTA is not necessarily mediated by dysphoric drug effects, then the paradox of drug-induced CTA conveniently disappears, although this resolution of the "paradox" may well appear rather too convenient!

The discussion above about the paradoxical nature of drug-induced CTA serves to highlight the poverty of our understanding of what a conditioned aversion is; just as the discussion of the methodology of CTA testing (section 1.2) highlights the complexity of the *apparently* simple (unitary) phenomenon of CTA. It is abundantly clear that CTA remains a poorly understood phenomenon, a point that is emphasized by controversy over the *pharmacological* specificity of the CTA procedure, which is discussed below.

4. Pharmacological Specificity of the Taste-Aversion Procedure

Rondeau et al. (1981) suggested that the CTA procedure is a good method for screening and classifying psychoactive agents because it is relatively simple and can be rapidly executed. This argument presupposes that the procedure shows substantial pharmacological specificity. However, as noted above (section 2.2) there has been a general tendency for workers investigating CTA to assume that drugs induce CTA by causing "nausea"/"malaise," which is generally presumed to be a nonspecific effect. In contrast, in some studies a degree of pharmacological specificity has been reported, since the actions of different drugs have been shown to be pharmacologically dissociated. We outline below evidence for and against the idea that drug-induced CTA shows pharmacological specificity.

4.1. Demonstrations of Drug-Specific Effects

Goudie et al. (1975) reported that pretreatment with the catecholamine-depleting agent alpha-methyltyrosine attenuated amphetamine-, but not lithium-induced, CTA. A similar effect was reported by Roberts and Fibiger (1975) after intraventricular treatment with 6-hydroxydopamine (6-OHDA). Similarly, Wagner et al. (1981) reported that depletion of central dopamine by intraventricular injection of 6-OHDA blocked methamphetamine-, but not lithium-induced, CTA. Such data indicate clearly that amphetamine-induced CTA is mediated by catecholamine systems (*see* Grupp, 1977; Lorden et al., 1980), which are not involved in lithium-induced CTA, suggesting that these aversions show a degree of pharmacological specificity. Such specificity may be related to the behaviorally specific CRs observed following treatment with these two agents (Parker, 1982). In similar fashion, Amit et al. (1977) reported that inhibition of catecholamine functioning attenuated morphine- and ethanol-induced CTA, but had no effect on the action of lithium, demonstrating again pharmacological specificity in the CTA procedure. Other evidence for specific effects in CTA research has been derived from studies of narcotic agonists and antagonists. Blair and Amit (1981) reported that lesions of the periaqueductal gray blocked morphine CTA, but had no effect on CTA induced by lithium, ethanol, or fenfluramine, suggesting that morphine CTA is specifically mediated by opiate receptors (which are located in the periaqueductal gray in high concentrations). This conclusion is supported by data indicating that naloxone attenuates morphine-induced CTA (Le Blanc and Cappell, 1975; Van der Kooy and Phillips, 1977). However, there is also evidence (Stolerman et al., 1978) that opiate *antagonists* induce CTA with a high degree of stereospecificity, indicating presumably that the CTA-inducing properties of antagonists are also mediated by actions at the opiate receptor.

Kumar et al. (1983) reported that nicotine-induced CTA also shows a degree of stereospecificity, suggesting that the effect may be mediated via a nicotinic receptor, a conclusion supported by the finding that the nicotinic antagonist mecamylamine blocked nicotine-induced CTA, but had no effect on an equipotent CTA induced by apomorphine, i.e., pharmacologically specific antagonism was observed. As a follow-up to these findings, Pratt and Stolerman (1983) reported that pimozide pretreatment blocked apomorphine CTA, but had no effect on an equipotent CTA induced by nicotine, again demonstrating the pharmacological specificity of drug-induced CTA.

In summary, many reports suggest that the actions of various drugs in the CTA procedure show a degree of pharmacological specificity.

4.2. Nonspecific Effects in the CTA Procedure

The strongest evidence against the idea that drug-specific actions mediate CTA comes from so-called "pretreatment studies," in which the actions of various drugs in the CTA procedure have been shown to be abolished by prior experience with either the drug subsequently used in CTA conditioning (e.g., Goudie et al., 1976) or with drugs from various other pharmacological classes, and even with nonpharmacological aversion-inducing treatments such as rotation (Braveman, 1975). There are many possible explanations for this well-documented phenomenon (Randich and LoLordo, 1979), including (i) the suggestion that some pretreatment effects in CTA studies are caused by the development of tolerance to aversive treatments, (ii) the interpretation of the effect in terms of associative interference by cues present during pretreatment that subsequently "block" taste/drug association on conditioning trials, (iii) the so-called "incremental illness" hypothesis, which postulates that if subjects are already "ill" at the time of taste/drug pairing (because of a prior drug treatment), then the taste will not be associated with a second aversive drug effect because it produces a relatively small increment of "illness," (iv) the so-called "unnatural-need state" hypothesis, which attributes the pretreatment effect to dependence induced by chronic drug treatment, which is presumed to attenuate the aversive drug effect when it is subsequently paired with a taste, since the drug alleviates withdrawal, and finally, (v) the "learned irrelevance/learned helplessness" hypothesis, which suggests that during chronic drug pretreatment, subjects learn that drug-induced states occur independently of their behavior; they therefore fail to learn to avoid a taste when it is subsequently a reliable predictor of an aversive drug state.

A detailed discussion of the large literature on pretreatment studies in CTA research is beyond the scope of this chapter. However, it should be clear from the discussion above that the actions of drugs in the CTA procedure could be attenuated by a variety of mechanisms, which may or may not develop independently of each other, and which may or may not have interactive and/or additive effects. Although superficially simple, pretreatment effects in CTA studies have consistently shown themselves to be complex phemonena. For example, there is evidence (Domjan and Siegel, 1983) that although preexposure to morphine attenuates both its aversive (CTA-inducing) and analgesic effects, different mechanisms are involved in these two processes (*see* also Stewart and Eikelboom, 1978). Attenuation of analgesia is mediated by environmentally specific tolerance (Siegel, 1976). However, the attenuation of morphine-induced CTA by prior drug experience is *not* environmentally specific and is therefore mediated by some other, as yet undefined, mechanism. Furthermore, a distinction has been drawn (Domjan, 1980) between "proximal" and "remote" pretreatment effects. The "proximal" pretreatment effect is short-lasting and only occurs if subsequent taste/drug pairing takes place within a few hours at most of drug preexposure. In contrast, the "remote" preexposure effect occurs even when prolonged periods (days) intervene between drug preexposure and subsequent taste/drug pairings. Different mechanisms are believed to mediate "proximal" and "remote" preexposure effects. The "proximal" preexposure effect is of particular significance for studies on the pharmacological specificity of drug-induced CTA. Domjan (1980) suggested that many studies investigating the pharmacological basis of drug-induced CTA have been confounded by nonspecific "proximal" preexposure effects that induced malaise, which subsequently interfered with the development of an association between taste and drug-induced illness (compare the "incremental illness" hypothesis described above). It certainly seems possible that such effects could confound CTA studies. For example, Brown et al. (1979) reports that "proximal" pretreatment with diazepam attenuated CTA induced by both itself and by morphine, i.e., a pharmacologically nonspecific pretreatment effect was observed that was possibly attributable to the type of "proximal" preexposure effect described by Domjan (1980). On the other hand, Kumar et al. (1983) and Pratt and Stolerman (1983) have provided reliable evidence for pharmacologically specific antagonist effects in studies involving "proximal" drug pretreatment in which nonspecific proximal preexposure effects might have been exected to occur. Thus, as described above, they reported that mecamylamine blocks nicotine CTA, but has no effect on an equipotent apomorphine-induced CTA, although pimozide blocks apomorphine CTA, but has no effect on an equipotent nicotine-induced CTA. The conditions under which "proximal" preexposure effects do and do not occur clearly need to be more closely defined. Previous research into the nature of preexposure effects in CTA studies suggests that this will not prove an easy task (Randich and LoLordo, 1979), since multiple mechanisms are almost certainly involved. However, demonstrations of preexposure effects have historically been important in supporting the belief that drug-induced CTA is a nonspecific phenomenon. For example, Braveman's (1975) demonstration that it is possible to attenuate rotation-induced CTA by "remote" pretreatment with either lithium, methyl-scopolamine, *or* amphetamine is difficult to account for in terms of pharmacologically specific mechanisms! Such data are much more easily reconciled with the belief that a common nonspecific mechanism, such as "nausea" or "illness," mediates CTA induced by all agents. However, as noted above, the "illness" interpretation of CTA is not without its weaknesses.

Further evidence that suggests, albeit indirectly, that drug-induced CTA is a nonspecific phenomenon comes from the general finding that it has proved virtually impossible to correlate the CTA-inducing potency of drugs with any other pharmacological actions (*see* Goudie and Newton, 1985). For example, in a study on the comparative potency of phenylethylamine-derived and related stimulant and anorectic drugs in the CTA paradigm, Booth et al. (1977) noted that the potency of these compounds in inducing CTA did not correlate with any specific neurochemical action or with stimulant potency. A subsequent study (Stolerman and D'Mello, 1978b) demonstrated that the aversive potency of such compounds also did not correlate with their adipsic effects. Similar data have been obtained by other authors working with related drugs. Greenshaw and Dourish (1984b) reported that the aversive potency of the structurally related compounds PEA and amphetamine (α-methyl-PEA) differed markedly. Likewise, Foltin and Schuster (1981) reported that the potency of cathinone (an amphetamine congener) relative to that of amphetamine in the CTA procedure was lower than that which would have been predicted on the basis of their comparative anorectic potency. We have recently replicated and considerably extended these data (Goudie et al., 1986; Goudie and Newton, 1985) by demonstrating that the aversive potency of cathinone relative to that of amphetamine does not correlate with the relative potency of these structurally related compounds in a very wide range of in vivo and in vitro assay procedures. Clearly, compounds can differ markedly in CTA potency when they are very closely related structurally and pharmacologically. This conclusion is supported by the report of Switzman et al. (1981), who noted that morphine was much more potent than heroin (diacetylmorphine) in the CTA procedure, but less potent in inducing analgesia. This observation is particularly striking since heroin is metabolized to morphine. Although attempts have been made to explain the comparative potency of structurally related compounds in the CTA procedure in terms of their pharmacokinetic profiles (Goudie et al., 1978; Goudie and Dickins, 1978; Switzman et al., 1981), it is clear, as discussed above, that pharmacokinetic factors alone do not readily predict the aversive potency of closely related compounds (*see* also D'Mello et al., 1981).

The CTA-inducing properties of drugs clearly do not correlate with other pharmacological actions, suggesting that this effect is perhaps a nonspecific one. However, it could be argued that an alternative way of conceptualizing these data is to suggest that the *pharmacology* of the CTA procedure needs further analysis to demonstrate specific drug effects. It is not, however, at all clear what pharmacological effect might correlate with aversive potency. The obvious candidate is gross behavioral "toxicity"; however, as discussed above, the gross behavioral effects of drugs also do not predict CTA potency (Greenshaw and Dourish, 1984b; Kallman et al., 1983; Barker et al., 1977). It is obvious that the CTA paradigm remains something of a pharmacological enigma!

What then is one to make of the pharmacological specificity of the CTA procedure? There is evidence for both drug specific and nonspecific actions in the CTA procedure. One way of resolving this apparent dilemma would be to suggest that drug-specific effects are involved in initial drug actions that all converge at a later stage on a final common pathway (e.g., the vomiting system) that has nonspecific actions common to all drugs. However, this conclusion is clearly weakened by the deficiencies described above in the evidence relating CTA to activation of the vomiting center. Perhaps the strongest conclusion that can be reached about the specificity of the CTA procedure at present is the relatively weak statement that in some circumstances drug-specific effects are observed, whereas in others nonspecific effects occur.

5. Implications of the Complexity of the CTA Procedure for Experimental Psychopharmacology

Recent years have seen a trend in experimental psychopharmacology toward attempts to specify whether behavioral effects of drugs are specific actions, or whether they simply reflect a more general process of behavioral disruption. A classic example of such work is that on drug-induced anorexia, which has demonstrated that the anorectic effects of amphetamine (in many ways the prototypical anorectic drug) are mediated, at least partially, by drug effects on response output rather than by a specific effect on hunger motivation (Blundell and Latham, 1982; *see* chapter by Cooper and Turkish in this volume). The need to demonstrate that drug effects on behavior are not caused by nonspecific actions is obvious, and the CTA paradigm has been used by a number of authors to attempt to rule out the possibility that observed effects are simply caused by drug-induced malaise. For example, Deutsch and Hardy (1977) and Deutsch (1981) have argued that the abilities of cholecystokinin and calcitonin to induce CTA argue against the putative roles of both of these agents as endogenous satiety hormones, since the apparent satiation these agents induce is possibly caused by malaise rather than a specific effect on satiety (*see* Wellman et al., 1981 for an analogous explanation of anorexia induced by phenylpropanolamine). A similar attempt to utilize the CTA paradigm to rule out nonspecific drug effects was put forward by McGlone et al. (1980), who argued that because both the antiaggressive effect of lithium and the CTA-inducing properties of this drug were abolished in rats by lesioning the area postrema, then the antiaggressive effect was caused by nonspecific malaise. However, these authors acknowledged the weakness of this analysis by noting that some CTA-inducing agents (e.g., apomorphine) actually enhance aggression. They suggested, therefore, that apomorphine must act on aggression in a different manner to lithium. However, this analysis begs more questions than it answers. The attempt to rule out nonspecific drug effects on the basis of drug-induced malaise is clearly tenuous at the least.

In all the examples discussed above, one poorly analyzed phenomenon (CTA) is effectively being used in an attempt to understand the mechanism(s) involved in other complex processes that are also poorly analyzed. A clear example of this type of theorizing was recently provided by Ettenberg et al. (1983), who argued that the putative memory-enhancing effects in animals of the hormone vasopressin are actually caused by aversive properties of vasopressin, which produces behavioral effects in tasks designed to test memory that are identical to those of lithium—a prototypical CTA-inducing agent. Ettenberg et al. (1983) consequently concluded that agents such as vasopressin and lithium may have apparent memory-enhancing properties by virtue of their aversive actions, which induce "arousal," facilitating performance in memory tasks. Ettenberg et al. (1983) are clearly attempting to analyze one complex process (pharmacological actions on memory) by utilizing another complex process (CTA) via a vague intervening variable ("arousal"). The weaknesses of such an analysis are obvious. However, the problem remains for the experimental psychopharmacologist that the question of the behavioral specificity of drug treatments is of such fundamental significance that it cannot be ignored. The use of the CTA paradigm to attempt to rule out nonspecific drug effects caused by "malaise" or "arousal" may perhaps be one of the *only* possible ways of attempting to address this important issue.

A further problem that relates to the use of the CTA procedure to analyze the specificity of drug effects is that because the determinants of drug potency in the CTA procedure are unclear, the procedure may in *some* cases be too sensitive and result in the rejection of useful drug treatments on the grounds that they have nonspecific effects. For example, it has been shown that in rats, the anorectic agent fenfluramine will induce potent CTA at a dose as low as 0.65 mg/kg (Booth et al., 1977). It is even possible that refinements of procedure (e.g., increasing the concentration of the fluid or the number of conditioning trials) could detect CTA at doses lower than 0.65 mg/kg. On the basis of such data, fenfluramine-induced anorexia might be attributed to nonspecific malaise induced by the drug. However, a large body of data suggests that in rats, fenfluramine has specific effects on eating behavior and on the neurochemical systems controlling food intake at doses much greater than 0.65 mg/kg (e.g., Blundell et al., 1976). Thus, the use of the CTA procedure as an index of nonspecific malaise would have resulted in the rejection of this drug as a putative anorectic agent. In fact, the compound has proved a useful clinical treatment for obesity and an important pharmacological tool for the analysis of behavioral and neurochemical mechanisms involved in food intake (Blundell and Latham, 1982) (*see* chapter by Cooper and Turkish in this volume).

In summary, despite the wealth of data available on actions of drugs in the CTA procedure, the effects of many agents in the procedure remain enigmatic. The basic paradigm is perhaps deceptively simple, and is certainly by no means as well understood as has frequently been assumed in the past. Considerable caution should therefore be exercised by individuals utilizing the procedure in an attempt to demonstrate the specificity of drug effects on behavior. The challenge for the future is clear—to analyze the CTA procedure in sufficient detail for it to be better understood in its own right and thereby to provide a better tool for the analysis of the specificity of other drug effects on behavior.

Note Added In Proof

We argued above (section 3) that all attempts to induce conditioned taste preferences with drugs have failed. Recent studies with narcotics (Mucha R. F. and Herz A., Motivational properties of kappa and mu opioid receptor agonists studied with place and taste preference conditioning. *Psychopharmacology* **86**, 274–280, 1985) indicate that this conclusion is no longer valid. However, the parametric conditions that allow for the demonstration of drug-induced conditioned taste preferences are completely unclear at present. The isolation of factors that allow taste preferences to be demonstrated could be of considerable significance for the development of theories of drug dependence and for the analysis of the reinforcing effects of drugs.

Acknowledgment

Thanks are due to Mrs. Dorothy Foulds for typing this chapter, probably better than I could myself, without complaint or interruption, from indecipherable and incomprehensible manuscript.

References

Amit Z., Levitan D. E., Brown Z. W., and Rogan F. (1977) Possible involvement of central factors in the mediation of conditioned taste aversion. *Neuropharmacology* **16**, 121–124.

Anderson C. E., Tilson H. A., and Mitchell C. L. (1982) Conditioned taste aversion following acutely administered acrylamide. *Neurobehav. Toxicol. Teratol.* **4**, 497–499.

Archer T., Sjoden P. O., Nilsson L. G., and Carter N. (1980). Exteroceptive context in taste-aversion conditioning and extinction: Odour, cage and bottle stimuli. *Q. J. Exp. Psychol.* **32,** 197–214.

Barker L. M., Smith J. C., and Suarez E. M. (1977) "Sickness" and the Backward Conditioning of Taste Aversions, in *Learning Mechanisms in Food Selection* (Barker L. M., Best M. R., and Domjan M., eds.), Baylor University Press, Waco, Texas.

Berger B. D. (1972) Conditioning of food aversions by injections of psychoactive drugs. *J. Comp. Physiol. Psychol.* **81,** 21–26.

Berger B. D., Wise C. D., and Stein L. (1973) Area postrema damage and bait shyness. *J. Comp. Physiol. Psychol.* **83,** 475–479.

Bernstein I. L. (1978) Learned taste aversions in children receiving chemotherapy. *Science* **200,** 1302–1303.

Bernstein I. L. and Goehler L. E. (1983a) Vagotomy produces learned food aversions. *Beh. Neurosci.* **97,** 585–594.

Bernstein I. L. and Goehler L. E. (1983b) Chronic lithium chloride infusions: Conditioned suppression of food intake and preference. *Beh. Neurosci.* **97,** 290–298.

Bernstein I. L. and Webster M. M. (1980) Learned taste aversions in humans. *Physiol. Behav.* **25,** 363–366.

Bernstein I. L., Goehler L. E., and Bouton M. E. (1983) Relative potency of foods and drinks as targets in aversion conditioning. *Beh. Neural Biol.* **37,** 134–148.

Berridge K., Grill H. J., and Norgren R. (1981) Relation of consummatory responses and preabsorptive insulin release to palatability and learned taste aversions. *J. Comp. Physiol. Psychol.* **94,** 363–382.

Blair R. and Amit Z. (1981) Morphine conditioned taste aversion reversed by periaqueductal gray lesion. *Pharmacol. Biochem. Behav.* **15,** 651–653.

Blundell J. E. and Latham C. J. (1982) Behavioural Pharmacology of Feeding in *Drugs and Appetite* (Silverstone T., ed.), Academic, New York.

Blundell J. E., Latham C. J., and Lesham M. B. (1976) Differences between the anorexic actions of amphetamine and fenfluramine—possible effects on hunger and satiety. *J. Pharm Pharmacol.* **28,** 471–477.

Bond N. W. and DiGiustio E. L. (1975) Amount of solution drunk is a factor in the establishment of taste aversion. *Anim. Learning Behav.* **3,** 81–84.

Booth D. A., D'Mello G. D., Pilcher C. W. T., and Stolerman I. P. (1977) Comparative potencies of amphetamine, fenfluramine and related compounds in taste aversion experiments in rats. Br. J. Pharmacol. **61,** 669–677.

Borison H. L. and Wang S. C. (1953) Physiology and pharmacology of vomiting. *Pharmacol. Rev.* **5,** 193–230.

Bradley R. M. and Mistretta C. M. (1971) Intravascular taste in rats as demonstrated by conditioned aversion to sodium saccharin. *J. Comp. Physiol. Psychol.* **75,** 186–189.

Braveman N. S. (1975) Formation of taste aversions in rats following prior exposure to sickness. *Learning Motiv.* **6,** 512–534.

Brown Z. W., Amit Z., Smith B., and Rockman G. (1979) Disruption of taste aversion learning by pretreatment with diazepam and morphine. *Pharmacol. Biochem. Behav.* **10,** 17–20.

Cairnie A. B. and Leach K. E. (1982) Dexamethasone: A potent blocker for rotation-induced taste aversion in rats. *Pharmacol. Biochem. Behav.* **17,** 305–311.

Cappell H. and Le Blanc A. E. (1971) Conditioned aversion to saccharin by single administration of *d*-amphetamine and mescaline. *Psychopharmacologia* **22,** 352–356.

Cappell H. and Le Blanc A. E. (1975) Conditioned aversion by psychoactive drugs: Does it have significance for an understanding of drug dependence? *Addict. Behav.* **1,** 55–64.

Cappell H. D. and Le Blanc A. E. (1977) Gustatory Avoidance Conditioning by Drugs of Abuse: Relationships to General Issues in Research on Drug Dependence, in *Food Aversion Learning* (Milgram N. W., Krames L. and Alloway T., eds.), Plenum, New York.

Cappell H. D., Le Blanc A. E., and Endrenyi L. (1973) Aversive conditioning by psychoactive drugs: Effects of morphine, alcohol and chlordiazepoxide. *Psychopharmacologia* **29,** 239–246.

Carey R. J. (1978) A comparison of food intake suppression produced by giving amphetamine as an aversion treatment versus as an anorexic treatment. *Psychopharmacology* **56,** 45–48.

Coil J. D. and Norgren R. (1981) Taste aversions conditioned with intravenous copper sulfate: Attenuation by ablation of the area postrema. *Brain Res.* **212,** 425–433.

Coil J. D., Hankins W. D., Jenden J. D., and Garcia J. (1978a) The attenuation of a specific cue-to-consequence association by antiemetic agents. *Psychopharmacology* **56,** 21–25.

Coil J. D., Rogers R. C., Garcia J., and Novin D. (1978b) Conditioned taste aversions: Vagal and circulatory mediation of the toxic unconditioned stimulus. *Behav. Biol.* **24,** 509–519.

Coussens W. R. (1974) Conditioned Taste Aversion: Route of Drug Administration, in *Drug Addiction: Neurobiology and Influences on Behavior* (Singh J. M. and Lal H., eds.), Symposia Specialists, Miami, Florida.

Crawford D. and Baker T. B. (1982) Alcohol dependence and taste-mediated learning in the rat. *Pharmacol. Biochem. Behav.* **16,** 253–261.

Cunningham C. L. (1978) Alcohol interacts with flavor during extinction of conditioned taste aversion. *Physiol. Psychol.* **6,** 510–516.

Cunningham C. L. (1979) Flavor and location aversions produced by ethanol. *Beh. Neural Biol.* **27,** 362–367.

Cunningham C. L. (1981) Spatial aversion conditioning with ethanol. *Pharmacol. Biochem. Behav.* **14,** 263–264.

Dantzer R. (1980) Conditioned taste aversion as an index of lead toxicity. *Pharmacol. Biochem. Behav.* **13,** 133–135.

Deutsch J. A. (1981) Calcitonin: Aversive effects in rats? *Science* **211,** 733.

Deutsch J. A. and Hardy W. T. (1977) Cholecystokinin produces bait shyness in rats. *Nature* **266,** 196.

Dickinson A., Nicholas D. J., and Adams C. D. (1983) The effect of the instrumental training contingency on susceptibility to reinforcer devaluation. *Q. J. Exp. Psychol.* **35B,** 35–51.

D'Mello G. D. and Stolerman I. P. (1978) Suppression of fixed interval responding by flavour–amphetamine pairings in rats. *Pharmacol. Biochem. Behav.* **9,** 395–398.

D'Mello G. D., Goldberg D. M., Goldberg S. R., and Stolerman I. P. (1981) Conditioned taste aversion and operant behavior in rats: Effects of cocaine, apomorphine and some long-acting derivatives. *J. Pharmacol. Exp. Ther.* **219,** 60–68.

D'Mello G. D., Stolerman I. P., Booth D. A., and Pilcher C. W. T. (1977) Factors affecting flavour aversions conditioned with amphetamine in rats. *Pharmacol. Biochem. Behav.* **7,** 185–190.

Domjan M. (1975) Attenuation and Enhancement of Neophobia for Edible Substances, in *Learning Mechanisms in Food Selection.* (Barker L. M., Best M. R., and Domjan M., eds.), Baylor University Press, Waco, Texas.

Domjan M., ed. (1980) Ingestional Aversion Learning: Unique and General Processes in *Advances in the Study of Behaviour,* vol. 11, Academic, New York.

Domjan M. and Siegel S. (1983) Attenuation of the aversive and analgesic effects of morphine by repeated administration: Different mechanisms. *Physiol. Psychol.* **11,** 155–158.

Domjan M. and Wilson N. E. (1972) Contribution of ingestive behaviors to taste-aversion learning in the rat. *J. Comp. Physiol. Psychol.* **80,** 403–412.

Domjan M., Foster K., and Gillan D. J. (1981) Effects of distribution of the drug unconditioned stimulus on taste-aversion learning. *Physiol. Behav.* **23,** 931–938.

Dourish C. T., Greenshaw A. J., and Boulton A. A. (1983) Deuterium substitution enhances the effects of β-phenylethylamine on spontaneous motor activity in the rat. *Pharmacol. Biochem. Behav.* **19,** 471–475.

Edwards R. C. and Ritter S. C. (1981) Ablation of the area postrema causes exaggerated consumption of preferred foods in the rat. *Brain Res.* **216,** 265–276.

Elkins R. L. (1974) Bait-shyness acquisition and resistance to extinction as functions of US exposure prior to conditioning. *Physiol. Psychol.* **2,** 341–343.

Etscorn F. (1980) Sucrose aversions in mice as a result of injected nicotine or passive tobacco smoke inhalation. *Bull. Psychon. Soc.* **15,** 54–56.

Etscorn F. and Parsons P. (1979) Taste aversion in mice using phencyclidine and ketamine as the aversive agents. *Bull. Psychon. Soc.* **14,** 19–21.

Ettenberg A., Garrett O. J., and Milner P. M. (1979) Effects of exteroceptive stimuli on conditioned taste preferences induced by self-stimulation in the rat. *Physiolog. Psychol.* **7,** 126–130.

Ettenberg A., Van der Kooy D., Le Moal M., Koob G. F. and Bloom F. E. (1983) Can aversive properties of (peripherally-injected) vasopressin account for its putative role in memory? *Beh. Brain Res.* **7,** 331–350.

Evans H. L. and Weiss B. L. (1978) Behavioral Toxicology, in *Contemporary Research in Behavioral Pharmacology* (Blackman D. E. and Sanger D. J., eds.), Plenum, New York.

Foltin R. W. and Schuster C. R. (1981) The effects of *dl*-cathinone in a gustatory avoidance paradigm. *Pharmacol. Biochem.*

Behav. **14,** 907–909.

Foltin R. W., Preston K. L., Wagner G. C., and Schuster C. R. (1981) The aversive stimulus properties of repeated infusions of cocaine. *Pharmacol. Biochem. Behav.* **15,** 71–74.

Gamzu E. (1977) The Multifaceted Nature of Taste-Aversion Inducing Agents: Is There a Common Factor?, in *Learning Mechanisms in Food Selection* (Barker L. M., Best M. R., and Domjan M., eds.), Baylor University Press, Waco, Texas.

Garb J. L. and Stunkard A. J. (1974) Taste aversions in man. *Am. J. Psychiat.* **131,** 1204–1207.

Garcia J. and Koelling R. A. (1966) Relation of cue to consequence in avoidance learning. *Psychon. Sci.* **4,** 123–124.

Garcia J., Ervin F. R., and Koelling R. A. (1967) Bait-shyness: A test for toxicity with N = 2. *Psychon. Sci.* **7,** 245–246.

Garcia J., Hankins W., and Rusiniak K. (1974) Behavioral regulation of the milieu interne in man and rat. *Science* **185,** 824–831.

Glowa J. R. and Barrett J. E. (1983) Response suppression by visual stimuli paired with postsession *d*-amphetamine injections in the pigeon. *J. Exp. Anal. Behav.* **39,** 165–173.

Goldberg S. R., Kelleher R. T., and Morse W. H. (1975) Second order schedules of drug injection. *Fed. Proc.* **34,** 1771–1776.

Goudie A. J. (1979) Aversive stimulus properties of drugs. *Neuropharmacology* **18,** 971–979.

Goudie A. J. and Dickins D. W. (1978) Nitrous oxide-induced conditioned taste aversions in rats: The role of duration of drug exposure and its relation to the taste aversion/self-administration "paradox." *Pharmacol. Biochem. Behav.* **9,** 587–592.

Goudie A. J. and Newton T. (1985) The puzzle of drug-induced conditioned taste aversion: Comparative studies with cathinone and amphetamine. *Psychopharmacology,* **87,** 328–333.

Goudie A. J., Atkinson J., Newton T., and Demellweek C. (1986) Discriminative and aversive actions of *dl*-cathinone and *d*-amphetamine in rats: Comparisons with effects on operant responding and water intake. *Psychopharmacology* **83,** 53.

Goudie A. J., Dickins D. W., and Thornton E. W. (1978) Cocaine-induced conditioned taste aversions in rats. *Pharmacol. Biochem. Behav.* **8,** 757–761.

Goudie A. J., Stolerman I. P., Demellweek C., and D'Mello G. D. (1982) Does conditioned nausea mediate drug-induced conditioned taste aversion? *Psychopharmacology* **78,** 277–281.

Goudie A. J., Thornton E. W., and Wheatley J. (1975) Attenuation by alpha-methyltyrosine of amphetamine-induced conditioned taste aversion. *Psychopharmacologia,* **45,** 119–123.

Goudie A. J., Thornton E. W., and Wheeler T. J. (1976) Drug pretreatment effects in drug induced taste aversions: Effects of dose and duration of pretreatment. *Pharmacol. Biochem. Behav.* **4,** 629–633.

Greenshaw A. J. and Buresova O. (1982) Learned taste aversion to saccharin following intraventricular or intraperitoneal administration of *d,l*-amphetamine. *Pharmacol. Biochem. Behav.* **17,** 1129–1133.

Greenshaw A. J. and Dourish C. T. (1984a) β-Phenylethylamine and *d*-Amphetamine: Differential Potency in the Conditioned Taste Aversion Paradigm, in *Neurobiology of the Trace Amines* (Boulton A., Baker G., Dewhurst W., and Sandler M., eds.), Humana, Clifton, New Jersey.

Greenshaw A. J. and Dourish C. T. (1984b) Differential aversive stimulus properties of β-phenylethylamine and of *d*-amphetamine. *Psychopharmacology* **82,** 189–193.

Grupp L. A. (1977) Effect of pimozide on the acquisition, maintenance and extinction of amphetamine induced conditioned taste aversion. *Psychopharmacology* **53,** 235–242.

Gustavson C. R. (1977) Comparative and Field Aspects of Learned Food Aversions, in *Learning Mechanisms in Food Selection* (Barker L. M., Best M. R., and Domjan M., eds.), *Baylor University Press, Waco, Texas.*

Hasegawa Y. and Matsuzawa T. (1981) Food-aversion conditioning in Japanese monkeys (*Macaca fuscata*): A dissociation of feeding in two separate situations. *Behav. Neural Biol.* **33,** 237–242.

Holman E. W. (1975) Some conditions for dissociation of consummatory and instrumental behavior in rats. *Learning Motiv.* **6,** 358–366.

Ionescu E. and Buresova O. (1977) Failure to elicit conditioned taste aversion by severe poisoning. *Pharmacol. Biochem. Behav.* **6,** 251–254.

Kallman M. J., Lynch M. R., and Landauer M. R. (1983) Taste

aversions to several halogenated hydrocarbons. *Neurobehav. Toxicol. Teratol.* **5**, 23–27.

Kiefer S. W., Cabral R. J., Rusiniak K. W., and Garcia J. (1980) Ethanol-induced flavor aversions in rats with subdiaphragmatic vagotomies. *Behav. Neural Biol.* **29**, 246–254.

Klauenberg B. J. and Sparber S. B. (1983) Behavioral toxicity of amphetamine is differentially affected by hot and cold water immersion stress. *Neurobehav. Toxicol. Teratol.* **5**, 83–90.

Krane R. V. (1980) Toxiphobia conditioning with exteroceptive cues. *Anim. Learning Behav.* **8**, 513–523.

Kresel J. J. and Barofsky I. (1979) Conditioned saccharin aversion development following administration of hypotensive agents. *Physiol. Behav.* **23**, 733–736.

Kumar R., Pratt J. A., and Stolerman I. P. (1983) Characteristics of conditioned taste aversion produced by nicotine in rats. *Br. J. Pharmacol.* **79**, 245–253.

Landaeur M. R., Lynch M. R., Balster R. L., and Kallman M. J. (1982) Trichloromethane-induced taste aversions in mice. *Neurobehav. Toxicol. Teratol.* **4**, 305–309.

Leander J. D. and Gau B. A. (1980) Flavor aversions rapidly produced by inorganic lead and triethyl tin. *Neurotoxicology* **1**, 635–642.

Le Blanc A. E. and Cappell H. (1975) Antagonism of morphine induced aversive conditioning by naloxone. *Pharmacol. Biochem. Behav.* **3**, 185–188.

Lorden J. F., Callahan M., and Dawson R. (1980) Depletion of central catecholamines alters amphetamine- and fenfluramine-induced taste aversions in the rat. *J. Comp. Physiol. Psychol.* **94**, 99–114.

MacPhail R. C. and Leander J. D. (1980) Flavor aversions induced by chlordimeform. *Neurobehav. Toxicol.* **2**, 363–365.

Marfaing-Jallat P. and Le Magnen J. (1979) Ethanol-induced aversion in ethanol dependent and normal rats. *Behav. Neural Biol.* **26**, 106–114.

Martin J. R., Cheng F. Y., and Novin D. (1978) Acquisition of learned taste aversions following bilateral subdiaphragmatic vagotomy in rats. *Physiol. Behav.* **21**, 13–17.

Martonyi B. and Valenstein E. S. (1971) On drinkometers: Problems and an inexpensive photocell solution. *Physiol. Behav.* **7**, 913–914.

Matsuzawa T. and Hasegawa Y. (1982) Food-aversion conditioning in Japanese monkeys (*Macca fuscata*): Suppression of key-pressing. *Behav. Neural Biol.* **36,** 298–303.

McGlone J. J., Ritter S., and Kelley K. (1980) The antiaggressive effect of lithium is abolished by area postrema lesion. *Physiol. Behav.* **24,** 1095–1100.

Miceli D., Marfaing-Jallat P., and Le Magnen J. (1980) Ethanol aversion induced by parenterally administered ethanol acting both as CS and UCS. *Physiol. Psychol.* **8,** 433–436.

Miller D. B. and Miller L. L. (1983) Bupropion, *d*-amphetamine and amitriptyline-induced conditioned taste aversion in rats: Dose effects. *Pharmacol. Biochem. Behav.* **18,** 737–740.

Mitchell D., Winter W., and Morisaki C. M. (1977) Conditioned taste aversions accompanied by geophagia: Evidence for the occurrence of "psychological" factors in the etiology of pica. *Psychosom. Med.* **39,** 402–412.

Miyagawa M., Honma T., Sato M., and Hasegawa H. (1984) Conditioned taste aversion induced by toluene administration in rats. *Neurobehav. Toxicol. Teratol.* **6,** 33–37.

Morrison G. R. and Collyer R. (1974) Taste mediated aversion to an exteroceptive stimulus following LiCl poisoning. *J. Comp. Physiol. Psychol.* **86,** 51–55.

Morse W. H. and Kelleher R. T. (1977). Determinants of Reinforcement and Punishment, in *Handbook of Operant Psychology* (Honig W. K. and Staddon J. E. R., eds.), Prentice-Hall, New Jersey.

Nachman M. and Hartley P. L. (1975) Role of illness in producing learned taste aversions in rats: A comparison of various rodenticides. *J. Comp. Physiol. Psychol.* **89,** 1010–1018.

Nachman M., Lester D., and Le Magnen J. (1970) Alcohol aversion in the rat: Behavioral assessment of noxious drug effects. *Science* **168,** 1244–1246.

Ossenkopp K-P. (1983a) Taste aversions conditioned with gamma radiation: Attenuation by area postrema lesions in rats. *Behav. Brain Res.* **7,** 297–305.

Ossenkopp K-P. (1983b) Area postrema lesions in rats enhance the magnitude of body rotation-induced conditioned taste aversions. *Behav. Neural Biol.* **38,** 82–96.

Parker L. A. (1982) Nonconsummatory and consummatory behavioral CRs elicited by lithium- and amphetamine-paired flavors. *Learning Motiv.* **13,** 281–303.

Parker L. A., Hutchinson S., and Riley A. L. (1982) Conditioned flavor aversions: A toxicity test of the anticholinesterase agent, physostigmine. *Neurobehav. Toxicol. Teratol.* **4,** 93–98.

Pelchat M. L., Grill H. J., Rozin P., and Jacobs J. (1983) Quality of acquired responses to tastes by *Rattus norvegicus* depends on type of associated discomfort. *J. Comp. Psychol.* **97,** 140–153.

Pilcher C. W. T. and Stolerman I. P. (1976) Conditioned flavor aversions for assessing precipitated morphine abstinence in rats. *Pharmacol. Biochem. Behav.* **4,** 159–163.

Pratt J. A. and Stolerman I. P. (1983) Specific effects of antagonists on conditioned taste aversions. *Neurosci. Lett.* Suppl. 14, S292.

Rabin B. M. and Hunt W. A. (1983) Effects of antiemetics on the acquisition and recall of radiation- and lithium chloride-induced conditioned taste aversions. *Pharmacol. Biochem. Behav.* **18,** 629–635.

Rabin B. M., Hunt W. A., and Lee J. (1983) Attenuation of radiation and drug-induced conditioned taste aversions following area postrema lesions in the rat. *Rad. Res.* **93,** 388–394.

Randich A. and LoLordo V. M. (1979) Associative and Nonassociative theories of the UCS preexposure phenomenon: Implications for Pavlovian conditioning. *Psychol. Bull.* **86,** 523–548.

Rappold V. A., Porter J. H., and Llewellyn G. C. (1984) Evaluation of the toxic effects of alfatoxin B_1 with a taste aversion paradigm in rats. *Neurobehav. Toxicol. Teratol.* **6,** 51–58.

Reicher M. A. and Holman E. W. (1977) Location preference and flavor aversion reinforced by amphetamine in rats. *Anim. Learning Behav.* **5,** 343–346.

Riley A. L. and Clarke C. M. (1977) Conditioned Taste Aversions: A Bibliography, in *Learning Mechanisms in Food Selection* (Barker L. M., Best M. R., and Domjan M., eds.), Baylor University Press, Waco, Texas.

Riley A. L. and Zellner D. A. (1978) Methylphenidate-induced conditioned taste aversion: An index of toxicity. *Physiol. Psychol.* **6,** 354–358.

Riley A. L., Jacobs W. J., and LoLordo V. M. (1978) Morphine-induced taste aversions: A consideration of parameters. *Physiol. Psychol.* **6,** 96–100.

Ritter S., McGlone J. J., and Kelley K. W. (1980) Absence of lithium-induced taste aversion after area postrema lesion. *Brain Res.* **201,** 501–506.

Roberts D. C. S. and Fibiger H. C. (1975) Attenuation of amphetamine-induced conditioned taste aversion following intraventricular 6-hydroxydopamine. *Neurosci. Lett.* **1,** 343–347.

Rondeau D. B., Jolicoeur F. B., Merket A. D., and Wayner M. J. (1981) Drugs and taste aversion. *Neurosci. Biobehav. Rev.* **5,** 279–294.

Rudy J. W. and Cheatle M. D. (1977) Odor-aversion learning in neonatal rats. *Science* **198,** 845–846.

Sanger D. J., Greenshaw A. J., Thompson I. P., and Mercer J. D. (1980) Learned taste aversion to saccharin produced by orally consumed *d*-amphetamine. *Pharmacol. Biochem. Behav.* **13,** 31–36.

Sherman J. E., Hickis C. F., Rice A. G., Rusinak K. W., and Garcia J. (1983) Preferences and aversions for stimuli paired with ethanol in hungry rats. *Anim. Learning Behav.* **11,** 101–106.

Sherman J. E., Roberts T., Roskam S. E., and Holman E. W. (1980) Temporal properties of the rewarding and aversive effects of amphetamine in rats. *Pharmacol. Biochem. Behav.* **13,** 597–589.

Siegel S. (1976) Morphine analgesic tolerance: Its situation specificity supports a Pavlovian conditioning model. *Science* **193,** 323–325.

Sjoden P-O., Archer T., and Carter N. (1979) Conditioned taste aversion induced by 2,4,5-trichlorophenoxyacetic acid. *Physiol. Psychol.* **7,** 93–96.

Smith D. F. (1983) Lithium and carbamazepine: Effects on learned taste aversion and open field behavior in rats. *Pharmacol. Biochem. Behav.* **18,** 483–488.

Smith S. G., Werner T. E., and Davis W. M. (1977) Alcohol-associated conditioned reinforcement. *Psychopharmacology* **53,** 223–226.

Spiker V. A. (1977) Taste aversion: A procedural analysis and an alternative paradigmatic classification. *Psychol. Rec.* **27,** 753–769.

Steiner S. S., Beer H., and Shaffer M. (1969) Escape from self-produced rates of brain stimulation. *Science* **163,** 90–91.

Stewart J. and Eikelboom R. (1978) Pre-exposure to morphine and the attenuation of conditioned taste aversion in rats. *Pharmacol. Biochem. Behav.* **9,** 639–645.

Stickrod G., Kimble D. P., and Smotherman W. P. (1982) In utero taste/odor aversion conditioning in the rat. *Physiol. Behav.* **28,** 5–7.

Stolerman I. P. and D'Mello G. D. (1978a) Amphetamine-induced taste aversion demonstrated with operant behavior. *Pharmacol. Biochem. Behav.* **8,** 107–111.

Stolerman I. P. and D'Mello G. D. (1978b) Amphetamine-induced hypodipsia and its implications for conditioned taste aversion in rats. *Pharmacol. Biochem. Behav.* 8, 333–338.

Stolerman I. P. and D'Mello G. D. (1981) Oral Self-Administration and the Relevance of Conditioned Taste Aversions, in *Advances in Behavioral Pharmacology* (Thompson T., Dews P. B., and McKim W. A., eds.), vol. 3, Academic, New York.

Stolerman I. P., Pilcher C. W. T., and D'Mello G. D. (1978) Stereospecific aversive property of narcotic antagonists in morphine-free rats. *Life Sci.* **22,** 1755–1762.

Switzman L., Amit Z., White N., and Fishman B. (1978) Novel Tasting Food Enhances Morphine Discriminability in Rats, in *Stimulus Properties of Drugs: Ten Years of Progress* (Colpaert F. C. and Rosecrans J. A., eds.), Elsevier North Holland Biomedical Press, Amsterdam.

Switzman L., Hunt T., and Amit Z. (1981) Heroin and morphine: Aversive and analgesic effects in rats. *Pharmacol. Biochem. Behav.* **15,** 755–759.

Testa T. J. and Ternes J. W. (1977) Specificity of Conditioning Mechanisms in the Modification of Food Preferences, in *Learning Mechanisms in Food Selection* (Barker L. M., Best M. R., and Domjan M., eds.), Baylor University Press, Waco, Texas.

Van der Kooy D. and Phillips A. G. (1977) Temporal analysis of naloxone attenuation of morphine-induced taste aversion. *Pharmacol. Biochem. Behav.* **6,** 637–641.

Van der Kooy D., Swerdlow N. R., and Koob G. F. (1983) Para-doxical reinforcing properties of apomorphine: Effects of nucleus accumbens and area postrema lesions. *Brain Res.* **259,** 111–118.

Vogel J. R. and Nathan B. A. (1975) Learned taste aversions induced by hypnotic drugs. *Pharmacol. Biochem. Behav.* **3,** 189–194.

Wagner G. C., Foltin R. W., Seiden L. S., and Schuster C. R. (1981) Dopamine depletion by 6-hydroxydopamine prevents conditioned taste aversion induced by methylamphetamine but not lithium chloride. *Pharmacol. Biochem. Behav.* **14,** 85–88.

Weijnen J. A. W. (1972) Current Licking: Lick Contingent Electrical Stimulation of the Tongue, in *Drinking Behavior: Oral Stimulation and Preference* (Weijnen J. A. M. and Mendelson J., eds.), Plenum, New York.

Wellman P. J. and Boissard C. G. (1981) Influence of fluid deprivation on the level of conditioned taste aversion induced by amphetamine in female rats. *Physiol. Psychol.* **9,** 281–284.

Wellman P. J., Malpas P. B., and Wikler K. C. (1981) Conditioned taste aversion and unconditioned suppression of water intake induced by phenylpropanolamine in rats. *Physiol. Psychol.* **9,** 203–207.

White N., Sklar L. S., and Amit Z. (1977) The reinforcing action of morphine and its paradoxical side effect. *Psychopharmacology* **52,** 63–66.

Wise R. A. (1982) Neuroleptics and operant behavior: The anhedonia hypothesis. *Behav. Brain Sci.* **5,** 39–87.

Wise R. A., Yokel R. A., and De Wit H. (1976) Both positive reinforcement and conditioned aversion from amphetamine and from apomorphine in rats. *Science* **191,** 1273–1274.

Zabik J. E. and Roache J. D. (1983) 5-Hydroxytryptophan-induced conditioned taste aversion to ethanol in the rat. *Pharmacol. Biochem. Behav.* **18,** 785–790.

Zahorik D. M. (1977) Associative and Non-associative Factors in Learned Food Preference, in *Learning Mechanisms in Food Selection* (Barker L. M., Best M. R., and Domjan M., eds.), Baylor University Press, Waco, Texas.

Measurement of Drug Effects on Stimulus Control

Linda A. Dykstra and
Raymond F. Genovese

1. Introduction

Operant behavior is defined as behavior that is maintained by its consequences. If a consequent event follows behavior only in the presence of certain discriminative stimuli (S^D), responding becomes differentiated with respect to the discriminative stimuli. When this occurs, it can be said that responding is under stimulus control (Terrace, 1966). In order to determine whether behavior is under stimulus control, a stimulus-generalization gradient is often obtained, i.e., the discriminative stimulus is varied systematically along some dimension, and responding is measured in the presence of several different values of the stimulus. Stimulus control is demonstrated when the probability of responding varies systematically as a function of different values of the stimulus (for a discussion of procedures for obtaining generalization gradients and interpreting them, *see* Rilling, 1977, and Ray and Sidman, 1970).

Numerous factors are important in the stimulus control of behavior. These include the subject's sensory systems and prior experience, the number and type of other stimuli in the environment, the method by which the stimulus came to control behavior, the nature of the response, and the nature of the reinforcer. Many of these factors are also known to alter drug effects on stimulus control. For example, if amphetamine alters behavior under the control of an auditory stimulus, this effect may be related to the dose of amphetamine, the intensity of the stimulus controlling behavior, and/or the schedule of reinforcement maintaining responding. Additional variables, such as the organism's prior pharmacological or behavioral history, may also contribute to the drug effect. In this chapter, emphasis will be placed on the many behavioral factors known to be important determinants of a drug's effect on stimulus control.

2. Procedures for Measuring Drug Effects on Stimulus Control

In this section a number of procedures that are used to investigate drug-induced changes in stimulus control will be discussed. These include multiple schedules, conditional discrimination procedures, classical conditioning procedures, and methods for determining thresholds. Discussion will be restricted to studies in which behavior is shown to be under stimulus control, i.e., studies demonstrating that changes in the physical parameters of the stimulus presumed to control behavior actually induce a change in that behavior. Studies in which a drug's effects are modulated by the presence of discriminative stimuli are discussed by Sanger in this volume.

Most of the studies in this chapter investigate control by visual and auditory stimuli; however, studies in which the cutaneous senses are examined will also be considered. The cutaneous senses are particularly interesting since they represent a number of qualities, such as cold, warmth, pressure, touch, pain, and vibration, all of which might be altered by drug administration. Of the many aspects of cutaneous sensory function, the one that will be discussed here is that of pain sensitivity.

2.1. Multiple Schedules

Early investigations of drug effects on stimulus control employed the multiple schedule of food presentation (Dews, 1955; Waller, 1961; Clarke and Steele, 1966). Under the multiple schedule, responding is maintained by at least two different schedule components, each signaled by a different discriminative stimulus. Thereby, different rates and patterns of responding are established in the presence of different stimuli. If, following drug administration, rates and patterns of responding under the two schedule components are no longer differentiated, it might be suggested that the drug diminished stimulus control of behavior. The problem with this interpretation, as pointed out by Dews (1971), is that drug-induced changes in rates of responding might be caused by factors unrelated to the control of responding by the discriminative stimuli. For example, the effects of amphetamine, as well as a number of other drugs, are related to the rate of responding that occurs prior to drug administration (*see* chapter by Sanger in this volume), and thus, it cannot be assumed that drug-induced alterations in schedule-controlled patterns of responding are stimulus-dependent. Because of this difficulty, multiple schedules are seldom used to examine drug-induced changes in stimulus control. Instead, emphasis is placed on procedures that attempt to minimize the contribution of rate dependencies to the measurement of drug-induced changes in stimulus control.

2.2. Conditional Discrimination Procedures

One way in which drug-induced changes in stimulus control can be assessed independently of changes in response rate is exemplified by the work of Katz (1982), using a conditional discrimination procedure. In this procedure, pigeons were trained to make one of two responses, depending on the stimulus condition. Stimulus control was assessed by comparing relative frequencies of the two responses independently of the rate at which each response occurred. Briefly, each chamber contained two keys that could be transilluminated with either a red or amber light. The position of the key color was switched randomly between two keys after each response. When the houselight was on, responses on the red key (S^D responses) produced food with a fixed-interval, 5-min schedule. Responses on the amber key did not produce food. When the houselight was off, responses on the amber key (S^D responses) produced food with a fixed-interval, 5-min schedule, and responses on the red key did not produce food. Thus, the key color that signaled reinforcement was conditional on the presence of the houselight. Rates of responding were measured within successive 1-min portions of the fixed interval. In addition, the relative frequency of responding on the two keys was examined under each condition.

The proportion of red key responses when the houselight was on (reinforced responses) was compared to the proportion of red key responses when the houselight was off (nonreinforced responses). This proportion was described with a measure of stimulus control used in signal detection analysis (*see* section 4 for a complete description of this analysis). Figure 1 shows control performance. It can be seen that whereas rates of responding increased throughout the fixed interval, stimulus control as measured by the proportion of reinforced to nonreinforced responses remained constant and was thus independent of rate of responding. Figure 2 shows that *d*-amphetamine, cocaine, pentobarbital, and promazine all altered rates of responding in a dose-dependent manner. Despite these alterations in rates of responding, stimulus control was only altered at doses that markedly decreased rates of responding.

Conditional discrimination procedures have also been used to examine different opioid agonists. Moerschbaecher and Thompson (1983) found that *n*-allyl-normetazocine disrupted stimulus control at doses that did not alter rates of responding. On the other hand, morphine and ethylketocyclazocine either did not alter stimulus control or did so only at doses that markedly decreased rates of responding.

Matching-to-sample procedures represent another type of conditional discrimination. Typically, a sample stimulus is presented, followed by two or more stimuli, one of which matches the original sample stimulus. The subject's task is to

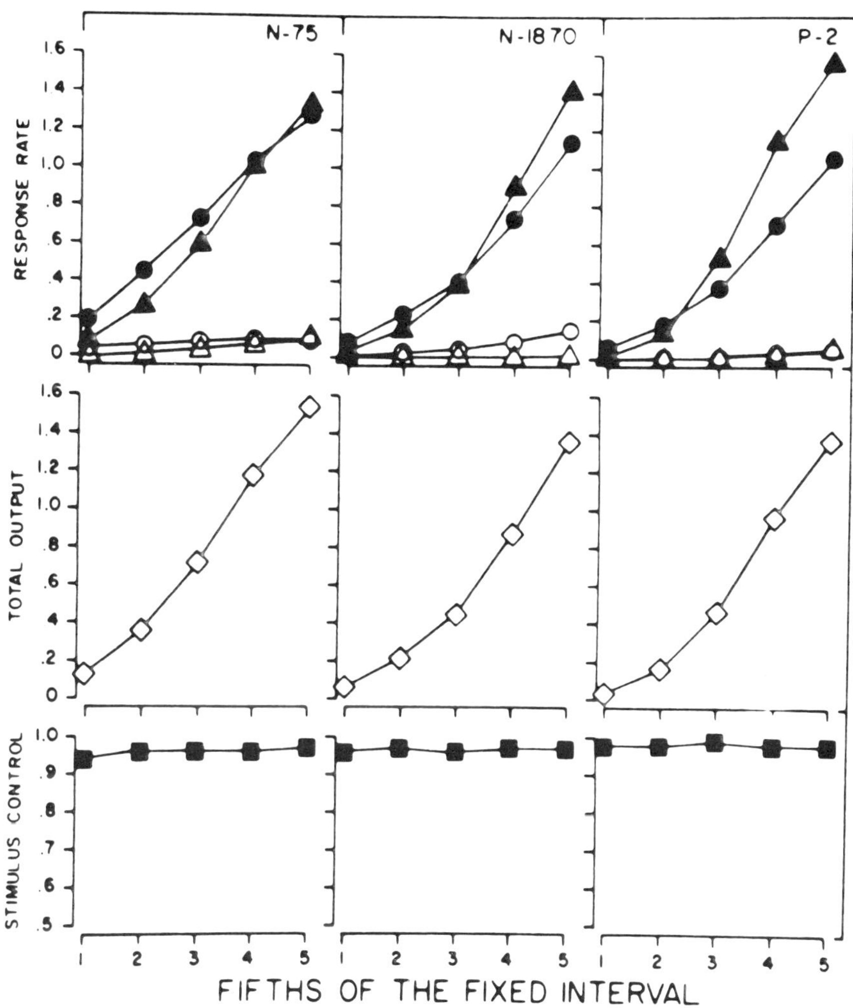

Fig. 1. Average control performances of individual pigeons in successive 1-min portions of the fixed-interval, 5-min schedule. Top panels: response rates (responses per second) with the houselight on (triangles) or off (circles). Filled symbols represent reinforced responding; open symbols represent responding that was not reinforced. Middle panels: average response rates, both reinforced and nonreinforced. Bottom panels: stimulus control (from Katz, 1982, with permission from author and publisher).

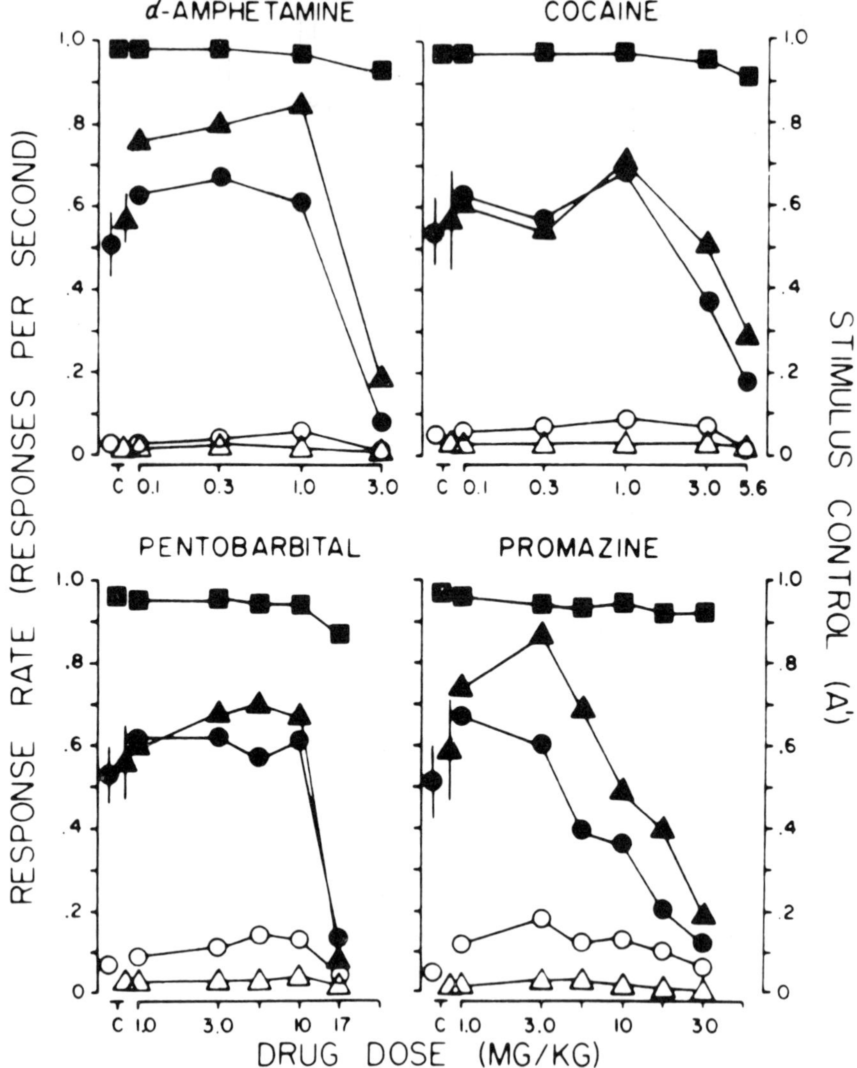

Fig. 2. Effects of *d*-amphetamine, cocaine, pentobarbital, and promazine on rates of responding and stimulus control (A^1) under the fixed-interval, 5-min schedule of reinforcement. Filled triangles, reinforced responding (red key, houselight on); filled circles, reinforced responding (amber key, houselight off); open triangles, nonreinforced responding (amber key, houselight on); open circles, nonreinforced responding (red key, houselight off); filled square, stimulus control. Each point is the mean of at least two observations in three pigeons except control points (above C), which are means of 4–10 control observations. Vertical bars about control points represent the mean of $+1$ SD (from Katz, 1982, with permission from author and publishers).

respond to the stimulus that matches the sample. Only a few investigations have used matching-to-sample procedures to examine drug effects on stimulus control; however, this procedure has been used more often to investigate the effects of drugs when a delay is introduced between the sample stimulus and the matching stimuli (*see* Heise and Milar, 1984, for a discussion of these studies).

2.3. *Classical Conditioning*

Although studies using classical conditioning procedures primarily concern the analysis of drug-induced changes in the acquisition of a conditioned response, studies of this type exemplify one way in which drug-induced changes in motor function can be separated from drug-induced changes in the manner in which a stimulus controls behavior. Within the classical conditioning paradigm, a stimulus (such as electrical shock) is first shown to elicit a response. The eliciting stimulus is then paired with another stimulus, which after being repeatedly presented in temporal proximity to the original stimulus also comes to elicit a response. Many drugs are known to alter this acquisition process. Moreover, numerous investigators have attempted to determine the mechanism whereby these changes take place. For example, Harvey et al. (1983) were interested in determining whether a drug's effect as observed within a conditioning paradigm was (1) caused by alteration in the acquisition of the conditioned response, and (2) related to drug-induced alterations in sensory or motor function.

In order to examine this question, they employed the rabbit nictitating membrane response. An electric shock was presented to the skin of the rabbit paraorbital region, producing eyeball retraction that resulted in the passive extension of the nictitating membrane. Prior to conditioning, the baseline frequency of this unconditioned response was very low (1–3 responses/h) and did not occur in the presence of stimuli such as a light or tone. After rabbits were observed for a period of time to obtain data on baseline frequency of membrane extension, conditioning was initiated. Conditioning consisted of several daily trials during which presentation of an electric shock (UCS) was preceded by a tone (CS). The number of membrane extensions that occurred after presentation of the conditioned stimulus, but prior to the unconditioned stimulus, was determined. As conditioning progressed, a greater percent of the membrane extensions occurred in the presence of the conditioned stimulus. Scopolamine (0.025–1.6 mg/kg) retarded this process in a dose-dependent manner.

In order to determine whether scopolamine's effects were caused by alterations in acquisition, a series of control experiments were run. The first control consisted of unpaired presentations of the tone and shock. Under these conditions, scopolamine did not alter the frequency of baseline responding, the frequency of responding to tone or light stimuli, or the amplitude of the response. Moreover, the frequency, latency, and amplitude of the nictitating membrane response was examined in the presence of varying intensities of the shock and tone. Figure 3 shows that scopolamine did not

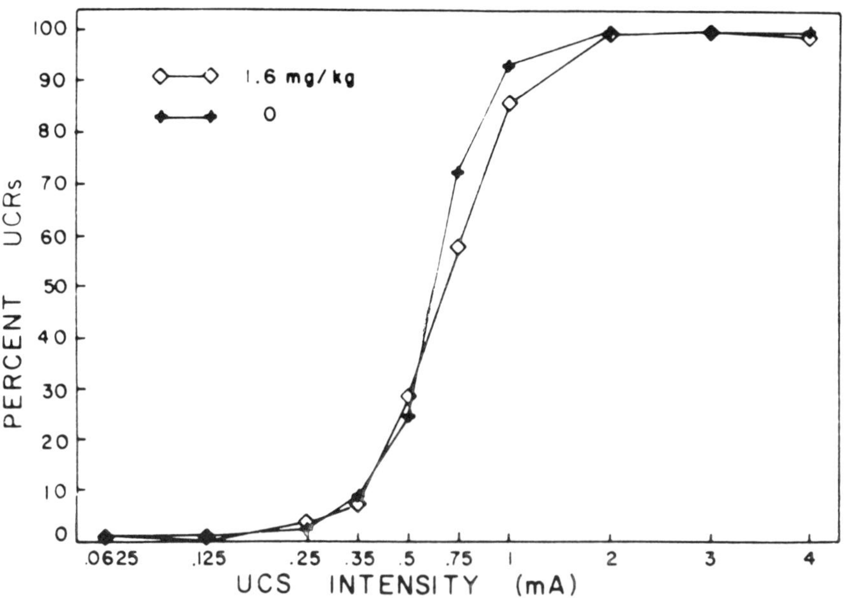

Fig. 3. Percent of unconditioned nictitating membrane responses as a function of shock intensity in the presence of saline (0) or 1.6 mg/kg scopolamine. Percentages were calculated on the basis of 10 presentations of each shock intensity. Each point is based on data from 12 rabbits (from Harvey et al., 1983, with permission from the authors and publisher).

alter the percent of unconditioned nictitating membrane response at any shock intensity. On the other hand, as shown in Fig. 4, scopolamine did reduce the percent of conditioned responses as a function of tone intensity. Thus, it was concluded that retardation in acquisition following scopolamine could not be attributed to alteration in the sensory processing of the shock or the motoric expression of the nictitating membrane response. On the other hand, scopolamine certainly altered control by the auditory stimulus. In this sense, scopolamine's effects are similar to those of haloperidol and morphine, which also retard the acquisition of the conditioned nictitating membrane response (Harvey and Gor-

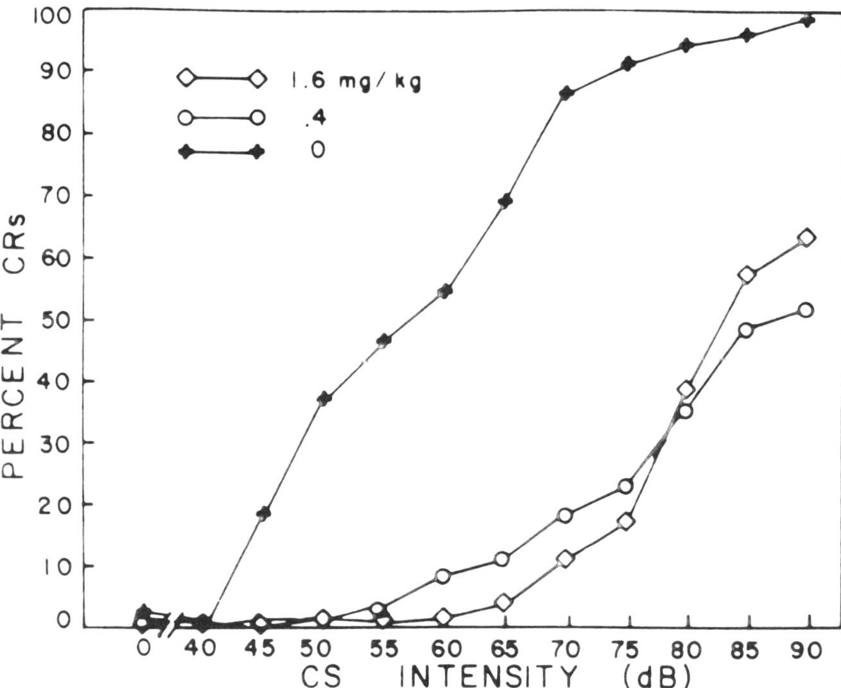

Fig. 4. Percent of conditioned nictitating membrane responses as a function of tone intensity in the presence of saline, 0.4 or 1.6 mg/kg scopolamine, administered 30–45 min before each session. Percentages were calculated on the basis of 15 presentations of each tone intensity. Each point is based on data from 12 rabbits (from Harvey et al., 1983, with permission from the authors and publisher).

mezano, 1981; Schindler et al., 1983), but different from LSD, which enhances acquisition of the conditioned response (Gimpl et al., 1979).

2.4. *Discrete Trial Procedures*

There are two general types of discrete trial procedures (Heise, 1975). In one, a stimulus is presented to an organism and a response occurs or not (go/no-go procedure). In the other procedure, a single response is reinforced in the presence of one discriminative stimulus and another response is reinforced in the presence of a different discriminative stimulus. This procedure is useful in studying drug effects on stimulus control because concomitant, nonspecific drug effects on response rate would presumably affect both responses equally. Thus, a two-choice discrete trial procedure might provide a measure of drug effects on stimulus control not confounded by drug effects upon response rates.

The discrete trial procedure has been used successfully in a number of contexts. For example, Evans (1975) examined the effects of scopolamine in monkeys trained to discriminate the shape of a visual stimulus projected on a key at various luminances. One of the most interesting aspects of Evans' study was the fact that he first demonstrated a relationship between the physical property of the stimulus (i.e., luminance) and the control of behavior. Thus, the effects of drug administration could be compared to effects induced by changing luminance. Briefly, as shown in Figs. 5 and 6, Evans found that as the luminance of the visual stimulus decreased, the percentage of correct discriminations also decreased. Similarly, scopolamine (15–60 mg/kg) induced dose-dependent decreases in correct discriminations that were dependent on stimulus intensity.

Discrete trial procedures have also been used to examine behavior under the control of temporal stimuli. In one study (Daniel and Thompson, 1980), pigeons were trained to respond on a red or green key, depending on whether the chamber was illuminated by a houselight for a short (4 s) or long (8 s) duration. When responding was examined at intermediate durations, a greater number of "long" responses

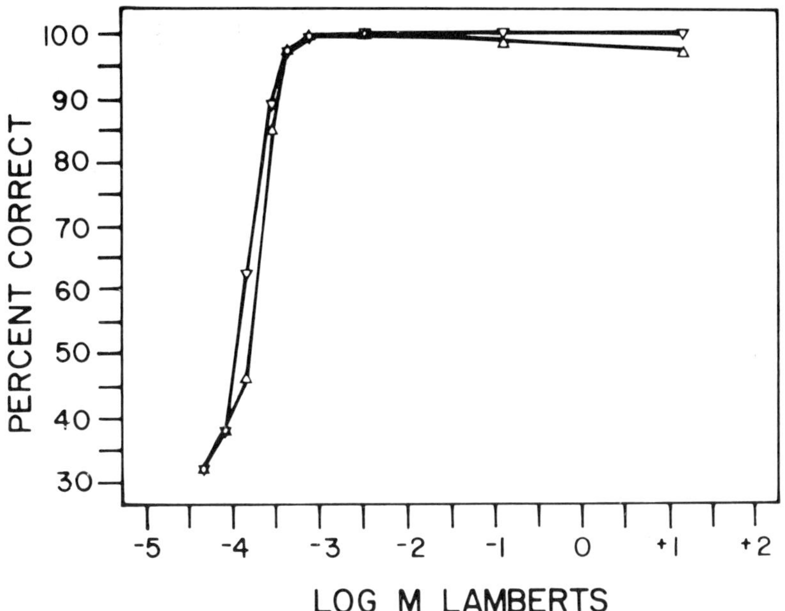

Fig. 5. Percentage of correct-form discriminations as a function of stimulus luminance. The *x*-axis shows the luminance in mL (milliLamberts). Each function represents data from a different monkey (from Evans, 1975, with permission from the authors and publisher).

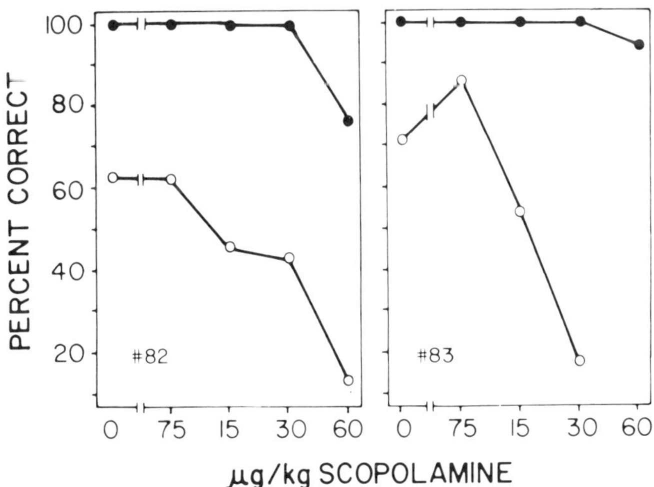

Fig. 6. Percentage of correct-form discriminations as a function of dose of scopolamine in two monkeys. Closed circles represent data obtained at a luminance of 10–0.9 mL; open circles represent data obtained at a luminance of 10–3.8 mL (from Evans, 1975, with permission from the authors and publisher).

occurred as the duration of the stimulus increased. ΔTetrahydrocannabinol (THC) (0.25–0.50 mg/kg) produced a dose-dependent decrease in responses controlled by the long-duration stimulus. Similar effects have been reported for THC in monkeys trained to discriminate between a visual stimulus with a duration of 100 s and 60, 80, or 90 s (Elsmore, 1972), and for amphetamine or methamphetamine in pigeons or rats trained to discriminate between stimuli of long and short durations (Stubbs and Thomas, 1974; Maricq et al., 1981).

In another series of studies, discrete trial procedures were used to examine discrimination of electric shock. Dykstra (1979a) examined morphine's effects in monkeys trained to discriminate between the presence and absence of shock by making one of two discrete responses (a right or a left lever-press). Responding was designated as correct if the monkey responded on the right lever when shock had been presented and on the left lever when shock had not been presented. Correct responses were followed by food on about 10% of the correct trials and incorrect responses were followed by a 20-s timeout period. Initially, monkeys were trained at a shock intensity of 0.35 mA and morphine's effects were examined. Then, to determine the lowest shock intensity at which this discrimination could be maintained, a psychophysical method of limits was examined. The results of this probe are shown in Fig. 7, in which it can be seen that the percentage of correct responses in the presence of shock increased as a function of shock intensity. Probes such as these are important because they indicate that the shock intensity maintained a controlling relationship over responding.

On the basis of these investigations, monkeys were then trained at an intensity determined to be close to their threshold (0.15 mA). After responding was stable at the lower shock intensity, the effects of morphine were examined. Morphine (0.3–1.0 mg/kg) decreased the percentage of correct responses in the presence of shock, but not in the absence of shock. These effects were accompanied by marked increases in time to respond both in the presence and the absence of shock; however, since discrete responses were measured, these changes in rate of responding did not interfere with the meas-

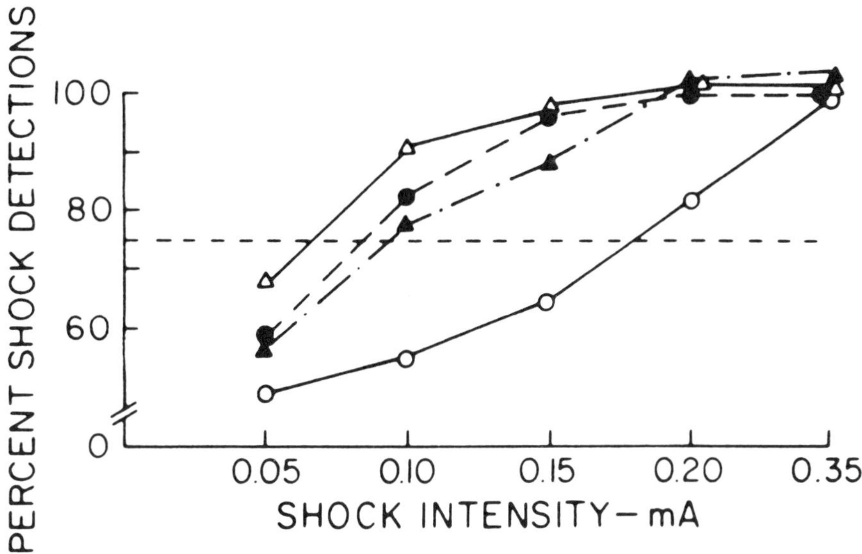

Fig. 7. Percent of shock detections as a function of shock intensity in four monkeys. Each point represents the mean of five sessions in each monkey (from Dykstra, 1979a).

ure of stimulus control. Other opioid analgesics, such as mcthadonc (0.3–1.0 mg/kg), nalorphinc (1.0–10.0 mg/kg), and cyclazocine (0.03–0.1 mg/kg), as well as the nonopioid analgesic levonantradol (0.017–0.03 mg/kg), also decreased correct responses in the presence but not the absence of shock (Dykstra, 1980, 1981). Moreover, in rats trained to respond differentially in the presence or absence of shock, morphine and other analgesics have similar effects (Lloyd et al., 1978; Poling et al., 1978; Hernandez and Appel, 1980).

Another notable feature of these data is that morphine's effects at the higher (0.35 mA) shock intensity were less than at the lower (0.05–0.15 mA) shock intensity, even though monkeys were about 90% correct at detecting both intensities. Other experiments also suggest that opioids alter discrimination of a low-intensity shock, but not of a high-intensity shock (Lloyd et al., 1978; Poling et al., 1978); however, this effect appears to be specific to situations in which the discrimination is between presence and absence of shock. In squirrel monkeys trained to discriminate between a high- and low-intensity shock (0.5 vs 0.1 mA), morphine decreased correct responses, but the extent to which it did so depended on the dose of morphine and not on the stimulus intensity (Genovese and Dykstra, 1984).

2.5. Threshold Measures

In most of the procedures described above, a discrimination was established between two stimuli, then drug effects were determined by examining responding in the presence of those stimuli. An alternative method for assessing drug effects on behavior under the control of discriminative stimuli is to determine the lowest value at which a stimulus can control behavior and then examine drug-induced alterations in this value. A study by Stebbins and Moody (1979) serves to illustrate this method. Food-deprived monkeys were trained to respond by holding a contact-sensitive plate for a period of 1–9 s until an acoustic stimulus was presented. If contact was broken after the tone had been presented, food was presented. If contact was broken prior to presentation of the tone, the trial was terminated without food delivery. The intensity at which monkeys responded 50% of the time was determined and described as the monkey's threshold. Drug-induced changes in this threshold were then measured and it was shown that daily treatment with the antibiotic kanamycin induced frequency-dependent deficits in the auditory threshold. A similar procedure has been used to examine the effects of pentobarbital upon auditory and visual thresholds in the baboon and squirrel monkey (Hienz et al., 1981; Delay et al., 1979).

In a modification of the threshold procedure, the value of the stimulus is changed on the basis of the organism's behavior (Blough, 1957). An example of this is the shock-titration procedure in which small increments in shock are programmed to occur at a specified interval and decrements in the shock intensity follow an appropriate response by the subject. The level at which the shock is maintained is often said to reflect tolerance for the shock. Presumably, drug-induced decreases in sensitivity to electric shock would induce an increase in the level at which the shock intensity is maintained.

In using procedures such as these, it is important to determine whether drug-induced changes in the intensity at which the shock is maintained reflect a change in response rate. For example, many drugs decrease response rate; thus alterations in shock intensity in the titration procedure may be caused by nonspecific decreases in rate of responding. Recently, a modification of the shock-titration procedure has been introduced that tends to minimize the contribution of decreases in rates of responding in determining the intensity at which shock is maintained (Dykstra, 1979b). In this procedure, shock is delivered during discrete shock periods. If responding does not occur during the shock period, shock intensity increases; however, if responding does occur, shock is terminated for a period of time (timeout period). At the end of the timeout period, the shock resumes at a lower intensity. Figure 8 shows a response record representative of

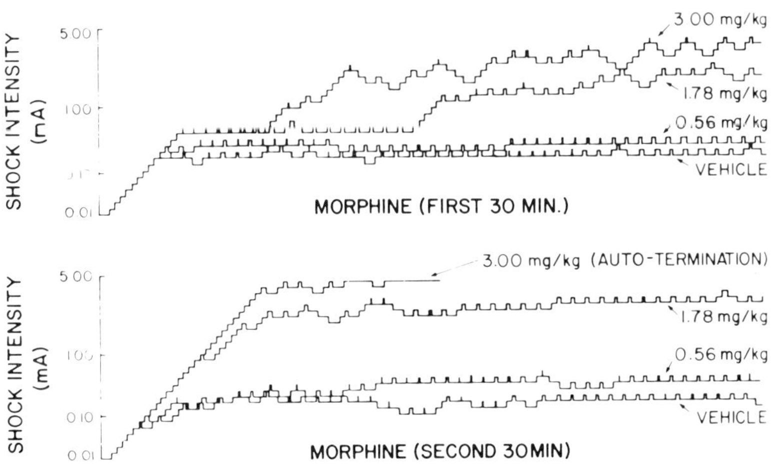

Fig. 8. Representative performance of one monkey under a shock titration schedule following vehicle or doses of morphine. Abscissa, time; ordinate, shock increments. The top set of records were obtained during the first 30 min of the session and the bottom set from the second 30 min of the session. The shock intensity reset to 0.01 mA at the beginning of the second 30-min period.

responding under the shock titration schedule. Under control conditions, the shock was maintained at a fairly constant level throughout the session; following morphine administration, this level increased in a dose-dependent manner. Many drugs have been shown to increase the intensity at which shock is maintained under this procedure, including morphine, pentazocine, cyclazocine, nantradol, ketocyclazocine, and ethylketocyclazocine (Dykstra, 1979b, 1983a,b). Moreover, it has been shown that increases in median shock level are not accompanied by decreases in rate of responding.

3. Behavioral Determinants of Drug Effects

It has been shown repeatedly that drug-induced alterations in behavior can be influenced by a number of behavioral as well as pharmacological variables. For example, drug effects are known to depend on the schedule and type of event that maintains responding (Kelleher and Morse, 1968), the behavioral history of the organism (Barrett, 1977; Barrett and Stanley, 1983), and the nature of the stimulus–reinforcer relationship (Spealman et al., 1978). In this section, behavioral variables that have been shown to determine the effects of drugs on behavior under stimulus control will be discussed.

3.1. Stimulus Variables

The fact that morphine's effects under the shock discrimination procedure described above depend on the intensity of the shock points to an important relationship that has been demonstrated repeatedly, i.e., stimulus intensity is an important determinant of a drug's effect on stimulus control. For example, in the Evans (1975) study discussed above, scopolamine's effects in monkeys trained to discriminate the shape of a visual stimulus depended on the luminance of the stimulus. At a low luminance, which produced 60–70% discrimination accuracy, scopolamine's effects were more marked than at a high luminance, which produced close to 100% accuracy. Similarly, the effects of both THC and amphetamine on a temporal discrimination depended on the duration of the stimulus controlling responding, with responding in the presence of long-duration stimuli being affected more than responding in the presence of short-duration stimuli (Daniel and Thompson, 1980; Stubbs and Thomas, 1974). Ksir and Slifer (1982) demonstrated a similar relationship in rats trained to discriminate the brightness of two keys. By varying the brightness of the key, rats responded at two levels of stimulus control within the same session. Under these conditions, *d*-amphetamine (0.5–2.0 mg/kg) and scopolamine (0.12–1.0 mg/kg) induced a greater decrement in stimulus control when the difference between the stimuli was decreased.

Thus, each of these studies demonstrate clearly that drug effects may be related to stimulus intensity. Nevertheless, the mechanism responsible for these differential effects is not clear. For example, differences may be caused by a number of factors, such as the level of accuracy or pattern of responding generated by different stimulus intensities.

The shock discrimination study described above (Dykstra, 1979a) indicates that physical intensity is an important factor in morphine's effect since both high (0.35 mA) and low (0.05–0.15 mA) shock intensities produced the same level of stimulus control (90% correct), yet morphine's effects were different under the two intensities.

A study by Katz (1983) addressed the question of whether pattern of responding or stimulus intensity is the determining factor in pentobarbital and promazine's effects on a visual conditional discrimination. As discussed above, Katz (1982) showed that pentobarbital and promazine did not alter stimulus control of behavior when control was established with a houselight intensity of 22.4 foot Lamberts (ftL). At this intensity, stimulus control was close to 100%. In a subsequent study, Katz (1983) examined houselight intensities that reduced stimulus control to 70%. Under these conditions, pentobarbital and promazine decreased stimulus control. In order to examine these effects further, Katz reexamined the effects of pentobarbital and promazine with the high-intensity houselight using a conjunctive schedule in which a certain number of incorrect responses was required for reinforcement. The number of incorrect responses required was adjusted so that the ratio of correct to incorrect responses was the same in the presence of the high-intensity houselight as in the presence of the low-intensity houselight. Figure 9 shows that pentobarbital and promazine did not alter stimulus control under this condition. Thus, Katz concluded that pentobarbital's and promazine's effects with the low-intensity houselight were related to the value of the stimulus rather than to the different pattern of responding generated by the low-intensity stimulus.

When qualitatively different stimuli are employed as consequences for behavior, they often control similar patterns and rates of responding; however, the effects of drugs on those behaviors have been shown to depend on the characteristics of the maintaining event. For example, the effects of chlordiazepoxide have been shown to depend on whether responding is maintained by food or shock (Barrett et al., 1981). In some instances then, the type of maintaining stimulus can function as a determinant of the behavioral effects of drugs. Although there has been considerable research examining drug effects on behavior maintained by qualitatively different consequences, there has not been similar emphasis on behavior controlled by different antecedent or discriminative stimuli that set the occasion for responding. This question has considerable application to investigations of the effects of analgesics. For example, it is not clear whether the effects of opioid analgesics are unique to noxious stimuli. One way to investigate this is to compare the effects of some analgesics on behavior that is differentially controlled by noxious or nonnoxious stimuli.

The work of Warren and Ison (1982) serves as an example. They made use of the startle response elicited by two different types of stimuli—an auditory or a shock stimulus. Previous work has shown that both of these stimuli readily elicit a startle response that can be measured indirectly by determining the intensity of the force applied to the floor of a holding cage by the rat's reflexive jump response. Figure 10 shows that morphine induced a greater decrease in the

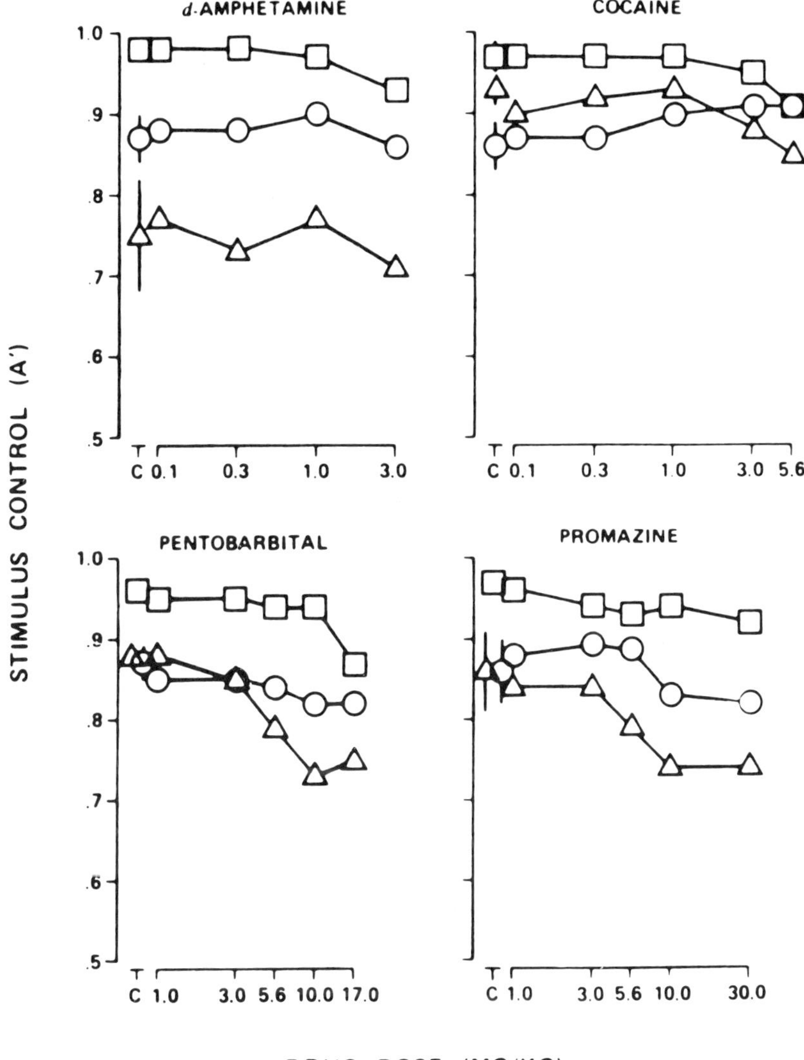

Fig. 9. Comparison of effects of *d*-amphetamine, cocaine, pentobarbital, and promazine on stimulus control under the fixed-interval schedule at a high- (squares) and low- (triangles) intensity houselight and under the conjunctive schedule at a high intensity houselight (circles). Stimulus control was highest under the fixed-interval schedule at the high-intensity houselight. Note that both pentobarbital and promazine selectively decreased stimulus control at the low-intensity houselight, but did not affect comparable values of stimulus control at a high-intensity houselight under the conjunctive schedule (from Katz, 1983, with permission of the authors and publisher).

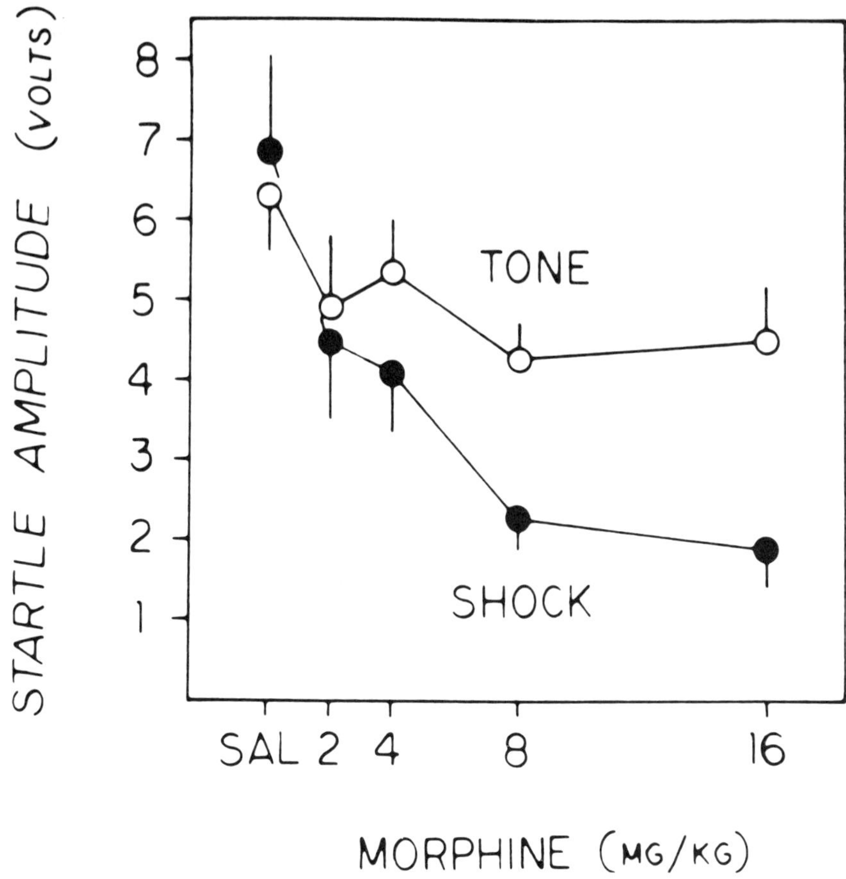

Fig. 10. Amplitude of the startle response elicited by a tone or a shock as a function of dose of morphine (from Warren and Ison, 1982, with permission of the authors and publisher).

response to shock than the response to the tone. Thus, it was concluded that the decrease in response force in the presence of the shock could not be attributed to a loss of motor function.

3.2. Response Variables

In addition to the stimulus variables discussed above, a number of other factors might be expected to influence drug effects on stimulus control. These include variables such as schedule of reinforcement, the characteristics of a response, and the relationship between the response and the discriminative stimulus. For example, Smith and McKearney (1977) have shown that morphine's effects under a titration procedure depend on the schedule employed. When a single response decreased shock by one increment, morphine did not alter responding; however, when 3–5 responses were required to produce a decrement in shock intensity, morphine induced dose-dependent alterations in responding. Differential effects have also been reported for morphine when shock increments occurred every 2 vs every 7.5 or 10 s. Under these conditions, morphine induced a greater increase in the intensity at which rats or squirrel monkeys maintained shock than when increments in shock intensity occured every 2 s (Weiss and Laties, 1961; Dykstra and McMillan, 1977).

Another response variable shown to contribute to a drug's effect is that of response bias or the subjects' tendency to engage in one response over another as the result of prior history or present reinforcement conditions. Signal-detection analysis, which has emphasized the contribution of response bias to drug effects on stimulus control, is discussed below.

4. Signal Detection Analysis

In discussing procedures used to measure drug effects on stimulus control, emphasis was placed on the way in which each of these procedures attempted to separate a drug's effect on rate of responding from its effects on stimulus control. Discrete trial procedures were shown to be particularly useful in this respect. Nevertheless, discrete trial procedures do not provide a way to examine how drug-induced changes in responding might interact with changes in stimulus control. Signal detection procedure differs from other stimulus control procedures in their emphasis on both sensory and response variables as important determinants of behavior. Within this context, sensory variables include the level of activity produced by a stimulus, and response variables include factors such as prior experience, reinforcement magnitude, and expectancies.

4.1. Introduction

In a typical signal detection experiment, an observer is trained to discriminate between the presence and absence of a low-intensity stimulus, such as a tone. Tone-present and tone-absent trials are presented in an unpredictable fashion, and on each trial the observer reports whether or not the tone was presented. Figure 11 shows two hypothetical curves that are useful in describing this situation. One curve (i.e., the noise distribution) represents sensory activity on trials when the tone is absent, i.e., random activity within the sensory sys-

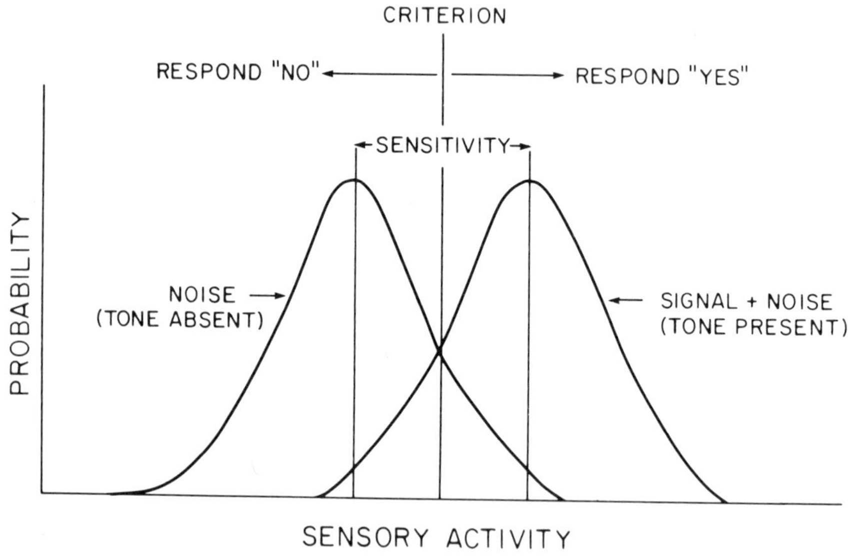

Fig. 11. Distributions of sensory activity representing data shown in Table 1. The distance between the mean of the noise distribution (from trials not containing the tone) and the mean of the signal-plus-noise distribution (from trials containing the tone) represents sensitivity. The criterion line represents the decision rule the subject established for responding "yes" or "no."

tem. The second curve, the signal-plus-noise distribution, represents sensory activity on trials when the tone is present. Two assumptions are made about this situation (Swets, 1961). First, sensory activity will vary on any given trial both when the tone is present and when the tone is absent. Second, in responding, the observer assesses the probability that the activity on any given trial resulted from noise alone or signal plus noise. It is important to note that this assessment must be made with some degree of uncertainty since the distributions of signal plus noise and noise alone overlap. Therefore, the observer is thought to make use of a decision rule or criterion such that when sensory activity exceeds a certain level, the observer responds "yes"; if sensory activity does not exceed that level, the observer responds "no." The criterion is thought to shift on the basis of response factors such as the consequences of a "yes" or "no" response.

Table 1 shows the four outcomes that occur within this situation. If a tone is presented and the observer responds "yes," then a hit is said to occur, whereas a "no" response following tone presentation is classified as a miss. On the other hand, on trials during which the tone is absent, a "yes" response is classified as a false alarm and a "no" response is classified as a correct rejection. From the hit rate and false alarm rate, statistical indices of sensitivity and response bias can be calculated. A common measure of sensitivity is d', which corresponds to the distance between the means of the noise and signal-plus-noise distributions. A common measure

Table 1

Hypothetical Results From a Signal Detection Experiment in Which a Subject Detects the Presence or Absence of a Tone

Trials	"Yes" response	"No" response
Trials with tone	0.80	0.20
Trials without tone	0.20 (false alarm rate)	0.80 (correct rejection rate)

of response bias is β, which corresponds to the ratio of the ordinates of the noise and signal-plus-noise distributions at the intersection of the criterion. Additional parametric and nonparametric measures of sensitivity and response bias can be derived (Pollack and Norman, 1964; Green and Swets, 1966; Grier, 1971; Clark, 1974; Appel and Dykstra, 1977).

A convenient way to represent sensitivity and response bias is with the receiver operating characteristic (ROC) curve shown in Fig. 12. The proportion of hits is shown on the ordinate and the proportion of false alarms is shown on the abscissa. Sensitivity is represented by the point at which the ROC curve intercepts the negative diagonal and/or by the area contained under the ROC curve. For example, a curve in the far upper-left portion of the graph would contain an area close to 100% and would represent a high degree of sensitivity, whereas the area contained under the major diagonal would be 50%, representing responding at a chance level. Bias is represented by the position of the point to the right or left of the negative diagonal. For illustrative purposes, five points are represented here. Points 1, 2, and 3 fall along the same ROC curve, indicating that each of these points represents the same sensitivity. Nevertheless, points 1, 2, and 3 are at different positions along the curve, indicating different biases. In reference to the signal and noise distributions shown in Fig. 11, points 1, 2, and 3 correspond to a shift in the criterion to the right (point 2) or left (point 3), whereas the distance between the means of the signal-plus-noise and the noise distributions has not changed. One situation that might be expected to produce data that correspond to points 1, 2, and 3 would be differential consequences for a hit or correct rejection.

In contrast to points 1, 2, and 3, points 4 and 5 correspond to a change in sensitivity, as reflected by their position on the negative diagonal. At points 4 and 5, the criterion remains constant and sensitivity changes. One situation that might be expected to produce data that correspond to point 4 would be a decrease in the volume of the tone, which would shift the signal-plus-noise distribution closer to the noise distribution. On the other hand, point 5 corresponds to

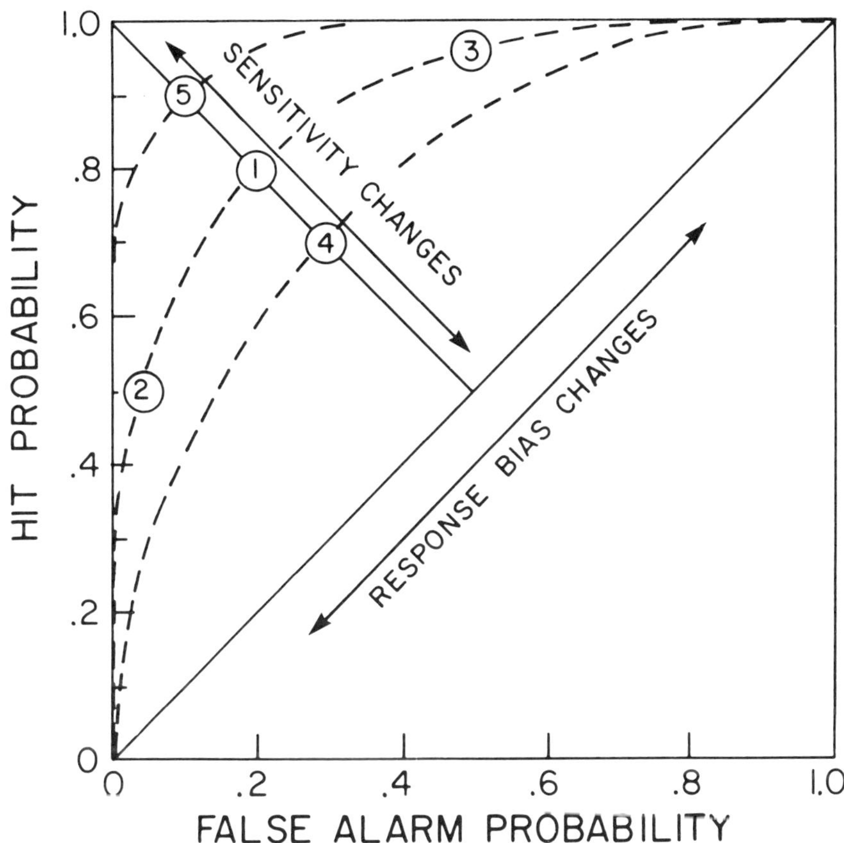

Fig. 12. Representation of receiver operating characteristic curves from a hypothetical signal-detection experiment. Points 1, 2, and 3 indicate three different values of bias at the same value of sensitivity. Points 1, 4, and 5 represent three different values of sensitivity at the same value of bias.

an increase in the volume of the tone, shifting the signal-plus-noise distribution further to the right of the noise distribution.

4.2. Representative Studies

Studies that have used signal detection analysis to examine drug effects on stimulus control generally replace the yes/no response of the human observer with a discrete response by the experimental animal, such as a right or left lever-press or a right or left turn in a T-maze. In each case, reinforcement follows appropriate responses on signal or noise trials. Moreover, discriminations are usually between two different signals (S1 and S2), each imposed on the noise distribution.

Dykstra and Appel (1974) used signal detection analysis to examine the behavior of rats under the control of an auditory stimulus. Rats were trained to respond differentially on two levers in the presence of tones of different frequencies. Correct responses were followed by milk and the number of correct responses required for reinforcement was varied. An ROC curve derived from the performance of one rat in this experiment is shown in Fig. 13. Sensitivity is shown by the point at which the ROC curves generated at each of the three different discriminations (2000 vs 5000 Hz; 3000 vs 4000 Hz; 3300 vs 3800 Hz) intercepted the negative diagonal. Sensitivity increased as the difference between the two tones increased. Moreover, bias as shown by position on the ROC curve changed as a function of reinforcement frequency. That is, when reinforcement probability was higher on the right lever (two correct responses produced food) than on the left lever (ten correct responses produced food), responding was biased toward the right lever. Data generated from this condition are on the left side of the ROC curve. Switching these probabilities moved the data to the right side of the curve. When lysergic acid diethylamide (LSD) (0.04–0.16 mg/kg) was administered, response bias changed, but sensitivity did not (data not shown). Thus, the effects of LSD were more similar to a change in reinforcement frequency than to a change in sensitivity. Similar results were reported for LSD in pigeons trained to discriminate the presence and absence of colored stimuli (Nielsen and Appel, 1983).

Signal-detection methods have also been used to determine whether drug-induced changes in stimulus control might simply be caused by an increase or decrease in response tendency. For example, there are numerous reports that scopolamine disrupts responding under stimulus control. Moreover,

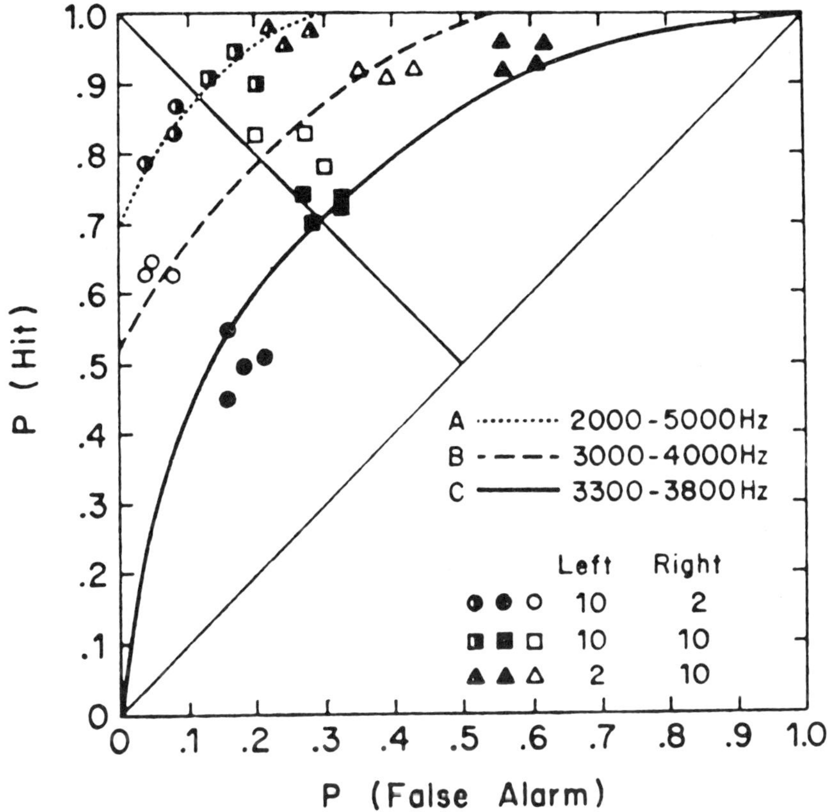

Fig. 13. Three receiver operating characteristic (ROC) curves for the performance of one rat at three different frequency discriminations. Hits were defined as responding on the left lever in the presence of a "high" tone, and false alarms were defined as responding on the left lever in the presence of a "low" tone. Each discrimination was observed under three different reinforcement conditions. In one condition, every tenth correct response on the left lever and every second correct response on the right lever was followed by milk presentation. In the second condition, every tenth correct response on the left lever and every tenth correct response on the right lever was reinforced with milk. The third condition was the opposite of the first condition. Curves were fitted to these points by inspection (from Dykstra and Appel, 1974, with permission of the publisher).

it has been suggested that these disruptions are a result of response factors (e.g., "response disinhibition") rather than changes in stimulus control. A study by Milar (1981) used signal-detection analysis to show that scopolamine altered stimulus control in rats trained to discriminate between a bright or dim light. In this experiment, a "yes" response was defined as a response on a lever and a "no" as a failure to respond. Within this context, scopolamine's effects could be examined separately on responding and nonresponding. If scopolamine's effects were caused by an increase in response probability, Milar argued that this would be reflected as a selective increase in "yes" responses. Milar first showed that responding was actually under control of the light. That is, changes in the intensity difference between the two stimuli produced changes in sensitivity. This author also showed that changes in reinforcement probability produced changes in response bias. When the difference between the stimuli was small, scopolamine (0.50 mg/kg) as well as physostigmine (0.05 mg/kg) decreased sensitivity but not bias.

Although this study suggests that scopolamine's effects under a visual discrimination are not caused by changes in response probability, other investigators have suggested that amphetamine's effects on behavior under stimulus control may be the result of changes in response probability (Robbins and Iversen, 1973). For example, Koek and Slangen (1983, 1984) used both a signal detection analysis as well as an analysis of response repetition to show that amphetamine disrupted performance under both an auditory and a visual discrimination by increasing response repetition.

4.3. Assessment of Analgesics

Perhaps the most compelling application of signal detection analysis is to the study of nociception and analgesia. In a stimulus control context, analgesia refers to the alteration of behavior under the control of noxious events. As with the effects of many drugs on stimulus control, alteration of behavior under the control of noxious stimuli is thought to involve at least two factors—those related to the stimulus and those related to the response. It has been emphasized repeatedly that a very important part of an analgesic's power lies in its ability to modify the response component of nociception. Thus, it seems particularly important to develop methods for directly studying both stimulus and response factors in drug-induced analgesia.

Signal detection is one method that attempts to distinguish between variables that determine an organism's sensitivity to stimuli, as well as variables that determine how an organism responds in the presence of those stimuli. When signal detection is used to examine nociception, response bias is interpreted by examining a subject's tendency to "describe" a stimulus as noxious, whereas sensitivity is determined by noting the accuracy with which a subject distinguishes between noxious stimuli of different intensities. Superficially, the interpretation of changes in sensitivity and response bias following administration of an analgesic appears to be straightforward, i.e., a reduction in sensitivity would indicate a reduction in the intensity of the noxious stimulus, whereas a change in response bias would reflect changes in a subject's tendency to describe the stimulus as noxious. Unfortunately, there are many theoretical and empirical issues that indicate that the situation is far more complex (McBurney, 1976; Rollman, 1977; 1980; Chapman, 1977; Jones, 1979; Velden, 1979; Coppola and Gracely, 1983). Since most applications of signal detection analysis to the investigation of analgesia have used human subjects, these will be discussed briefly as background for the animal studies that follow (for a more thorough discussion of this work, *see* reviews from Clark, 1974; Lloyd and Appel, 1976; Grossberg and Grant, 1978).

Clark (1969) found that the administration of a placebo described to subjects as a potent analgesic sharply decreased the number of stimuli classified as "painful," suggesting that the placebo had altered the subject's sensitivity. Signal detection analysis, however, showed that the sole effect of the placebo was to alter the subject's response bias (or tendency to classify a stimulus as "painful"), whereas sensitivity remained unchanged. On the other hand, in subjects trained to discriminate between the presence and absence of different intensities of a radiant heat stimulus, nitrous oxide (33%) decreased sensitivity and altered response bias such that the number of times a stimulus was labeled "painful" was decreased. Moreover, diazepam had no effect under these conditions (Chapman et al., 1973, 1975; Chapman and Feather, 1973). In summary, these studies suggest that placebos alter response bias, whereas an analgesic such as nitrous oxide alters both bias and sensitivity.

Signal-detection analysis has also been used to examine behavior under the control of noxious stimuli in nonhuman organisms. In these studies, sensitivity is assessed by examining discrimination between noxious stimuli, and response bias is assessed by the presence or absence of a response such as a lever-press or a turn in a T-maze. For example, Lineberry and Kulics (1978) trained monkeys to press a lever in the presence of two intensities of electric shock. Hits were defined as a response (lever-press) following presentation of an 8.0-mA shock; correct rejections were defined as the withholding of a response following presentation of a 7.0-mA shock. Morphine (0.125–0.5 mg/kg) and diazepam (0.062–0.25 mg/kg) had no effect on sensitivity in this situation, whereas both drugs increased response bias. Similarly, morphine and diazepam altered response bias, but did not consistently alter sensitivity in a procedure in which monkeys escaped a shock presented at different intensities. Responses following a high-intensity shock were classified as hits, and responses following a low-intensity shock were classified as false alarms (Lineberry and Kulics, 1978, 1980).

In another series of studies (Grilly and Genovese, 1979; Grilly, 1981; Grilly et al., 1980), rats were trained to turn right or left in a T-maze, depending on whether a high- or low-intensity shock had been presented. Decreasing the difference between the shocks decreased sensitivity, as measured by correct turns in the T-maze. Response bias was altered by varying reinforcement magnitude or stimulus probability. Under these conditions, signal detection analysis indicated that morphine decreased sensitivity to the shock, but did not consistently alter response bias. Hernandez and Appel (1980) reported a similar effect with morphine in rats trained to discriminate between the presence and absence of shock.

There are numerous differences between the studies discussed above that might account for the discrepant results. Lineberry and Kulics used rhesus monkeys and a go/no-go procedure, whereas rats and a two-response procedure were used in the other studies. Moreover, the nature of the discrimination differed. In the Hernandez and Appel study, the discrimination was between the presence and absence of shock, whereas in the other studies the discrimination was between two different shock intensities. Although procedural variables may account for the different findings, discrepant results such as these also raise doubts about the appropriateness of signal detection analysis in this context. One problem concerns the unique aspects of noxious stimuli. When stimuli such as electric shock and radiant heat are examined, a case can certainly be made for their noxiousness, provided the intensity employed is high enough. Nevertheless, stimuli such as these can have other attributes, and unless one clearly determines what aspect of these stimuli is controlling responding, it is difficult to interpret a drug effect as relating only to the noxiousness of the stimuli. Moreover, it cannot be assumed that analgesics only alter behavior under the control of noxious stimuli. For example, morphine has been shown to alter stimulus control involving auditory (Hernandez and Appel, 1979; Koek and Slangen, 1983), as well as visual stimuli (Grilly et al., 1980; Koek and Slangen, 1984).

Even if stimuli can be specified as purely noxious, considerable difficulty still remains in the interpretation of changes in sensitivity. This might be best illustrated by reference to Fig. 11. Although the abscissa in Fig. 11 represents sensory activity, a decrease in sensory activity may not accompany analgesia. Furthermore, sensitivity is usually measured by noting the accuracy with which a subject distinguishes between high and low stimulus intensities. Under these conditions, drug administration could alter both high- and low-intensity stimuli, but not the magnitude of the difference between the two stimuli. If both noise and signal-plus-noise distributions are moved to the left to the same extent, a change in sensitivity would not occur. Thus a decrease in sensitivity is neither necessary nor sufficient to indicate that analgesia has occurred (Rollman, 1977, 1980).

5. Summary

This chapter has emphasized the importance of behavioral variables as determinants of a drug's effect on stimulus control. For example, the results of a number of studies indicate that the magnitude of a drug's effect on stimulus control is a function of the degree to which a stimulus controls behavior. Moreover, degree of stimulus control often relates to intensity of the discriminative stimulus. The importance of considering drug-induced changes in response rate as a potential confounding factor when interpreting drug effects on stimulus control was also discussed, along with numerous procedures for minimizing this problem. Moreover, it was shown that signal-detection analysis could be used to examine both stimulus and response variables as determinants of a drug's effect on stimulus control.

As a result of the emphasis that many investigators have placed on behavioral variables, generalizations are beginning to emerge about the effects of selected drugs on stimulus control. For example, it has been shown under a number of different conditions that amphetamine alters behavior under the control of temporal stimuli. Moreover, it appears that the effects of amphetamine (or methamphetamine) in this context are similar to a decrease in the duration of the discriminative stimulus. A similar case is also emerging for THC. It has also been shown that morphine and a number of other opioid analgesics selectively alter behavior under the control of electric shock, although it is still not clear whether these effects are caused by the noxious qualities of shock or response variables. Unfortunately, the application of signal detection analysis has not clarified this issue. General observations are also beginning to emerge about scopolamine, which has been shown repeatedly to alter behavior controlled by visual, auditory, and temporal stimuli.

Thus, it is clear that careful attention to the contribution of both behavioral and pharmacological variables in the assessment of drug effects on stimulus control is beginning to produce some important general principles.

References

Appel J. B. and Dykstra L. A. (1977) Drugs, Discrimination and Signal Detection Theory, in *Advances in Behavioral Pharmacology* (Thompson T. and Dews P. B., eds.), Academic, New York.

Barrett J. E. (1977) Behavioral history as a determinant of the effects of *d*-amphetamine on punished behavior. *Science* **198,** 67–69.

Barrett J. E. and Stanley J. A. (1983) Prior behavioral experience can reverse the effects of morphine. *Psychopharmacology* **81,** 107–110.

Barrett J. E., Valentine J. O., and Katz J. L. (1981) Effects of chlordiazepoxide and *d*-amphetamine on responding of squirrel monkeys maintained under concurrent or second-order schedules or response-produced food or electric shock presentation. *J. Pharmacol. Exp. Ther.* **219,** 199–206.

Blough D. S. (1957) Effect of lysergic acid diethylamide on absolute visual threshold of the pigeon. *Science* **126,** 304–305.

Chapman C. R. (1977) Sensory decision theory methods in pain research: A reply to Rollman. *Pain* **3,** 295–305.

Chapman C. R. and Feather B. W. (1973) Effects of diazepam on human pain tolerance and pain sensitivity. *Psychosom. Med.* **35,** 330–340.

Chapman C. R., Murphy T. M., and Butler S. H. (1973) Analgesic strength of 33 percent nitrous oxide: A signal detection theory evaluation. *Science* **179,** 1246–1248.

Chapman C. R., Gehrig J. D., and Wilson M. E. (1975) Acupuncture compared with 33 percent nitrous oxide for dental analgesia: A sensory decision theory evaluation. *Anesthesiology* **42,** 532–537.

Clark W. C. (1969) Sensory-decision theory analysis of the placebo effect on the criterion for pain and thermal sensitivity (*d'*). *J. Abnorm. Psychol.* **74,** 363–371.

Clark F. C. and Steele B. J. (1966) Effects of *d*-amphetamine on performance under a multiple schedule in the rat. *Psychopharmacologia* **9**, 157–169.

Clark W. C. (1974) Pain sensitivity and the report of pain: An introduction to sensory decision theory. *Anesthesiology* **40**, 272–287.

Coppola R. and Gracely R. H. (1983) Where is the noise in SDT pain assessment? *Pain* **17**, 257–266.

Daniel S. A. and Thompson T. (1980) Methadone-induced attenuation of the effects of Δ^9-tetrahydrocannabinol on temporal discrimination in pigeons. *J. Pharmacol. Exp. Ther.* **213**, 247–253.

Delay E. R., Steiner N. O., and Isaac W. (1979) Effects of *d*-amphetamine and methylphenidate upon auditory threshold in the squirrel monkey. *Pharmacol. Biochem. Behav.* **10**, 861–864.

Dews P. B. (1955) Studies on behavior. II. The effects of pentobarbital, methamphetamine and scopolamine on performances in pigeons involving discriminations. *J. Pharmacol. Exp. Ther.* **115**, 380–389.

Dews P. B. (1971) Commentary, in *Behavioral Analysis of Drug Action* (Harvey J. A., ed.), Scott, Foresman, Glenview, Illinois.

Dykstra L. A. (1979a) Effects of morphine, diazepam, and chlorpromazine on discrimination of electric shock. *J. Pharmacol. Exp. Ther.* **209**, 297–303.

Dykstra L. A. (1979b) Effects of morphine, pentazocine and cyclazocine alone and in combination with naloxone on electric shock titration in the squirrel monkey. *J. Pharmacol. Exp. Ther.* **211**, 722–732.

Dykstra L. A. (1980) Discrimination of electric shock: Effects of some opioid and nonopioid drugs. *J. Pharmacol. Exp. Ther.* **213**, 234–240.

Dykstra L. A. (1981) Effects of morphine, levonantradol, and *n*-methyl levonantradol on shock intensity discrimination. *J. Clin. Pharmacol.* **21**, 341S–347S.

Dykstra L. A. (1983a) Electric shock titration in squirrel monkeys following administration of nantradol, levonantradol, or *n*-methyl levonantradol. *Psychopharmacology* **79**, 322–324.

Dykstra L. A. (1983b) Effects of ketocyclazocine and ethylketocyclazocine on electric shock titration. *Eur. J. Pharmacol.* **94**, 19–26.

Dykstra L. A. and Appel J. B. (1974) Effects of LSD on auditory perception: A signal detection analysis. *Psychopharmacologia* **34**, 289–307.

Dykstra L. A. and McMillan D. E. (1977) Electric shock titration: Effects of morphine, methadone, pentazocine, nalorphine, naloxone, diazepam and amphetamine. *J. Pharmacol. Exp. Ther.* **202**, 660–669.

Elsmore T. F. (1972) Effects of delta-9-tetrahydrocannabinol on temporal and auditory discrimination performances of monkeys. *Psychopharmacologia* **26**, 62–72.

Evans H. L. (1975) Scopolamine effects on visual discrimination: Modifications related to stimulus control. *J. Pharmacol. Exp. Ther.* **195**, 105–113.

Genovese R. F. and Dykstra L. A. (1984) Effects of morphine, clonidine and intensity change on electric-shock discrimination. *J. Exp. Anal. Behav.* **41**, 309–317.

Gimpl M. P., Gormezano I., and Harvey J. A. (1979) Effects of LSD on learning as measured by classical conditioning of the rabbit nictitating membrane response. *J. Pharmacol. Exp. Ther.* **208**, 330–334.

Green D. M. and Swets J. A. (1966) Signal detection theory and psychophysics. John Wiley, New York.

Grier J. B. (1971) Nonparametric indexes for sensitivity and bias: computing formulas. *Psychol. Bull.* **75**, 424–429.

Grilly D. M. (1981) A signal detection analysis of morphine effects on the response bias of rats in a two-shock discrimination task. *Life Sci.* **28**, 1883–1888.

Grilly D. M. and Genovese R. F. (1979) Assessment of shock discrimination in rats with signal detection theory. *Perception and Psychophysics* **25**, 466–472.

Grilly D. M., Genovese R. F., and Nowak M. J. (1980) Effects of morphine, d-amphetamine, and pentobarbital on shock and light discrimination performance in rats. *Psychopharmacology* **70**, 213–217.

Grossberg J. M. and Grant B. F. (1978) Clinical psychophysics: Applications of ratio scaling and signal detection methods to research on pain, fear, drugs and medical decision making. *Psychol. Bull.* **85**, 1154–1176.

Harvey J. A. and Gormezano I. (1981) Effects of haloperidol and pimozide on classical conditioning of the rabbit nictitating membrane response. *J. Pharmacol. Exp. Ther.* **218**, 712–719.

Harvey J. A., Gormezano I., and Cool-Hauser V. A. (1983) Effects of scopolamine and methylscopolamine on classical conditioning of the rabbit nictitating membrane response. *J. Pharmacol. Exp. Ther.* **225**, 42–49.

Heise G. A. (1975) Discrete trial analysis of drug action. *Fed. Proc.* **34**, 1898–1903.

Heise G. A. and Milar K. S. (1984) Drugs and Stimulus Control, in *Handbook of Psychopharmacology* vol. 18 (Iversen L. L., Iversen S. D., Snyder S. H., eds.), Plenum, New York.

Hernandez L. L. and Appel J. B. (1979) An analysis of some perceptual effects of morphine, chlorpromazine and LSD. *Psychopharmacology* **60**, 125–130.

Hernandez L. L. and Appel J. B. (1980) Effects of pentazocine and other opiates on shock detection in the rat: Involvement of opiate and dopamine receptors. *Psychopharmacology* **67**, 155–163.

Hienz R. D., Lukas S. E., and Brady J. V. (1981) The effects of pentobarbital upon auditory and visual thresholds in the baboon. *Pharmacol. Biochem. Behav.* **15**, 799–805.

Jones B. (1979) Signal detection theory and pain research. *Pain* **7**, 305–312.

Katz J. L. (1982) Effects of drugs on stimulus control of behavior. I. Independent assessment of effects on response rates and stimulus control. *J. Pharmacol. Exp. Ther.* **223**, 617–623.

Katz J. L. (1983) Effects of drugs on stimulus control of behavior. II. Degree of stimulus control as a determinant of effect. *J. Pharmacol. Exp. Ther.* **226**, 756–763.

Kelleher R. T. and Morse W. H. (1968) Determinants of the specificity of behavioral effects of drugs. *Ergeb. Physiol. Biol. Chem. Exp. Pharmakol.* **60**, 1–56.

Koek W. and Slangen J. L. (1983) Effects of *d*-amphetamine and morphine on discrimination: Signal detection analysis and assessment of response repetition in the performance deficits. *Psychopharmacology* **80**, 125–128.

Koek W. and Slangen J. L. (1984) Effects of *d*-amphetamine and morphine on delayed discrimination: Signal detection analysis and assessment of response repetition in the performance deficits. *Psychopharmacology* **83**, 346–350.

Ksir C. and Slifer B. (1982) Drug effects on discrimination performance at two levels of stimulus control. *Psychopharmacology* **76**, 286–290.

Lineberry C. G. and Kulics A. T. (1978) The effects of diazepam, morphine and lidocaine on nociception in rhesus monkeys: A signal detection analysis. *J. Pharmacol. Exp. Ther.* **205**, 302–310.

Lineberry C. G. and Kulics A. T. (1980) Morphine effects on escape in the rhesus monkey. *Neuropharmacology* **19**, 107–110.

Lloyd M. A. and Appel J. B. (1976) Signal detection theory and the psychophysics of pain: An introduction and review. *Psychosom. Med.* **38**, 79–94.

Lloyd M. A., Appel J. B., and McGowan III, W. T. (1978) Effects of morphine and chlorpromazine on the detection of shock. *Psychopharmacology* **58**, 241–246.

Maricq A. V., Roberts S., and Church R. M. (1981) Methamphetamine and time estimation. *J. Exp. Psych.: Animal Behav. Process.* **7**, 18–30.

McBurney D. H. (1976) Signal detection theory and pain (letter to the editor). *Anesthesiology* **44**, 356–359.

Milar K. S. (1981) Cholinergic drug effects on visual discriminations: A signal detection analysis. *Psychopharmacology* **74**, 383–388.

Moerschbaecher J. M. and Thompson D. M. (1983) Differential effects of prototype opioid agonists on the acquisition of conditional discriminations in monkeys. *J. Pharmacol. Exp. Ther.* **226**, 738–748.

Nielsen E. B. and Appel J. B. (1983) The effects of drugs on the discrimination of color following a variable delay period: A signal detection analysis. *Psychopharmacology* **80**, 24–28.

Poling A., Simmons M. A., and Appel J. B. (1978) Morphine and shock detection: Effects on shock intensity. *Comm. Psychopharmacol.* **2**, 333–336.

Pollack I. and Norman D. A. (1964) A non-parametric analysis of recognition experiments. *Psychon. Sci.* **1**, 125–126.

Ray B. A. and Sidman M. (1970) Reinforcement Schedules and Stimulus Control, in *The Theory of Reinforcement Schedules* (Schoenfeld W. N., ed.), Appleton-Century-Crofts, New York.

Rilling M. (1977) Stimulus Control and Inhibitory Processes, in *Handbook of Operant Behavior* (Honig W. D. and Staddon J E. R., eds.), Prentice-Hall, Englewood Cliffs, New Jersey.

Robbins T. W. and Iversen S. D. (1973) Amphetamine-induced disruption of temporal discrimination by response disinhibition. *Nature* **245**, 191–192.

Rollman G. B. (1977) Signal detection theory measurement of pain: A review and critique. *Pain* **3**, 187–211.

Rollman G. B. (1980) On the utility of signal detection theory pain measures. *Pain* **9**, 375–379.

Schindler C. W., Gormezano I., and Harvey J. A. (1983) Effect of morphine on acquisition of the classically conditioned nictitating membrane response of the rabbit. *J. Pharmacol. Exp. Ther.* **227**, 639–643.

Smith J. B. and McKearney J. W. (1977) Effects of morphine, methadone, nalorphine and naloxone on responding under schedules of electric shock titration. *J. Pharmacol. Exp. Ther.* **220**, 508–515.

Spealman R. D., Katz J. L., and Witkin J. M. (1978) Drug effects on responding maintained by stimulus-reinforcer and response-reinforcer contingencies. *J. Exp. Anal. Behav.* **30**, 187–196.

Stebbins W. C. and Moody D. B. (1979) Comparative behavioral toxicology. *Neurobehav. Toxicol.* **1** (suppl. 1), 33–44.

Stubbs D. A. and Thomas J. R. (1974) Discrimination of stimulus duration and *d*-amphetamine in pigeons: A psychophysical analysis. *Psychopharmacologia* **36**, 313–322.

Swets J. A. (1961) Detection theory and psychophysics: A review. *Psychometrika* **26**, 49–63.

Terrace H. S. (1966) Stimulus Control, in *Operant Behavior: Areas of Research and Application* (Honig W. K., ed.), Appleton-Century Crofts, New York.

Velden M. (1979) Does signal detection methodology allow to measure discrimination, but not pain? (letter to editor). *Pain* **7**, 377–378.

Waller M. B. (1961) Effects of chronically administered chlorpromazine on multiple-schedule performance. *J. Exp. Anal. Behav.* **4**, 351–359.

Warren P. H. and Ison J. R. (1982) Selective action of morphine on reflex expression to nociceptive stimulation in the rat: A contribution to the assessment of analgesia. *Pharmacol. Biochem. Behav.* **16**, 869–874.

Weiss B. and Laties V. G. (1961) Changes in pain tolerance and other behavior produced by salicylates. *J. Pharmacol. Exp. Ther.* **131,** 120–129.

Drug Discrimination Learning

CUE PROPERTIES OF DRUGS

Torbjörn U. C. Järbe

1. Introduction

In his tales of travels in the Far East, Marco Polo describes how the "Old Man on the Mountain" (Hassan Sabbah, year 1090, and followers) recruited loyal warriors, the assassins, to faithfully obey and follow their master. According to the tale, the old man invited the potential warrior to a delicious dinner in his fortress. A drug (hashish?) had been mixed with the food, and while intoxicated, the guest was transferred to a magnificent garden to enjoy "paradise." After once again being drugged and brought back to the old man, the guest was assured of a return to paradise if he served the old man faithfully. Having "experienced" paradise, the assassins became feared enemies of anyone who opposed the will of their master. This story is an early account reminiscent of what was later described as dissociative learning. Siegel (1982) has summarized other accounts of the phenomenon, for example "the well-known case of the Irish porter who, having lost a package when drunk, got drunk again and remembered where he had left it."

The report that a leg flexion conditioned response in dogs was elicited only when the state appropriate for the initial learning or conditioning was reinstated, i.e., curare or no drug (Girden and Culler, 1937), marks the beginning of the experimental analysis of dissociation of learning, or state-dependent learning (SDL) as it is more commonly called today. SDL implies that a response learned in one condition ("state") is specific to that condition and that the response will be performed poorly or not at all when tested in other states, i.e., a transfer failure because of dissociated learning.

A new approach to the study of the state-dependency concept was achieved with the introduction of drug-discrimination learning (DDL) techniques during the sixties. These techniques include use of the T-maze and three-compartment, shock–escape tasks (e.g., Overton, 1966, 1967), as well as operant procedures (e.g., Harris and Balster, 1968; Kubena and Barry, 1969; Morrison and Stephenson, 1969) to be described in some detail later. With the use of DDL procedures, a shift in emphasis from an interest in dissociation or SDL phenomena *per se* to pharmacology has been evident. This chapter will further this trend, treating DDL as one of the procedures of psychopharmacology in the broadest sense. The recent upsurge in the number of articles on DDL attests to its significance as a major contribution to psychophar-macology (Fig. 1). A bibliography on DDL reports, covering the period of 1951–1982, has been compiled by Stolerman et al. (1982).

2. Discrimination and Generalization

Discrimination learning may be either the successive or simultaneous presentation of stimuli with differential rein-forcement with the objective being to narrow the control of the response class to one stimulus value. Therefore, the prere-quisite for discrimination is an ability to differentiate stimuli and the choice between alternative responses. Discriminative stimuli have usually been defined as external events occasion-ing reactions at exteroceptive receptors of different sensory systems, or as drive stimuli such as thirst, hunger, and proprioceptive stimuli. To this list we now add drug effects as discriminative stimuli.

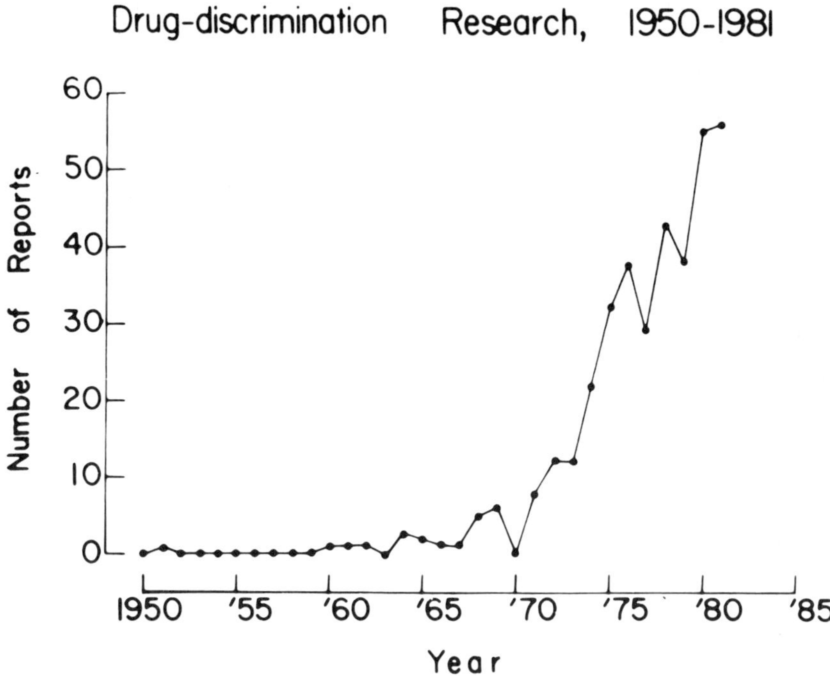

Fig. 1. Growth of the literature on drug discrimination over 30 yr since the first report appeared. Abstracts, research papers, reviews, and books were included to produce this diagram (from Stolerman et al., 1982; reprinted with permission of publisher and author).

A stimulus gradient is evident when responses conditioned to one stimulus are also elicited by other stimuli of the same dimension after a discrimination between a pair of training stimuli has been established. The nature and shape of such stimulus gradients are determined both by the conditioning history and the tests actually constructed for demonstrating the generalization (Heinemann and Chase, 1975; Honig and Urcuioli, 1981). Thus, the concept of generalization implies that stimuli can control behavior without ever having been involved in the original conditioning process. These two measures, discrimination and generalization, are the basis of a discrimination experiment.

3. Methods for Establishing Drug-Discriminative Control Over Behavior

3.1. T-Maze, Two-Choice Procedure

As noted earlier, T-maze, two-choice procedures were common in the early days of drug discrimination research. Although both positive and negative reinforcers have been used, most researchers employing these procedures use negative reinforcement (mostly shock).

In a typical training session in a T-maze shock–escape task, the rat is placed in the start (center) alley where shock is already on, delivered through a grid floor. To escape the aversive stimulation, the rat must turn to the "correct" side alley, left or right. Which side is correct is determined by the experimenter and depends on whether the rat is pretreated with a drug or trained nondrugged, i.e., a discrimination between the presence versus the absence of a particular dose of a certain training compound. The side alley permitting escape always correlates in a one-to-one fashion with the presence or absence of the training drug stimulus and the training conditions usually alternate between days (e.g., drug, D, training, turn left; nondrug, N, training, turn right; D, N; D, N; and so on). The daily first choice is the measure of discriminative control; a total of 5–10 trials per training session is usually run, one session per day for 5 d/wk. Of course, one can also subject animals to discrimination between two different compounds, or two different doses of the same drug.

Test sessions are the same as in the example given above, except that escape is possible through either side alley and only one trial is usually run. Examples of this procedure can be found in Overton (1966), Järbe and Henriksson (1974), Järbe (1976), and Romano et al. (1981). Other maze systems were described by Winter (1978).

3.2. Operant Procedures

Most DDL experiments today follow Skinnerian principles. Here the choice is between two levers (with rodents and monkeys) or pecking keys (with pigeons), but there are great variations in the schedules of reinforcement used, type of reinforcer, and test procedure (reward or extinction) employed.

An operant box may differ in various ways (size, shape, and location of manipulanda, levers, pecking keys, or reward facilities, and so forth). Varying such characteristics of the operant chamber, Overton (1978a) concluded that for rats (a) placement of dispenser at some distance from the levers will slow acquisition; (b) insertion of a barrier between levers is disadvantageous; (c) the sensory environment of each lever must clearly separate it from other levers; (d) location of a reward dispenser close to each lever may speed early discrimination training; and (e) the size of the discrimination box is not critical.

3.2.1. Two-Choice Procedures

The versatility and flexibility of the operant methodology offers distinct advantages over the methods described previously. In an early procedural report, Kubena and Barry (1969) arued in favor of test situations in which animals emit several responses before reinforcement feedback, rather than a single test choice, as in the T-maze. Other early DDL experiments using operant methodology were those of Harris and Balster (1968) and Morrison and Stephenson (1969); the former workers used positive reinforcement, but with different reinforcement contingencies in effect on the two levers, and the latter study combined positive reinforcement and punishment (shock). The latter procedures have not been used in DDL research recently; the common practice today is to instead use the same schedule of reinforcement on both manipulanda, whether fixed ratio (FR), variable ratio (VR), variable interval (VI), or differential responding of low rate (DRL) (*see* the chapter by Sanger in this volume). Combinations of schedules have also been utilized, such as VI-FR, i.e., the first section of the program is a VI followed by FR for the remainder of the session (e.g., Stolerman and D'Mello, 1981; Kock and Slangen, 1982a,b). The potential advantage of such an arrangement is that one is able to assess discriminative control over behavior over somewhat extended time-periods.

However, comparing the distribution of responses under the two schedule components, Stolerman and D'Mello (1981) found very similar results using amphetamine as the discriminative cue. Overton (1979a) compared some programs in terms of how fast rats reached a criterion of performing eight correct first-trial choices out of 10 consecutive training sessions (8/10 criterion), as well as the resulting asymptotic discrimination performance using phenobarbital as the discriminative stimulus. Among the schedules of reinforcement examined (DRL, FR, and VI), contingencies based on FR were the most efficient in these respects. Similar results were reported by Chance et al. (1977) using nicotine as the discriminative cue under contingencies of VI, DRL, and FR reinforcement. Comparing VI and DRL in terms of speed of acquisition of three discriminations, namely, N vs pentobarbital (15 mg/kg), N vs *l*-amphetamine (1 mg/kg), and pentobarbital vs amphetamine, all three discriminations occurred more rapidly in the DRL condition. However, neither the degree of stimulus control at asymptote, nor the drug or the dose generalization gradients were significantly different under the two schedules (Richards, 1978). Nonetheless, the VI schedule may have the advantage of permitting the researcher to observe generalization effects of a magnitude higher than that of the training drug dose, since the asymptote is usually substantially less than 100% (Barry and Krimmer, 1978).

A regular FR schedule is preferred by many workers; the FR value usually ranges between 10 and 32. Several ways of testing are possible with this approach. Colpaert (1978a) argues that the task is basically of a nominal, "all-or-nothing" character, and animals are trained according to a "win–stay, lose–shift" principle. In tests, the lever on which animals first accumulate 10 responses (FR 10) is designated the selected lever, and subsequent rewards are made contingent upon pressing that lever for the rest of the session. The major datum therefore is the number of animals selecting a particular lever. Variations of rewarded test procedures are those in which animals can obtain rewards from both manipulanda, regardless of which manipulandum is initially selected (e.g., Herling et al., 1980; Järbe, 1981; Järbe et al., 1981a), thus questioning a strictly nominal character of DDL generalization experiments.

Other researchers prefer tests in extinction, arguing that rewarded tests may alter the discrimination and therefore confound future tests. Hence, tests end without reward after 10 responses have accumulated on one of the two manipulanda, or when another preset number of responses has been emitted (*see* Winter, 1978, for references.)

There are no explicit comparisons available on the influence of reinforcement in tests, other than the demonstration that rats not being rewarded for pressing the appropriate lever when tested with the training stimuli will eventually press the other lever (Colpaert, 1977a; Schechter, 1981). In long-term experiments using either fentanyl or cocaine as cues in drug vs saline discriminations, the median dose (ED_{50}) estimates from many dose-generalization tests did not disclose systematic variation as a function of time, and hence experience with rewarded tests (Colpaert et al., 1978).

In order to obtain several choices in a single animal and test sessions not confounded by reinforcement feedback, McMillan et al. (1982) designed a second-order color-tracking procedure. In this procedure, training sessions ended after 10 rewards, with each reward requiring 10 FR-5 segments, whereas tests ended after one reward. The pharmacological specificity of a slightly modified version of this set-up was validated in a subsequent report (McMillan et al., 1982).

An "extended-schedule transfer test" was designed by Schechter (1981) to assess the perseverance or strength of generalization effects. In tests, rats were observed to accumulate 10 lever-presses on one of the two levers ("selected lever"), but the session did not end until the rat switched side and pressed the initially nonpreferred lever 10 times. Therefore, the persistence with which the animal pressed the initially selected lever was taken as a measure of the strength of drug-stimulus control (*see* also Winter, 1981).

Instead of positive reinforcement, Shannon and Holtzman (1976) trained rats in a discriminative discrete-trial procedure to avoid or escape shock. The box contained three levers, two of which were mounted on one wall of the chamber and the third on the opposite wall. Start of a trial was signaled by the onset of the houselight and, if the rat emitted the correct behavioral sequence, i.e., first gave the "observing response" (third lever) followed by a response on the appropriate training lever, the trial ended. If wrong, intermittent shocks were delivered until the correct sequence had occurred or the trial ended. Each session consisted of 21 trials equally spaced throughout the 30-min sessions.

Although lever-pressing or key-pecking are the more common behaviors brought under drug discriminative stimulus control in the operant chamber, other possibilities have been explored: Krimmer et al. (1978) used head-turns (left or right) in otherwise restrained rats as the dependent variable for a pentobarbital-saline discrimination. D'Mello and Stolerman (1978) used licking of distilled water from two spatially separated drinking tubes as the two responses in an otherwise ordinary amphetamine–saline discrimination. In comparison to this spatial task, a flavor task (location of drinking tubes varied across sessions) yielded only a slight, nonsignificant trend toward discriminative control. In a third experiment, a composite of spatial and flavor cues was examined and it was found that all conditioning accrued to the spatial stimuli and none to the flavors. As an adjunct to response selection, De Witte (1982a) emphasized the use of response latency to detect differences between pre- and post-treatment effects not necessarily evident from the selection index alone.

3.2.2. Three-Choice Procedures

The earliest attempt to train a three-choice discrimination was reported by Overton (1967) using a maze with three different "safe" boxes (left, middle, right), each corresponding to the three training conditions, namely, atropine, pentobarbital, and saline. The discriminative control achieved in the rats was modest. Subsequent work has utilized operant boxes. White and Holtzman (1981, 1983a,b) employed the previously described discrete-trial, shock-avoidance procedure in which three rather than two levers were mounted on the front wall. In the mornings, the rats were trained with vehicle, and drug training took place in the afternoons, one drug per day. The drug stimuli investigated together with saline were either phencyclidine and cyclazocine, or morphine and cyclazocine at doses previously found to produce comparable effects. Leberer and Fowler (1977) used amphetamine, pentobarbital, and saline as the discriminative conditions for pigeons on a VR schedule of reinforcement. In a similar setup, Järbe and Swedberg (1982) reported that pigeons discriminated between (1) 0.25 mg/kg of delta-9-tetrahydrocannabinol (Δ^9-THC), 4 mg/kg of pentobarbital, and vehicle, and (2) 0.50 mg/kg of Δ^9-THC, 8 mg/kg of pentobarbital, and vehicle; the two pigeons had originally been trained on a pentobarbital vs Δ^9-THC discrimination (Järbe and Ohlin, 1979). Other three-choice discriminations from this laboratory involve (1) LSD, Δ^9-THC, and vehicle, (2) morphine, Δ^9-THC, and vehicle, and (3) morphine, cocaine, and vehicle (unpublished). These discriminations involved two drug stimuli of different qualitative character and the vehicle. Other possible three-choice discriminations, such as that between different doses of the same drug, have not as yet received experimental attention (Järbe and Swedberg, 1982). Overton (1978a) has discussed features of the experimental chamber for possible three- and four-choice tasks.

3.3. *Time-Saving Aspects*

Drug-discrimination learning experiments are generally fairly time-consuming, involving both discrimination training and a testing phase. Initial training often takes several weeks, and thereafter animals are usually tested once or twice per week, provided good discriminative control is maintained during the intervening training sessions. To achieve control rapidly, it is advantageous to introduce drug-discriminative training early in the experiment (Overton, 1979a), and to use an initial "errorless" shaping procedure (e.g., Swedberg and Järbe, 1982), i.e., responding on the "state"-inappropriate manipulandum is prevented, for example, by having the inappropriate lever retracted (with rats) or by covering the wrong pecking key with tape (with pigeons) during the initial discrimination training. The schedule of reinforcement is also important, with variations of FR schedules generally being most efficient both in terms of speed of acquisition, as well as asymptotic performance (Overton, 1979a).

To achieve better response control with low doses of drugs, it may be beneficial to initiate training with a higher dose and then successively decrease the amount administered. Such a procedure was used by Overton (1979b) to have rats discriminate fairly small doses; drugs and dosages are indicated in Fig. 2.

Colpaert et al. (1980a,b) trained rats to discriminate between the opioid fentanyl and saline either according to progressively decreasing dosages (1980a), or in a more conventional manner in which different groups were given different doses from the outset of discrimination training (1980b). The former protocol yielded steeper dose-generalization gradients after low training doses, indicating enhanced stimulus control with the progressively decreasing schedule.

The dosing protocol that is implemented, however, affects the outcome of the "step-by-step" dosage schedule. Thus, Swedberg and Järbe (1982) observed that escalation of the opiate antagonist naltrexone (together with morphine) in threefold steps (0.01, 0.03, and so on) resulted in deterioration of stimulus control at lower naltrexone doses than when the pigeons received smaller escalations of naltrexone (0.01, 0.02, 0.03, and so on); the pigeons had been trained to discriminate morphine (5.6 mg/kg) from saline. Additionally, in another experiment the least discriminable dose of morphine was lower for a separate group of pigeons given naltrexone (0.3 mg/kg) after morphine (5.6 mg/kg) training sessions, as compared to saline postsession-treated birds (Swedberg and Järbe, 1982). Enhanced sensitivity to the morphine cue caused by the postsession naltrexone treatment was thus indicated, the reason for which being discussed by Swedberg and Järbe (1982).

To reduce the number of sessions needed to complete a dose–response curve, Bertalmio et al. (1982) and McMillan et al. (1982) designed cumulative dosing procedures for drug

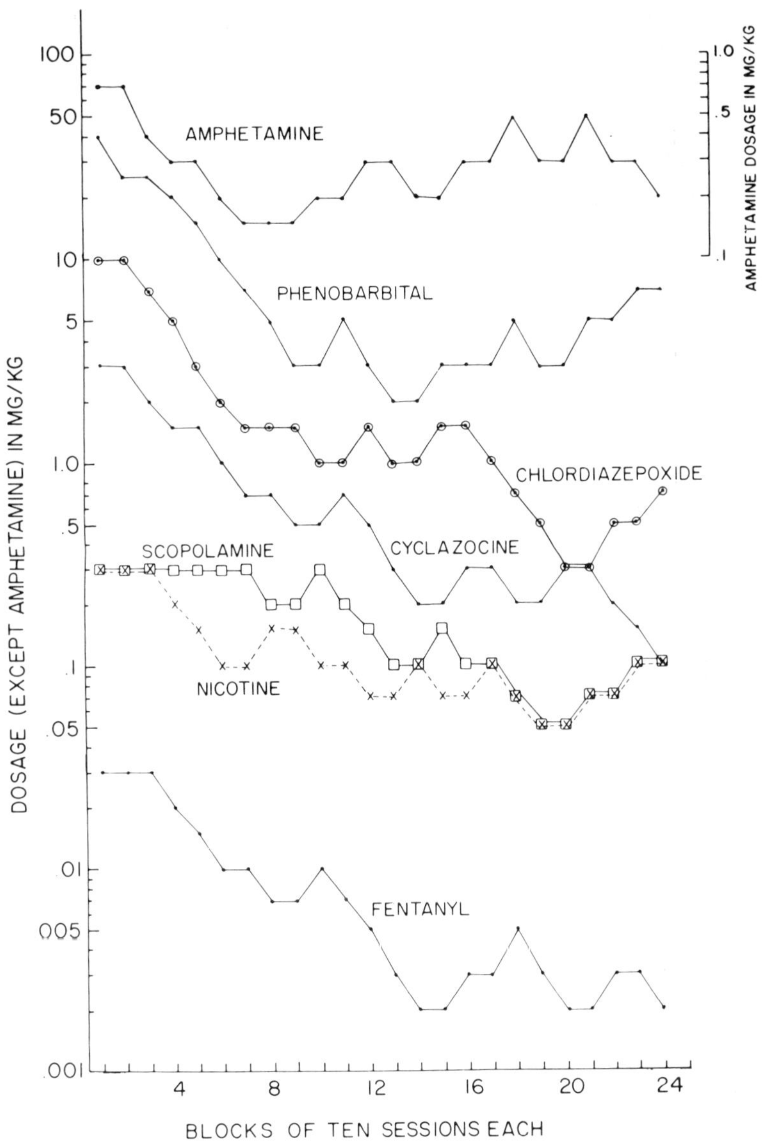

Fig. 2. Rats were required to press bar 1 when drugged and bar 2 when not drugged. Training dosage was decreased whenever this discrimination was learned and increased whenever the discrimination was not learned for 20 consecutive sessions. The plots show training dosages for seven individual rats during successive blocks of 10 sessions. Note the displaced ordinate for amphetamine (from Overton, 1979b; reprinted with permission of publisher and author).

generalization testing in a manner reminiscent of those used during in vitro analysis of drug action. This is not a new idea in psychopharmacology (Boren, 1966), but the experience is still limited.

Nevertheless, the generalization curves from cumulative dosing and separate tests in monkeys and pigeons, respectively, were very similar in the DDL studies of Bertalmio et al. (1982) and McMillan et al. (1982); the data for pigeons are illustrated in Fig. 3.

In discussing the utility of the cumulative-dosing procedure, Bertalmio et al. (1982) emphasized several factors, such as the number of doses for the generalization gradient, the number of intervening training sessions, and the pharmacokinetics of the drugs being evaluated. With respect to the latter point, the cumulative-dosing protocol probably works best with drugs that have a rapid onset and a long duration of effect. The procedure seems especially suited for experiments in which the dependent variable concerns a shift in dose–response curves (i.e., drug antagonism, supersensitivity, or tolerance) and the time for the preparation in itself is limited, such as intravenous, intraventricular, and intracerebral administration preparations.

In a similar vein, Järbe et al. (1981a) described a "repeated-tests procedure" for assessing the time-course of compounds after a single administration, in this particular case cannabinoids. Thus, rats trained to discriminate between Δ^9-THC and vehicle were administered a certain amount of the test drug and then tested at four successive intervals (30, 60, 120, and 240 min postadministration) after a single injection of the training drug, as well as a THC homolog. The curves so generated, in comparison to results from the conventional procedure (one dose and interval per test session), were almost identical (*see* Fig. 4). Other researchers have also evaluated the time-course of drugs repeatedly, but offered no comparative data (e.g., Haug and Götestam, 1982).

3.4. Summary

This section describes various procedures employed for DDL, variations of the FR, with the two-choice procedure

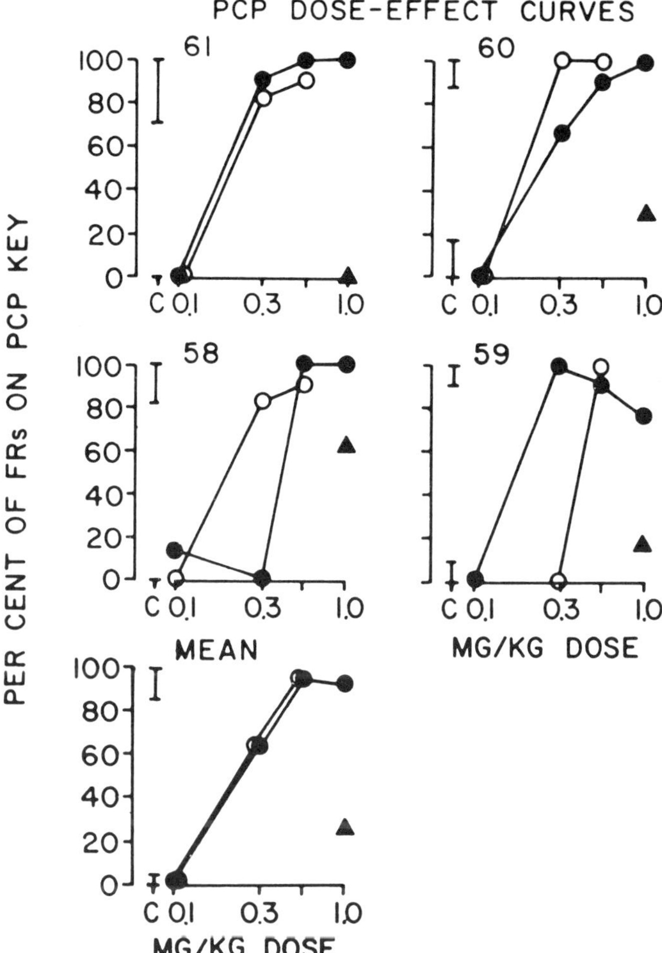

Fig. 3. Dose–effect curves for PCP. Abscissa: dose, log scale. Ordinate: percent of FRs completed on the PCP key following various PCP doses. Brackets at C show the range of percentages of the FRs completed on the PCP key after the training dose and after saline. Birds 58 and 61 made all responses on the green key (saline key) after saline injections. Filled points show the PCP dose–effect curve when single PCP doses were substituted during a session. Unfilled points show the PCP dose–effect curve with the cumulative dosing procedure. Injection-test intervals were 15 min. Triangles indicate tests conducted 4 h after administration of 1.0 mg/kg of PCP. The upper four frames show individual birds and the lowest frame shows the group dose effect curve (from McMillan et al., 1982; reprinted with permission from publisher and author).

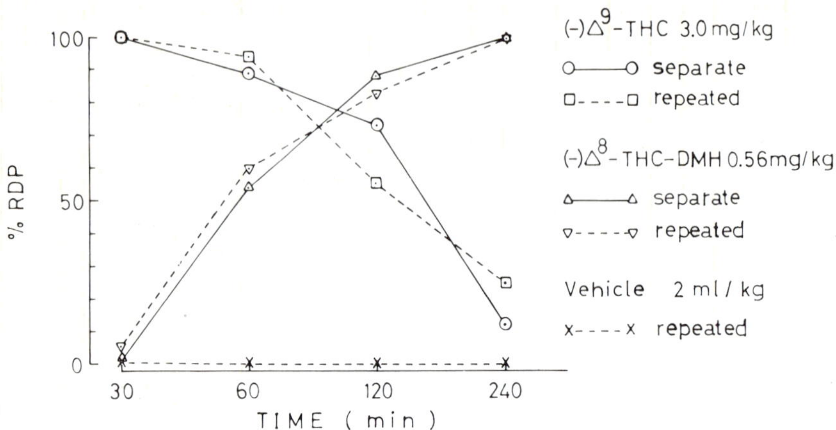

Fig. 4. The effects of separate and repeated tests of 3 mg/kg of $(-)\Delta^9$-THC and 0.56 mg/kg of $(-)\Delta^8$-THC-DMH at several intervals after injection. The animals were trained to discriminate between 3 mg/kg of $(-)\Delta^9$-THC and the vehicle, injected ip 30 min prior to sessions. Abscissa: time in min since injection until testing. Ordinate: mean responses on drug $[(-)\Delta^9$-THC]-appropriate position (%RDP). Separate tests, one at a time, were conducted on different days, whereas the repeated tests took place the same day after a single injection. Testing $(-)\Delta^9$-THC 3.0 mg/ kg; ◯——◯ separate; --- repeated. $(-)\Delta^8$-THC-DMH 0.56 mg/kg; Δ——Δ separate; Δ---Δ repeated. Vehicle 2 mg/kg; x---x repeated (from Järbe et al., 1981a; reprinted with permission from publisher and author).

motivated by hunger or thirst being most common today. An alternative is avoidance or escape from shock. Recently, De Witte (1982b) described the use of intracranial stimulation as the reinforcer in an ethanol-saline discrimination. Examples of three-choice procedures are also presented.

To improve discriminative stimulus control with low doses, progressively decreasing dose protocols have been devised. Cumulative-dosing procedures may be used to generate a dose–response curve (generalization gradient) in a single day. For the time-course of drugs, data are accumulating to suggest that animals can be tested repeatedly after a single injection to produce reliable time-course estimates.

4. Properties of Discriminative Drug Stimuli

Research on the discriminative stimulus properties of drugs has progressed considerably during the last decade. This section will focus on concepts used to denote DDL phenomena and the relevant experimental data.

4.1. Discriminability

The term discriminability was introduced by Overton (1971) to denote the finding that drugs differed in their ability to exert response control in a T-maze (see below). In discussing discriminability, Winter (1978) and Schuster and Balster (1977) have made an important distinction between efficacy and potency. Two drugs may differ in potency but can be equally efficacious in bringing about a given effect, e.g., higher doses of phenobarbital are required to produce discriminative control comparable to that of pentobarbital, but in other respects the two drugs appear similar. Reduced efficacy would be evinced when a drug at any dose does not produce the same end-result as the reference drug.

To measure discriminability of drugs, three approaches have been commonly used, i.e., speed of learning, asymptotic accuracy, and generalization tests (*see* section 4.2 for a discussion of the latter). Since this has been discussed previously at some length, a few examples will suffice to indicate that drug discriminability is not an invariable property of drugs (Colpaert, 1982; Schuster and Balster, 1977; Winter, 1978).

4.1.1. Speed of Learning

On the basis of the number of training sessions needed to reach an 8/10 criterion in a T-maze task, Overton (1971) categorized drugs in terms of the "degree of dissociation" displayed into strong, moderate, and weak or nonexisting. Barbiturates, alchol, and similar CNS sedative drugs belong to the first category, since discriminative control of behavior was achieved rapidly with these agents. Moderate dissociation occurred, for example, with anticholinergics, whereas chlorpromazine, imipramine, and peripherally acting drugs such as gallamine constituted the third category. Thus, animals trained with agents from the latter group reached criterion only after extensive training or not at all; the cut-off was 60 training sessions. Such a classification rests on the assumption that drugs possess "inherent" discriminability valid across tasks and species, and that the session-to-criterion reflects this property adequately. With the growth of DDL data from procedures other than the T-maze shock–escape task, it has become increasingly apparent that such a position is not tenable. For example, CNS motor stimulants such as amphetamine and cocaine produce discriminative control slowly in T-maze shock–escape tasts (Järbe and Kroon-Järbe, 1983; Overton, 1982a), whereas discriminative control may develop fairly rapidly in other procedures (e.g., Colpaert et al., 1978; Järbe and Kroon-Järbe, 1983; Leberer and Fowler, 1977).

4.1.2. Asymptotic Accuracy

The discriminability index here is reflected by the response control achieved after extensive training. Thus, if the discriminative control (percent correct) noted after a drug at any dose is less than the reference drug, the former can be said to induce less efficacious stimuli than the reference compound with that particular procedure (Schuster and Balster, 1977). To illustrate the relativity of this discriminability index, Järbe and Swedberg (1981; unpublished data) trained gerbils to discriminate between 15 mg/kg of pentobarbital and chlordiazepoxide (5, 10, or 20 mg/kg) from the outset of the discrimination training. Animals trained with 5 and 20 mg/kg of chlordiazepoxide gave evidence of drug discriminative control, whereas gerbils trained with 10 mg/kg performed about 50% or less correct first-trial choices during the 66 training days. Hence, 10 mg/kg of chlordiazepoxide and 15 mg/kg of pentobarbital seemed to induce qualitatively similar stimulus effects. However, two other groups of gerbils were trained to discriminate between either of two doses of chlordiazepoxide (20 or 30 mg/kg) and successively increasing doses of pentobarbital (range: 5–20 mg/kg). Drug-discriminative control (>80% correct first-trial responding) was achieved at all the doses examined. Thus, neither asymptotic accuracy nor substitution testing will produce an invariable measure of discriminability.

Based on signal-detection analysis (SDA), Colpaert (1978a) suggested the index d' (a measure of the sensitivity process) as a measure of discriminability both for the acquisition of DDL, and for asymptotic accuracy. The utility of this measure (as well as response bias) will depend on whether or not the assumptions of SDA can be met; for some, but not all, of the drugs analyzed, this was the case (Colpaert, 1978a).

4.2. Generalization

4.2.1. Quantitative Aspects

Animals trained to discriminate a certain dose of a particular training drug will emit progressively fewer drug responses in tests with lower doses, thereby producing a dose–response curve, i.e., a generalization gradient in the terminology of experimental psychology. Such a gradient allows the researcher to estimate a slope-function and a median effective dose (ED_{50}). Commonly used procedures to estimate ED_{50} values are those of Barry (1974), Finney (1976), and Litchfield and Wilcoxon (1949).

The family of best-fitting linear functions for dose-generalization effects in rats trained with different doses of the narcotic fentanyl, shown in Fig. 5, reveal their relation to the training dose and the ED_{50} value (Colpaert, 1982). A shallowing of the gradient with lower training doses has also been reported for other drugs (e.g., Stolerman and D'Mello, 1981). As with external stimuli, the slope may indicate stimulus specificity. Thus, greater specificity is assumed for the higher training doses.

However, this relationship does not seem to hold for all drugs. Colpaert and Janssen (1982a) trained rats to discriminate between saline and different doses of cocaine (range:

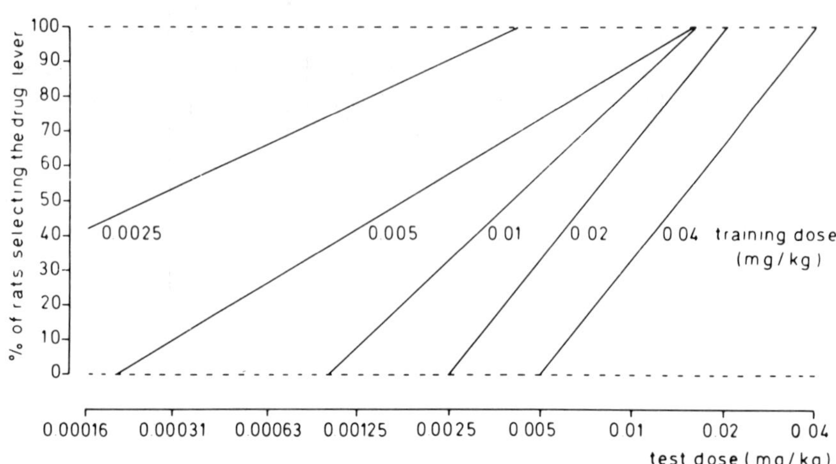

Fig. 5. The effect of fentanyl training dose on the slope of the fentanyl generalization gradient. Ordinate: percent of rats selecting the drug lever. Abscissa: test dose of fentanyl. The lines represent best-fitting linear functions in log-linear coordinates (from Colpaert, 1982; reprinted with permission of publisher and author).

0.63–10 mg/kg), and found the intermediate 2.5 mg/kg dose to yield the steepest dose generalization gradient.

Rats trained to differentiate between two doses of a drug will demonstrate the steepest gradient. In a study by Colpaert and Janssen (1982b), two parameters, dose ratio and absolute dose level, of fentanyl dose–dose discrimination were studied. Dose ratio refers to the high dose/low dose ratio; the ratios examined were 2, 4, 8, and 16 in four groups of animals. Absolute dose level refers to the amount for the "high-dose" condition; the higher training dose was progressively lowered from 0.04 to 0.00125 mg/kg. The training and the test doses are listed in Fig. 6, which shows the generalization gradients at the six training levels examined per group as functions of dose ratios and absolute dose levels, respectively. As with the fentanyl–saline discrimination (Fig. 5), slope was proportional to absolute dose, i.e., a flattening of the gradient occurred as a result of lowering the training doses. Dose ratio acted to steepen the gradients, with the most marked effects seen with the lowest dose ratio; hence, dose ratio 2 at an absolute dose level of 0.04 mg/kg yielded the highest ED_{50} value.

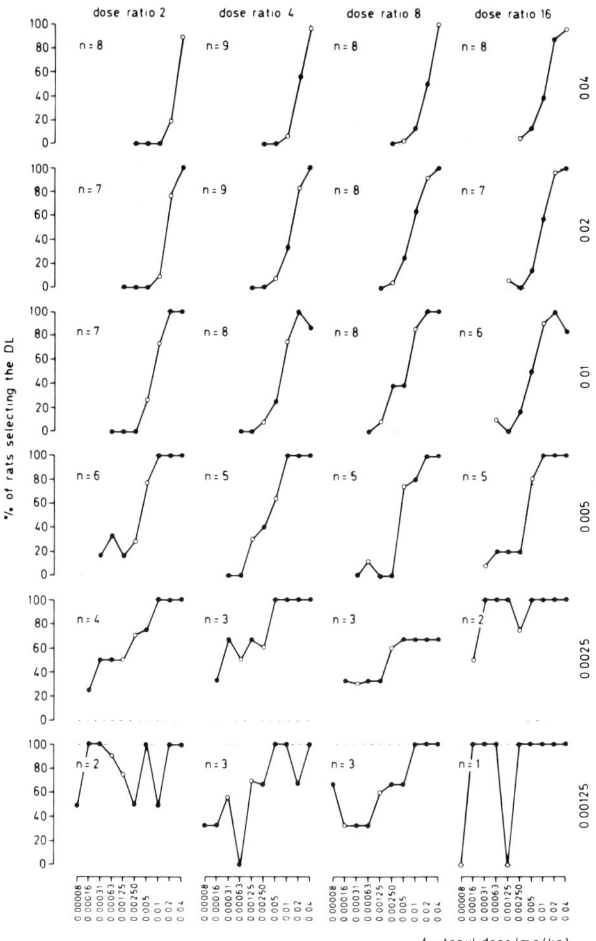

Fig. 6. Stimulus generalization gradient of fentanyl in rats trained to discriminate a higher from a lower training dose of fentanyl. The dose ratio of the higher to the lower training dose differed among each of four groups of subjects (values 2–16). Ordinate: percentage of rats selecting the lever that was appropriate to the higher training dose conditions. Abscissa: dose of fentanyl in mg/kg; n in each graph represents the number of animals. The numerals at the right of each row of graphs indicate the higher of the two fentanyl doses (in mg/kg) that the animals were to discriminate. Closed symbols pertain to stimulus generalization test data. Open symbols are used for the two training doses; their value was derived from the animals' discriminative performance at that particular discriminandum (from Colpaert and Janssen, 1982b; reprinted with permission of publisher and author).

Furthermore, in comparison to a fentanyl (0.04 mg/kg) vs saline discrimination, substantially less naloxone was needed to reverse the 0.02 vs 0.04 mg/kg fentanyl discrimination (Colpaert, 1982). From these and other data, Colpaert (1982) concluded that opioid discrimination experiments are variable, ranging from less specificity (associated with sensitivity to agonist activity) to greater specificity (enhancing sensitivity to antagonist action) (*see* also section 4.2.4).

Most work on stimulus control in experimental psychology suggests an inverted U-shaped generalization curve, i.e., stimulus control is at its maximum for the training value and fairly symmetrical generalization decrements surround the peak (Honig and Urcuioli, 1981). However, in DDL research, sigmoid (S-shaped) generalization gradients are generally observed (Järbe and Swedberg, 1982). The seeming discrepancy is more apparent than real. Common types of stimuli investigated in experimental psychology are wave length, tonal frequency, and so on, whereas the drug in DDL research is to be regarded as a composite stimulus, similar to that of brightness or sound intensity, for example; the "sensory" generalization curves in the latter case are similar in shape to those generally produced by drug stimuli (Heinemann and Chase, 1975; Järbe and Swedberg, 1982).

4.2.2. Qualitative Aspects

The response conditioned to a drug is specific to the drug class, as shown by research in the seventies. Hence, the response generalizes to pharmacologically-related agents, but not to dissimilar drugs. Classification of drugs according to discriminative stimulus properties produces the traditional general categories, such as hypnotic/sedatives (barbiturates, benzodiazepines, and to some extent alcohols), opiates (morphine, fentanyl, and so on), dissociative anesthetics (phencyclidine, ketamine), motor stimulants (amphetamine, cocaine, and to some extent apomorphine), psychedelics (LSD, mescaline), cannabinoids (Δ^9- and Δ^8-THC), cholinergic agonists (nicotine, arecholine), and antagonists (mecamylamine, atropine). This list does not cover all the drug categories examined, but rather presents groups of compounds often studied in DDL experiments. For overviews, *see* Colpaert and Rosecrans (1978), Colpaert and Slangen (1982), Ho et al. (1978), and Lal (1977a).

There are, however, also differences in the stimulus properties within these broader groups that may be made subject to discriminative conditioning. Opioids and sedatives provide good examples. Hence, drugs acting preferentially at postulated receptor sites associated with endogenous "opioid" substances may range from pure agonists, such as morphine or fentanyl, to antagonists, such as naloxone and naltrexone. There is no generalization between these agonists and antagonists (e.g., Carter and Leander, 1982; Colpaert, 1978b). However, the situation is more complicated with compounds exerting both agonist and antagonist activity to varying degrees. Models of multiple opiate receptors with that of Iwamoto and Martin (1981) being the most influential, provided the conceptual framework for much recent experimentation with mixed agonist/antagonist opioids. DDL studies with such compounds were recently summarized by Holtzman (1982), who concluded that opioids can be placed in three main groups depending on the following criteria; (1) the extent to which their stimulus effects in rats and squirrel monkeys resemble those of morphine, cyclazocine, and phencyclidine, and (2) the sensitivity of their stimulus effects to antagonism by naloxone and naltrexone. That the "hallucinogenic" agent phencyclidine shares stimulus properties with certain opioid psychotomimetics is a truly novel finding using DDL procedures. As a reflection of the complexity of action of these compounds and the resolving capacity of DDL techniques, it was recently shown that animals can also be conditioned to concurrently discriminate between cyclazocine, phencyclidine, and saline in a three-choice situation (White and Holtzman, 1983b).

With respect to sedative-hypnotics, antagonism tests have played a less prominent role for discerning various subclasses than for the opioids. Prior to the availability of the specific benzodiazepine antagonist Ro 15-1788, analeptics such as bemegride and to less extent pentylenetetrazol (PTZ) were the only known substances to block discriminations based on sedative/hypnotic agents (e.g., Barry and Krimmer, 1978; Colpaert, 1977b; Järbe, 1976). Tests with bemegride differentiated between diazepam and pentobarbital on the one hand and alcohol on the other hand (Järbe, 1976, 1977; Järbe and McMillan, 1983; however, *see* also Barry and Krimmer, 1978), corroborating other findings that generalizations between barbiturates and ethanol are not always found (e.g., Barry and Krimmer, 1978; York, 1978). In addition, ethanol is fairly easily discriminated from pentobarbital, chlordiazepoxide, and chlormethiazole in drug vs drug discrimination procedures (Barry and Krimmer, 1977; Järbe and Swedberg, 1981; Overton, 1977; Swedberg et al., 1978), whereas differential responding with appropriately matched doses is more difficult to establish between pentobarbital and chlordiazepoxide (Barry and Krimmer, 1978; Järbe and Swedberg, 1981). In fact, a clear differentiation between the two latter compounds was achieved only after applying a "successive approximation procedure" (Järbe and Swedberg, 1981; unpublished data), as described earlier (*see* section 4.1.2).

Although in most instances generalization is observed between barbiturates and benzodiazepines, Ro 15-1788 separates the two classes of compounds. Thus, in animals trained to discriminate between diazepam and vehicle, the diazepam cue was antagonized by Ro 15-1788, whereas the pentobarbital generalization was not. In addition, in rats trained to discriminate between pentobarbital and saline, Ro 15-1788 blocked the diazepam generalization, but not the pentobarbital discrimination (Herling and Shannon, 1982; *see* also Young and Dewey, 1982). A parallel situation exists for gerbils discriminating between either chlordiazepoxide and saline or ethanol and saline (Hiltunen et al., 1983). It should furthermore be noted that the degree of overlap between CNS depressants may depend on the procedure used; the similarity is suggested to be greater in shock–escape than in food-approach tasks (Barry and Krimmer, 1978).

The work with opioids and sedative/hypnotics serves to generally illustrate the methods and strategies used to discern similarities and differences in the stimulus attributes of drugs.

Thus, susceptibility to antagonism, drug vs drug discrimination techniques, and the use of different training drugs from within a broader drug category have proved useful in this endeavor. Recent procedural variations include "extended-transfer testing" (Schechter and Lovano, 1982), multiple-drug training (i.e., the discrimination between one particular drug vs several other drugs, rather than the vehicle condition) (Overton, 1982b), dose–dose discrimination (Colpaert, 1982; Järbe and Swedberg, 1982; Koek and Slangen, 1982a), and the discrimination of opiate antagonists in narcotic-dependent animals (Gellert and Holtzman, 1979; Valentino et al., 1983).

4.2.3. Time-Course of the Drug Stimulus

Since drugs have a gradual onset, a plateau effect, and a gradual elimination, the intensity and perhaps the quality of the drug stimulus may change during the course of drug action. Commonly, only one injection-test interval is examined. Recent data by Schechter and Lovano (1982) suggest that under certain conditions ethanol can induce qualitatively different stimulus effects depending on the injection-test interval.

Järbe (1981) compared gradients for cocaine and two supposedly longer-acting homologs (WIN 35,428 and 35,065-2), and found no marked differences in the duration of action in terms of cocaine-like stimulus effect. The generalization gradients are shown in Fig. 7; norcocaine, a metabolite of cocaine, was also tested. To reconcile these results with earlier data (*see* Järbe, 1981), it was proposed that even though there was complete generalization, the pharmacological action of cocaine and the WIN compounds may not be identical. It must be remembered that the conditioned response will generalize from the training drug (cocaine) only to the extent that the test drugs (WIN compounds) mimic the stimulus effects of the drug-training cue.

It is hoped that the time-course of the drug stimulus will be considered more often in the future than it has in the past. Implementation of the "repeated tests procedure" (Järbe et al., 1981a, 1985) reduces the time required to assess the onset and duration of a drug's cue effects.

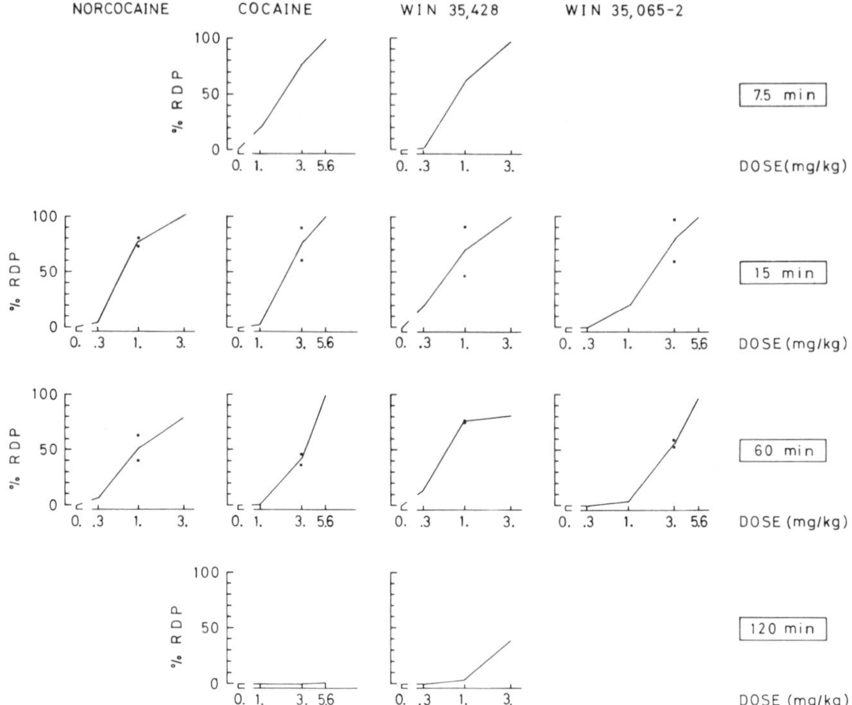

Fig. 7. Substitution tests with different doses of cocaine, norcocaine, WIN 35,428, and WIN 35,065-2 in cocaine-trained pigeons. The pigeons were trained to discriminate between the presence or absence of effects induced by cocaine HCl 5.6 mg/kg. Abscissa: dose in mg/kg. Ordinate, percent responses on drug (cocaine) appropriate position (% RDP); doses as the salts (cocaine and the WIN compounds) or the base (norcocaine). All curves are based on the mean results from five pigeons and all data points were determined on separate days. The means for some of the data points (i.e., 15 and 60 min pi) are based on the average performance of the birds during two different test occasions, as shown separately. The birds averaged ($\pm$ SEM) 99.7(0.14)% and 0.0 (0.0)% cocaine appropriate responses, respectively, during the initial six-reward segment of the regular cocaine and saline training sessions preceding the test data shown above (from Järbe, 1981; reprinted with permission from publisher and author).

4.2.4. Overinclusiveness and Specificity

"Transfer test overinclusiveness" denotes the phenomenon that generalization may occur to substances whose effects are only moderately similar to the training compound

(Overton, 1974). The degree of overinclusiveness will depend on the specificity of the drug-discrimination preparation. Pharmacological specificity refers to the degree of response generalization from the training-drug stimulus to other drug stimuli (Colpaert, 1982). Therefore, specificity may be viewed as the inverse of overinclusiveness. One important determinant is the training dose used. Often, the lower the training dose, the more common the overinclusiveness or, alternatively, the less the specificity (e.g., Colpaert et al., 1980b; Shannon and Holtzman, 1979).

Experimentally manipulated reinforcement density can markedly influence the shape of the drug–dose generalization gradients, generalization to other drugs, as well as the antagonism by naloxone of the fentanyl cue (Colpaert and Janssen, 1981; Koek and Slangen, 1982b). In general, the lower the reinforcement density associated with the fentanyl training condition, the more likely the animal was to choose the alternative condition. Thus, Koek and Slangen (1982b) observed a linear relationship between the proportion of reinforcements obtained during drug sessions and the ED_{50} value inthe fentanyl dose generalization. The latter results are summarized in Fig. 8. Apart from the possibility of manipulating the specificity of DDL experiments, another implication from these data seems to be that drug-induced rate changes *per se* might influence the discrimination, and hence the generalization tests.

Apparently the degree of specificity (or overinclusiveness) can be experimentally manipulated; again, stimulus properties of drugs are not invariant. Once acknowledging this, experiments can be designed to emphasize either of the concepts.

4.3. Origin of the Stimulus

4.3.1. Central vs Peripheral Mediation

Although various DDL techniques may differ in sensitivity, all centrally-acting drugs have been found to be capable of controlling choice behavior. Early studies failed to establish peripherally-acting drugs as discriminative cues,

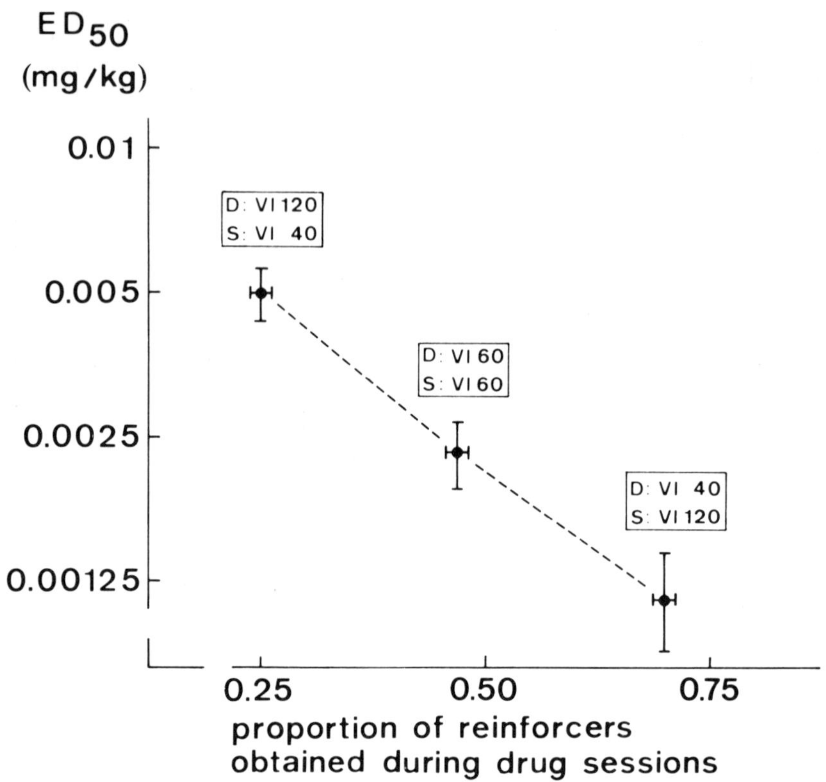

Fig. 8. Mean ED_{50} (± 1 SEM) of the fentanyl generalization gradient as a function of the mean (± 1 SEM) proportion of reinforcers obtained during drug sessions. The inserts show the mean value of the variable-interval (VI) component of the reinforcement schedule (in s), which was used during drug (D) and saline (S) sessions (from Koek and Slangen, 1982b; reprinted with permission from publisher and author).

indicating a central locus for the mediation of DDL. Data on the peripherally-acting drug isopropamide suggested, however, that CNS action is not a prerequisite for DDL (Colpaert, 1977a). Furthermore, the response learned in the presence of a low dose of *d,l*-amphetamine (0.16 mg/kg) generalized to the peripherally-acting drug *p*-hydroxyamphetamine, but not to a high dose of *d,l*-amphetamine (5 mg/kg), suggesting a peripheral origin of this discrimination and a qualitative difference between the peripherally- and centrally-mediated drug cues (Colpaert, 1977a).

On the other hand, a discriminative response conditioned to a CNS-acting compound has generally been found to neither generalize to peripherally-acting agents, nor to be blocked by peripheral antagonists; there are several examples concerning, for example, cholinergic and anticholinergic drugs (e.g., Rosecrans and Meltzer, 1981).

4.3.2. Sensory Mediation

Various mechanisms, such as stimulation of sensory pathways and modification of sensory input, have been proposed to explain the nature of the stimulus; e.g., altered visual perception could be the physiological substrate. Yet blinded rats learned a pentobarbital–saline discrimination almost as rapidly as controls; likewise, DDL was not appreciably changed by olfactory bulbectomy (Overton, 1978b). Although more work is needed, available data do not indicate any particular sensory modality or anatomical structure as the mediator for DDL (Lal, 1977b; Overton, 1978b). For individual drugs, specific areas and neuronal connections have been implicated (e.g., D'Mello, 1981; Barrett et al., 1982).

4.4. Summary

Drug stimuli are defined both qualitatively (type of drug) and quantitatively (the intensity or magnitude of alterations induced by the drug dose). The specificity of a DDL experiment is determined by several factors, such as type of drug and the dose used, type of discrimination (e.g., dose–dose, as compared to drug–no drug discrimination), and conditioning procedures (reinforcement density, type of schedule, and task). Thus, drug stimuli are not invariant. No specific sensory or anatomical mediator has been identified as responsible for DDL; direct CNS action is not a prerequisite for DDL.

5. Research Applications

Behavioral pharmacology is an interdisciplinary approach based on psychology and pharmacology. Many of the concepts used in DDL research are borrowed from the subdiscipline of experimental psychology concerned with conditioning and learning in regard to sensory modalities. Thus, DDL adds a new dimension to the study of stimulus control through the use of chemical "interoceptive" stimuli. To those trained in the medical sciences, mechanisms of drug action and aspects of bioassay methodology may be of more interest than the analysis of learning mechanisms *per se.*

5.1. Drug Classification

DDL techniques allow determinations of commonalities and differences in the perceptible qualities of drug-induced stimuli; thus, compounds can be categorized into various major drug classes according to their stimulus attributes. Specific pharmacological tools (antagonists, agonists, uptake and synthesis inhibitors, and neurotoxins) can be employed to characterize mediating neuropharmacological substrates [type of receptor and mechanism(s) of action]. For example, the commonality of the stimulus effects of CNS motor stimulants has been related to dopaminergic transmission as evinced by cross-generalization between stimulants and antagonism by haloperidol, even though the modes of action may differ; pretreatment with alpha-methyl-*p*-tyrosine attenuates the amphetamine cue, but not that of cocaine, the latter rather being attenuated by reserpine (Silverman and Ho, 1977) [for further examples, *see* Colpaert and Rosecrans (1978); Colpaert and Slangen (1982)]. A recent study by Barrett et al. (1982) demonstrated the utility of blocking peripheral side effects when establishing a discrimination between the presence and absence of L-5-hydroxytryptophan, the immediate precursor of serotonin; a similar approach seems appropriate if and when L-Dopa, the immediate precursor of dopamine, is investigated with DDL techniques.

5.2. Disease Models

Another interesting aspect of DDL techniques concerns their application as models or bioassays for disease states. This and other ideas were discussed by Lal (1977b), who recently developed an animal DDL model for assessing anxiogenic and anxiolytic properties of drugs. Lal and Shearman (1982) concluded that in rats trained to discriminate between a subconvulsive dose of PTZ and saline (1) only anxiogenic drugs, such as bemegride and high-dose cocaine, but not other motor stimulants and convulsants, produce PTZ-like stimulus effects; (2) only anxiolytics (benzodiazepines, meprobamate, barbiturates, and valproic acid), but not other anticonvulsants and depressants, block the PTZ stimulus; and (3) the PTZ discrimination may be a model for neurogenic anxiety.

More recently, Emmett-Oglesby et al. (1983) used the PTZ-discrimination model to detect withdrawal from diazepam. Other proposals by Lal (1977b), such as bioassays for "blood-pressure," "fever," "depression," and so on have not received enough experimental attention to allow a critical evaluation of their utility. A two-lever choice procedure as a bioassay of sweeteners was recently proposed by Shearman et al. (1981).

Weissman (1976) reported that arthritic as compared to nonarthritic rats more easily discriminated aspirin from no drug, suggesting that physiological imbalance can facilitate discrimination of certain agents. The state of morphine withdrawal distress presumably was the discriminative stimulus in the studies by Gellert and Holtzman (1979) and Valentino et al. (1983); altered sensitivity to antagonist action in morphine-dependent animals was indicated by the rather low doses of naltrexone effective as discriminative cues.

5.3. Context and Drug Stimuli

Although most experiments have emphasized the pharmacological aspects of DDL, some recent work was framed in terms of conditioning and learning. Thus, conditioning pro-

cedures pertaining to the concepts of overshadowing, blocking, and conditional discrimination (for definitions, *see*
Heinemann and Chase, 1975; Honig and Urcuioli, 1981)
using combinations of sensory and drug-induced stimuli have
been found to differentially effect drug stimuli (e.g., Colpaert,
1978b; Järbe et al. 1981b; 1983a,b; Krimmer et al., 1982). For
example, Järbe et al. (1983a) trained rats in a T-maze to
discriminate between the presence and absence of pentobarbital, the two conditions being consistently paired with the
presence and absence of light in the experimental room,
respectively. When pentobarbital training sessions were conducted, the light was on, whereas saline training occurred in
darkness. When tested with different doses of pentobarbital
with the light on, the pentobarbital/light associated side of
the maze was chosen more often than when the same tests
were conducted with the lights out. Therefore, the animals
were more "sensitive" to diminishing drug cues when tested
in the drug-appropriate environment (i.e., with the light on)
than when tested in the non-drug-appropriate exteroceptive
condition (i.e., with the lights out). The dose–generalization
gradients of nonpaired controls were intermediate to those of
the paired groups. These and other data (Järbe and Johansson, 1984) suggest that there is no dissociative barrier between
drug stimuli and exteroceptive stimuli, but rather that they
interact to control behavior. Such conditioning also appears
relevant for the analysis of drug discriminative stimuli in
addictive behavior (e.g., Harris and Balster, 1970).

These are only a few examples of research applications
in different areas of interest. No doubt there are many more
areas in which DDL techniques can contribute to scientific
progress. Recent examples concern behavioral teratology/
toxicology (Haenlein et al., 1983; Zenick and Goldsmith,
1981) and medicinal chemistry (Glennon and Rosecrans,
1982).

6. A Schematic View of DDL

Two aspects of the drug stimulus governing a DDL
experiment have been described; a qualitative and a quantita-

tive dimension. Quality reflects drug class and quantity reflects the magnitude of effect evoked by a particular dose. A general concept of DDL was recently proposed by Järbe and Swedberg (1982). The following is an excerpt of that article; specific experimental data will not be recapitulated here. The quantitative dimension includes discriminations between a drug and no drug (D vs N), and discriminations between one dose and another of the same compound (D_1 vs D_2). The qualitative dimension is comprised by discrimination between different drugs (D_A vs D_B). Discriminations in three-choice settings, it was argued, constitute composites of the above cases. Experimental data available today concern the discrimination between two qualitatively different drugs and the no-drug condition (N vs D_A vs D_B); other possible three-choice discriminations have been discussed by Järbe and Swedberg (1982). The N vs D, D_A vs D_B, and N vs D_A vs D_B discriminations may be schematically visualized as depicted in Fig. 9. The circled areas represent the stimulus properties of a training drug, separated from the rest of the perceptual space. The notation R stands for the response associated with the respective training conditions.

6.1. Drug vs No Drug

In the N vs D case, one response, R_A (e.g., pressing left lever), will become associated with drug training and the other response, R_N (pressing right lever), will be associated with no-drug training through differential reinforcement conditioning. Assuming no "N cues," no-drug represents the absence of the cue effects as defined by D_A. Hence, this represents a discrimination between the presence and absence of the stimulus effects induced by the training-drug dosage. Logically, drug stimuli not matching the D_A stimulus or cue will be generalized with its absence, i.e., the N category. Therefore, the lack of generalization simply means that the induced effects were not sufficiently similar to those of D_A, but it does not carry any information as to whether the test compound itself has discriminative properties or not. This may be self-evident, but has nevertheless been overlooked in

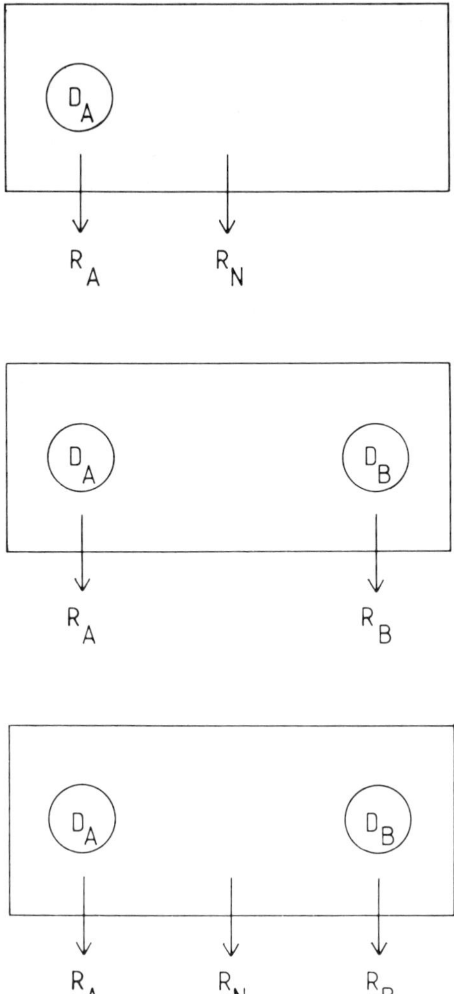

Fig. 9. Schematic outline of the N vs D discrimination (top section). D_A, a particular dose of a certain training drug; N, no drug (i.e., absence of D_A); R, response. Schematic outline of the D_A vs D_B discrimination (middle section). D_A, a particular dose of a certain training drug; D_B, a particular dose of another training drug, pharmacologically different from D_A; R, response. Schematic outline of the N vs D_A vs D_B discrimination (bottom section). D_A, a particular dose of a certain training drug; D_B, a particular dose of another training drug, pharmacologically different from D_A; N, no drug (i.e., absence of either D_A or D_B; R, response) (modified from Järbe and Swedberg, 1982; with permission from publisher and author).

many reports in the past; it is particularly relevant to testing for antagonism. Thus, when the drug stimulus is challenged with a presumed antagonist, the animals may behave as if no drug had been administered; such a pattern of results is shown in Fig. 10 for three groups of gerbils trained to discriminate between either of three doses of morphine and

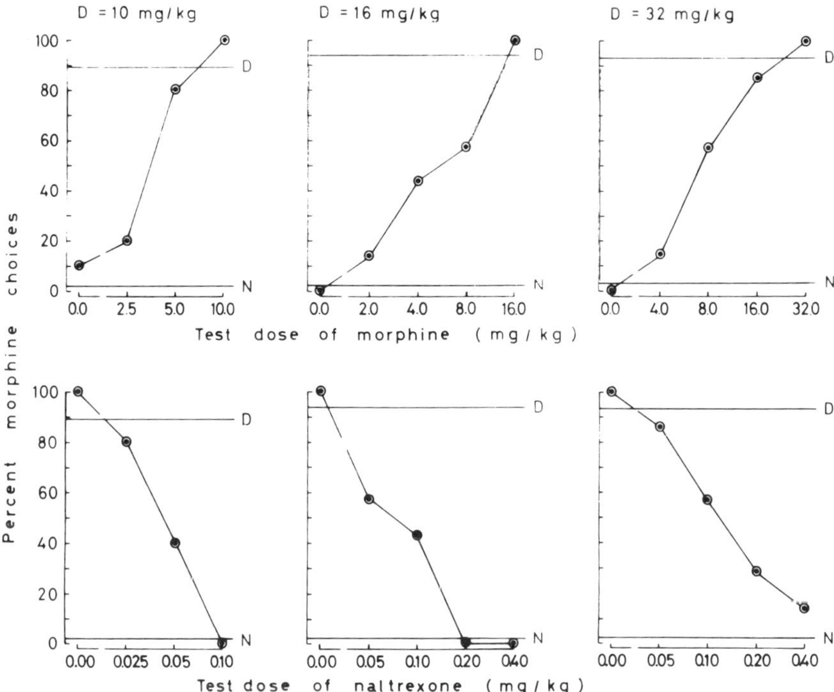

Fig. 10. Generalization and antagonism of the morphine cue. Ordinate: percent choices into morphine "correct" arm of a T-maze. Abscissa: upper portion, doses of morphine; lower portion, doses of naltrexone in conjunction with 10, 16, and 32 mg/kg of morphine, respectively. Injection-test interval was 60 min, and treatments were given in a single injection (4 mL/kg). Horizontal lines: percent first-trial choices into morphine-associated side of maze during morphine (D) and nondrug (N) training session for this test period. Training doses of morphine used are indicated at top of figure (from Järbe and Rollenhagen, 1978; reprinted with permission of publisher and author).

saline as described by Järbe and Rollenhagen (1978). This, however, does not imply lack of any pharmacological effects, because the drug combination may contain cues not previously attended to by the animal. This has been referred to as the "third-state hypothesis" (of antagonism results), the nature of which has been elaborated upon in several reports from this laboratory (e.g., Järbe et al., 1979; Swedberg and Järbe, 1982; see also Winter, 1978).

To determine if the challenge test results represent a no-drug state or a new "third state," animals may be subjected to discrimination training between the drug combination and its vehicle. If discriminated, we conclude that the antagonism produces a "third state." Such tests have been performed both in gerbils and pigeons with combinations of morphine and naltrexone (Järbe et al., 1979; Swedberg and Järbe, 1982). Although data in general do not support a "third state" interpretation with appropriately matched doses, the amounts of naltrexone required to abolish the discrimination were higher than those needed in the challenge tests.

6.2. Drug vs Drug

A discrimination between two pharmacologically different agents (D_A and D_B) is depicted in the middle section of Fig. 9. The outcome of this discrimination depends on the relative salience of the two training stimuli. Assuming equal salience, the dose–generalization gradients will be flatter than those generated in the N vs D and D_1 vs D_2 situations. Based on the assumption that stimuli sharing no elements with the training drug stimuli will induce random responding, saline may be used as an index of relative salience, with unequal salience being indicated by an extreme distribution of responses to the manipulandum associated with the less salient stimulus. Inequality in salience is also expected to steepen the generalization gradient of the more salient drug stimulus.

As an example, Järbe and Ohlin (1979) trained three groups of pigeons to discriminate between either (1) pentobarbital and vehicle; (2) Δ^9-THC and vehicle, or (3) pentobarbital and Δ^9-THC. The dose generalization gradients are shown in Fig. 11. Sections C and D pertain to the D_A vs D_B case; the other two sections represent the two N vs D discriminations.

The D_A vs D_B discrimination has been employed to determine whether two substances evincing cross-generalization indeed produce identical stimulus effects. The common practice has been to select doses of each drug assumed to be of equal salience, subject the animals to discrimination training, and, if discriminative control is achieved, proceed to generalization testing to determine whether the discrimination was caused by intensity differences, or if a qualitative aspect can be invoked. An alternative is to start with an N vs D_A discrimination and thereafter gradually fade in the new drug (D_B). If discriminative control is maintained throughout all training doses of D_B, a qualitative difference between D_A and D_B is inferred (*see* section 4.1.2 for an example).

6.3. Three-Choice Discrimination

Discriminations involving three different manipulanda and three separate training stimuli are sparse, probably because of the extensive training required (*see* section 3.2.2 for references). The three-choice discrimination for which data are available concerns N vs D_A vs D_B, i.e., the discrimination between two pharmacologically different drugs and vehicle. A schematic representation of this case is shown in the bottom section of Fig. 9.

The research by White and Holtzman (1981; 1983a,b) illustrates one potential use of this three-choice discrimination. Thus, compounds with overlapping pharmacological activity, such as that found among opioids, for example, can be used as the training stimuli, thereby enhancing the dissimilarities between the two agents. Although it is too early to make general statements about the resolving capacity of three-choice DDL, the results presented by White and Holtzman are reassuring.

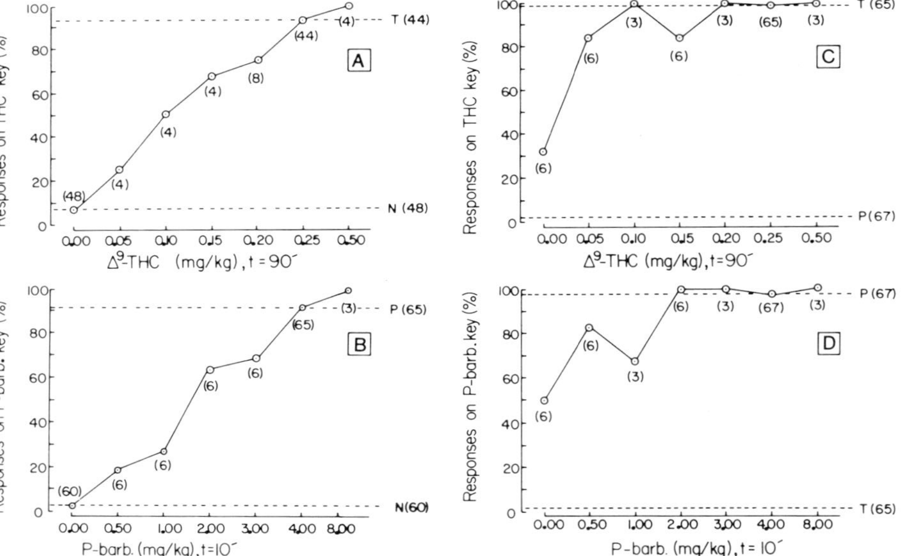

Fig. 11. Dose generalization gradients for pigeons trained a N vs D (two groups) or a D_A vs D_B discrimination (one group). The discriminative conditions for the two N vs D discriminations were, respectively: delta-9-tetrahydrocannabinol (Δ^9-THC, training dosage of 0.25 mg/kg) vs vehicle, injected im 90 min prior to sessions (two birds, graph A), and pentobarbital sodium (*P*-barb., training dosage of 4.0 mg/kg) vs vehicle, injected im 10 min prior to sessions (three birds, graph B). The third group (D_A vs D_B) was trained to discriminate between delta-9-THC and pentobarbital, injected im at the time intevals indicated above (three birds; graphs C and D). Numerals within brackets indicate the number of tests on which data points are based. Each bird performed 10 pecking responses per test. Dotted horizontal lines represent percent of "correct" responding during training sessions. ED_{50} values were, respectively: 0.10 mg/kg of delta-9-THC (graph A) and 1.60 mg/kg of pentobarbital (graph B); [from Järbe and Swedberg, 1982 (modified from Järbe and Ohlin, 1979); reprinted with permission from publisher and author].

This schematic presentation serves to connect the various discriminations referred to in the text, and it is hoped that the relationships between them should be more clear. As noted earlier, several factors determine a DDL experiment. These include the training dosage, the relationship between dosages, kind of drugs used, and the reinforcement contingencies. All these factors codetermine specificity, and, hence, the degree of discrimination and generalization obtained.

7. Epilog

In a short overview such as this, it is possible neither to deal with every aspect of the subject matter, nor to give credit to all relevant reports. The intent of this chapter is to bring together information concerning methods and strategies used to study discriminative stimulus properties of drugs. Thus, procedures for DDL are presented, emphasizing time-saving aspects. Concepts denoting DDL phenomena are discussed, and specificity/overinclusiveness emerge as one pair of key concepts. Although DDL is now considered a generally accepted behavioral analysis, it must be acknowledged that many issues need further clarification and, therefore, the search for controlling variables should continue in order to improve the resolving capacity of DDL techniques. This chapter is an introductory invitation to such endeavors.

Acknowledgments

Preparation of this chapter was supported by research grants from the Swedish Research Councils of FRN (83/126), HSFR (670/83), and MFR (5717-04), as well as the Faculty of Social Sciences, University of Uppsala, Sweden. For many helpful discussions and comments on previous drafts of this article I thank my collegue M. D. B. Swedberg. E. Enefjord and M. Lubandi excellently typed the manuscript. Technical assistance was provided by G. Ohlin and other members at the Department of Psychology, University of Uppsala, Sweden. I also thank the following publishers for allowing reprinting of figures: American Association for the Advancement of Science, Janssen Research Foundation, Macmillan Press (Scientific and Medical Division), Society for the Experimental Analysis of Behavior, and Springer-Verlag. This chapter is dedicated to the late professor I. Dureman.

References

Barrett R. J., Blackshear M. A., and Sanders-Bush E. (1982) Discriminative stimulus properties of 1-5-hydroxytryptophan: Behavioral evidence for multiple serotonin receptors. *Psychopharmacology* **76,** 29–35.

Barry III, H. (1974) Classification of drugs according to their discriminable effects in rats. *Fed. Proc.* **33,** 1814–1824.

Barry III, H. and Krimmer E. C. (1977) Discriminable Stimuli Produced by Alcohol and Other CNS Depressants, in *Discriminative Stimulus Properties of Drugs* (Lal H., ed.), Plenum, New York.

Barry III, H. and Krimmer E. C. (1978) Similarities and Differences in Discriminative Stimulus Effects of Chlordiazepoxide, Pentobarbital, Ethanol and Other Sedatives, in *Stimulus Properties of Drugs: Ten Years of Progress* (Colpaert F. C. and Rosecrans J. A., eds.), Elsevier, Amsterdam.

Bertalmio A. J., Herling S., Hampton R. Y., Winger G., and Woods J. H. (1982) A procedure for rapid evaluation of the discriminative stimulus effects of drugs. *J. Pharmacol. Meth.* **7,** 289–299.

Boren J. J. (1966) The Study of Drugs With Operant Techniques, in *Operant Behavior: Areas of Research and Application* (Honig W. K., ed.), Appleton-Century-Crofts, New York.

Carter R. B. and Leander J. D. (1982) Discriminative stimulus properties of naloxone. *Psychopharmacology* **77,** 305–308.

Chance W. T., Murfin D., Krynock C. M., and Rosecrans J. A. (1977) A description of the nicotine stimulus and tests of its generalization to amphetamine. *Psychopharmacology* **55,** 19–26.

Colpaert F. C. (1977a) Drug-Produced Cues and States: Some Theoretical and Methodological Inferences, in *Discriminative Stimulus Properties of Drugs* (Lal H., ed.), Plenum, New York.

Colpaert F. C. (1977b) Discriminative Stimulus Properties of Benzodiazepines and Barbiturates, in *Discriminative Stimulus Properties of Drugs* (Lal H., ed.), Plenum, New York.

Colpaert F. C. (1978a) Some Properties of Drugs as Physiological Signals: The FR Procedure and Signal Detection Theory, in *Stimulus Properties of Drugs: Ten Years of Progress* (Colpaert F. C. and Rosecrans J. A., eds.), Elsevier, Amsterdam.

Colpaert F. C. (1978b) Discriminative stimulus properties of narcotic analgesic drugs. *Pharmacol. Biochem. Bheav.* **9,** 863–887.

Colpaert F. C. (1982) The Pharmacological Specificity of Opiate Drug Discrimination, in *Drug Discrimination: Applications in CNS Pharmacology* (Colpaert F. C. and Slangen J. L., eds.), Elsevier, Amsterdam.

Colpaert F. C. and Janssen P. A. J. (1981) Factors regulating drug cue sensitivity: The effect of frustrative non-reward in fentanyl–saline discrimination. *Arch. Int. Pharmacodyn. Ther.* **254,** 241–251.

Colpaert F. C. and Janssen P. A. J. (1982a) Factors regulating drug cue sensitivity: Limits of discriminability and the role of progressively decreasing training dose in cocaine–saline discrimination. *Neuropharmacology* **21,** 1187–1194.

Colpaert F. C. and Janssen P. A. J. (1982b) Factors regulating drug cue sensitivity: the effects of dose ratio and absolute dose level in the case of fentanyl dose–dose discrimination. *Arch. Int. Pharmacodyn. Ther.* **258,** 283–299.

Colpaert F. C. and Rosecrans J. A., eds. (1978) *Stimulus Properties of Drugs: Ten Years of Progress.* Elsevier, Amsterdam.

Colpaert F. C. and Slangen J. L., eds. (1982) *Drug Discrimination: Applications in CNS Pharmacology.* Elsevier, Amsterdam.

Colpaert F. C., Niemegeers C. J. E., and Janssen P. A. J. (1978) Factors Regulating Drug Cue Sensitivity. A Long-Term Study on the Cocaine Cue, in *Stimulus Properties of Drugs: Ten Years of Progress* (Colpaert F. C. and Rosecrans J. A., eds.), Elsevier, Amsterdam.

Colpaert F. C., Niemegeers C. J. E., and Janssen P. A. J. (1980a) Factors regulating drug cue sensitivity: Limits of discriminability and the role of a progressively decreasing training dose in fentanyl–saline discrimination. *J. Pharmacol. Exp. Ther.* **212,** 474–480.

Colpaert F. C., Niemegeers C. J. E., and Janssen P. A. J. (1980b) Factors regulating drug cue sensitivity: The effect of training dose in fentanyl–saline discrimination. *Neuropharmacology* **19,** 705–713.

DeWitte P. H. (1982a) Response Latency as the Dependent Variable in Discrimination Procedures, in *Drug Discrimination: Applications in CNS Pharmacology* (Colpaert F. C. and Slangen J. L., eds.), Elsevier, Amsterdam.

DeWitte P. H. (1982b) Brain stimulation as the reinforcer in alcohol–saline discrimination. *Pharmacol. Biochem. Behav.* **17,** 1093–1096.

D'Mello G. D. (1981) A comparison of some behavioural effects of amphetamine and electrical brain stimulation of the mesolimbic dopamine system in rats. *Psychopharmacology* **75,** 184–192.

D'Mello G. D. and Stolerman I. P. (1978) Methodological Issues in Drug-Discrimination Research, in *Stimulus Properties of Drugs: Ten Years of Progress* (Colpaert F. C. and Rosecrans J. A., eds.), Elsevier, Amsterdam.

Emmett-Oglesby M. W., Spencer Jr., D. G., Elmesallamy F., and Lal H. (1983) The pentylenetetrazol model of anxietyt detects withdrawal from diazepam in rats. *Life Sci.* **33,** 161–168.

Finney D. A. (1976) A computer program for parallel line bioassays. *J. Pharmacol. Exp. Ther.* **198,** 497–506.

Gellert V. F. and Holtzman S. G. (1979) Discriminative stimulus effects of naltrexone in the morphine-dependent rat. *J. Pharmacol. Exp. Ther.* **211,** 596–605.

Girden E. and Culler E. A. (1937) Conditioned responses in curarized striate muscles in dogs. *J. Comp. Psychol.* **23,** 261–274.

Glennon R. A. and Rosecrans J. A. (1982) Indolealkylamine and phenylamine hallucinogens: A brief overview. *Neurosci. Biobehav. Rev.* **6,** 489–497.

Haenlein M., Caul W. F., Barrett R. J., and Michaelis R. C. (1983) Discrimination of serotonergic drugs is unaltered in rats prenatally exposed to ethanol. *Neurobehav. Toxicol. Teratol.* **5,** 475–478.

Harris R. T. and Balster R. L. (1968) Discriminative control by *d,l*-amphetamine and saline of lever choice and response patterning. *Psychon. Sci.* **10,** 105–106.

Harris R. T. and Balster R. L. (1970) An Analysis of Psychological Dependence, in *Drug Dependence* (Harris R. T., McIsaac W. M., and Schuster C. R., eds.), Univ. Texas Press, Austin.

Haug T. and Götestam K. G. (1982) Onset and offset of the diazepam stimulus complex. *Pharmacol. Biochem. Behav.* **17,** 1171–1174.

Heinemann E. G. and Chase S. (1975) Stimulus Generalization, in *Conditioning and Behavior Theory* (Estes W. K., ed.), LEA, Hillsdale.

Herling S. and Shannon H. E. (1982) Ro 15-1788 antagonizes the discriminative stimulus effects of diazepam in rats but not similar effects of pentobarbital. *Life Sci.* **31,** 2105–2112.

Herling S., Coale E. H., Valentino R. J., Hein D. W., and Woods J. H. (1980) Narcotic discrimination in pigeons. *J. Pharmacol. Exp. Ther.* **214,** 139–146.

Hiltunen A. J., Järbe T. U. C., and Swedberg M. D. B. (1983) Drug discrimination studies with ethanol and benzodiazepines. *Acta Pharmacol. Toxicol.* **53,** SII (abstract no. 37).

Ho B. T., Richards III, W., and Chute D. L., eds. (1978) *Drug Discrimination and State Dependent Learning.* Academic, New York.

Holtzman S. G. (1982) Discriminative Stimulus Properties of Opioids in the Rat and Squirrel Monkey, in *Drug Discrimination: Applications in CNS Pharmacology* (Colpaert F. C. and Slangen J. L., eds.), Elsevier, Amsterdam.

Honig W. K. and Urcuioli P. J. (1981) The legacy of Gutman and Kalish (1956); 25 years of research on stimulus generalization. *J. Exp. Anal. Behav.* **36,** 405–445.

Iwamoto E. T. and Martin W. R. (1981) Multiple opioid receptors. *Med. Res. Rev.* **1,** 411–440.

Järbe T. U. C. (1976) Characteristics of pentobarbital discrimination in the gerbil: Transfer and antagonism. *Psychopharmacology* **49,** 33–40.

Järbe T. U. C. (1977) Alcohol-discrimination in gerbils: Interactions with bemegride, DH-524 amphetamine, and delta-9-THC. *Arch. Int. Pharmacodyn. Ther.* **227,** 118–129.

Järbe T. U. C. (1981) Cocaine cue in pigeons: Time course studies and generalization to structurally related compounds (norcocaine, WIN 35, 428 and 35,065-2) and (+)-amphetamine. *Br. J. Pharmacol.* **73,** 843–852.

Järbe T. U. C. and Henriksson B. G. (1974) Discriminative response control produced with hashish, tetrahydrocannabinols (delta-8-THC and delta-9-THC), and other drugs. *Psychopharmacologia* **40**, 1–16.

Järbe T. U. C. and Johansson B. (1984) Interaction between drug discriminative stimuli and exteroceptive signals. *Behav. Neurosci.* **98**, 686–694.

Järbe T. U. C. and Kroon-Järbe E. R. (1983) Discriminability and procedure: Effects of cocaine and *d*-amphetamine. *Psychol. Rep.* **52**, 611–616.

Järbe T. U. C. and McMillan D. E. (1983) Interaction of the discriminative stimulus properties of diazepam and ethanol in pigeons. *Pharmacol. Biochem. Behav.* **18**, 73–80.

Järbe T. U. C. and Ohlin G. C. (1979) Discriminative effects of combinations of delta-9-tetrahydrocannabinol and pentobarbital in pigeons. *Psychopharmacology* **63**, 233–239.

Järbe T. U. C. and Rollenhagen C. (1978) Morphine as a discriminative cue in gerbils: Drug generalization and antagonism. *Psychopharmacology* **58**, 271–275.

Järbe T. U. C. and Swedberg M. D. B. (1982) A Conceptualization of Drug Discrimination Learning, in *Drug Discrimination: Applications in CNS Pharmacology* (Colpaert F. C. and Slangen J. L., eds.), Elsevier, Amsterdam.

Järbe T. U. C. and Swedberg M. D. B. (1981) Differences in the stimulus effects of CNS depressant substances as evidenced by drug vs drug discrimination techniques. *Acta. Pharmacol. Toxicol.* **49**, SIV (abstract no. 45).

Järbe T. U. C., Laaksonen T., and Svensson R. (1983a) Influence of exteroceptive contextual conditions upon internal drug stimulus control. *Psychopharmacology* **80**, 31–34.

Järbe T. U. C., Svensson R.,and Laaksonen T. (1983b) Conditioning of a discriminative drug stimulus: Overshadowing and blocking like procedures. *Scand. J. Psychol.* **24**, 325–330.

Järbe T. U. C., Swedberg M. D. B., and Mechoulam R. (1981a) A repeated tests procedure to assess onset and duration of the cue properties of (−)-delta-9-THC, (−)-delta-8-THC-DMH and (+)-delta-8-THC. *Psychopharmacology* **75**, 152–157.

Järbe T. U. C., Sterner U., and Hjerpe C. (1981b) Conditioning of an interoceptive drug stimulus to different exteroceptive contexts. *Psychopharmacology* **73**, 23–26.

Järbe T. U. C., Loman P., and Swedberg M. D. B. (1979) Evidence supporting lack of discriminative stimulus properties of a combination of naltrexone and morphine. *Pharmacol. Biochem. Behav.* **10,** 493–497.

Järbe T. U. C., Swedberg M. D. B., Hiltunen A. J., and Mechoulam R. (1985) Drug discrimination techniques for assessing structure activity relationships of cannabimimetics. *Acta Physiol. Scand.* **124,** 185 (Supplementum 542).

Koek W. and Slangen J. L. (1982a) The role of fentanyl training dose and of the alternative stimulus condition in drug generalization. *Psychopharmacology* **76,** 149–156.

Koek W. and Slangen J. L. (1982b) Effects of Reinforcement Differences Between Drug and Saline Sessions on Discriminative Stimulus Properties of Fentanyl, in *Drug Discrimination: Applications in CNS Pharmacology* (Colpaert F. C. and Slangen J. L., eds.), Elsevier, Amsterdam.

Krimmer E. C., Barry III, H., and Coltrin D. (1978) Antagonism of Pentobarbital Discriminative Stimulus by Bemegride in Immobilized Rats, in *Stimulus Properties of Drugs: Ten Years of Progress* (Colpaert F. C. and Rosecrans J. A., eds.), Elsevier, Amsterdam.

Krimmer E. C., Benson B. J., McGuire M., and Barry III, H. (1982) Conditional Sensory Stimuli During Morphine Discrimination, in *Drug Discrimination: Applications in CNS Pharmacology* (Colpaert F. C. and Slangen J. L., eds.), Elsevier, Amsterdam.

Kubena R. K. and Barry III, H. (1969) Two procedures for training differential responses to alcohol and nondrug conditions. *J. Pharmacol. Sci.* **58,** 99–101.

Lal H., ed. (1977a) *Discriminative Stimulus Properties of Drugs.* Plenum, New York.

Lal H. (1977b) Drug Induced Discriminable Stimuli: Past Research and Future Perspectives, in *Discriminative Stimulus Properties of Drugs* (Lal H., ed.), Plenum, New York.

Lal H. and Shearman G. T. (1982) Attenuation of chemically induced anxiogenic stimuli as a novel method for evaluating anxiolytic drugs: A comparison of clonazepam with other benzodiazepines. *Drug Dev. Res.* **S1,** 127–134.

Leberer M. R. and Fowler S. C. (1977) Drug discrimination and generalization in pigeons. *Pharmacol. Biochem. Behav.* **7,** 483–486.

Litchfield J. T. and Wilcoxon F. (1949) A simplified method of evaluating dose-effect experiments. *J. Pharmacol. Exp. Ther.* **96,** 99–113.

McMillan D. E. (1982) Generalization of the discriminative stimulus properties of phencyclidine to other drugs in the pigeon using color tracking under second-order schedules. *Psychopharmacology* **78,** 131–134.

McMillan D. E., Cole-Fullenwider D. A., Hardwick W. C., and Wenger G. R. (1982) Phencyclidine discrimination in the pigeon using color tracking under second-order schedules. *J. Exp. Anal. Behav.* **37,** 143–147.

Morrison C. F. and Stephenson J. A. (1969) Nicotine injections as the conditioned stimulus in discrimination learning. *Psychopharmacologia* **15,** 351–360.

Overton D. A. (1966) State-dependent learning produced by depressant and atropine-like drugs. *Psychopharmacologia* **10,** 6–31.

Overton D. A. (1967) Differential responding in a three-choice maze controlled by three drug states. *Psychopharmacologia* **11,** 376–378.

Overton D. A. (1971) Discriminative Control of Behavior by Drug States, in *Stimulus Properties of Drugs* (Thompson T. and Pickens R., eds.), Appleton-Century Crofts, New York.

Overton D. A. (1974) Experimental methods for the study of state-dependent learning. *Fed. Proc.* **33,** 1800–1813.

Overton D. A. (1977) Comparison of ethanol, pentobarbital and phenobarbital using drug vs drug discrimination training. *Psychopharmacology* **53,** 195–199.

Overton D. A. (1978a) Influence of Training Compartment Design on Performance in the Two-Bar Drug Discrimination Task: A Methodological Report, in *Stimulus Properties of Drugs: Ten Years of Progress* (Colpaert F. C. and Rosecrans J. A., eds.), Elsevier, Amsterdam.

Overton D. A. (1978b) Major Theories of State Dependent Learning, in *Drug Discrimination and State Dependent Learning* (Ho B. T., Richards III, D. W., and Chute D. L., eds.), Academic, New York.

Overton D. A. (1979a) Influence of shaping procedures and schedules of reinforcement on performance in the two-bar drug discrimination task: A methodological report. *Psychopharmacology* **65,** 291–298.

Overton D. A. (1979b) Drug discrimination training with progressively lowered doses. *Science* **205,** 720–721.

Overton D. A. (1982a) Comparison of the degree of discriminability of various drugs using the T-maze drug discrimination paradigm. *Psychopharmacology* **76,** 385–395.

Overton D. A. (1982b) Multiple drug training as a method for increasing the specificity of the drug discrimination procedure. *J. Pharmacol. Exp. Ther.* **221,** 166–172.

Richards III, D. W. (1978) A Functional Analysis of the Discriminative Stimulus Properties of Amphetamine and Pentobartical, in *Drug Discrimination and State Dependent Learning* (Ho B. T., Richards III, D. W., and Chute D. L., eds.), Academic, New York.

Romano C., Goldstein A., and Jewell N. P. (1981) Characterization of the receptor mediating the nicotine discriminative stimulus. *Psychopharmacology* **74,** 310–315.

Rosecrans J. A. and Meltzer L. T. (1981) Central sites and mechanisms of action of nicotine. *Neurosci. Biobehav. Rev.* **5,** 497–501.

Schechter M. D. (1981) Extended schedule transfer of ethanol discrimination. *Pharmacol. Biochem. Behav.* **14,** 23–25.

Schechter M. D. and Lovano D. M. (1982) Time-course of action of ethanol upon a stimulant–depressant continuum. *Arch. Int. Pharmacodyn. Ther.* **260,** 189–195.

Schuster C. R. and Balster R. L. (1977) The Discriminative Stimulus Properties of Drugs, in *Advances in Behavioral Pharmacology,* vol. 1 (Thompson T. and Dews P. B., eds.), Academic, New York.

Shannon H. E. and Holtzman S. G. (1976) Evaluation of the discriminative effects of morphine in the rat. *J. Pharmacol. Exp. Ther.* **198,** 54–65.

Shannon H. E. and Holtzman S. G. (1979) Morphine training dose: A determinant of stimulus generalization to narcotic antagonists in the rat. *Psychopharmacology* **61,** 239–244.

Shearman G. T., Cafaro M. P.,Lal H., and Howard J. L. (1981) Saccharin-taste discrimination by two-lever choice; A rat bioassay for sweeteners. *Drug. Dev. Res.* **1,** 145–150.

Siegel S. (1982) Drug Dissociation in the Nineteenth Century, in *Drug Discrimination: Applications in CNS Pharmacology* (Colpaert F. C. and Slangen J. L., eds.), Elsevier, Amsterdam.

Silverman P. B. and Ho B. T. (1977) Characterization of Discriminative Response Control by Psychomotor Stimulants, in *Discriminative Stimulus Properties of Drugs* (Lal H., ed.), Plenum, New York.

Stolerman I. P. and D'Mello G. D. (1981) Role of training conditions in discrimination of central nervous system stimulants in rats. *Psychopharmacology* **73**, 295–303.

Stolerman I. P., Baldy R. E., and Shine P. J. (1982) Drug Discrimination Procedure: A Bibliography, in *Drug Discrimination: Applications in CNS Pharmacology* (Colpaert F. C. and Slangen J. L., eds.), Elsevier, Amsterdam.

Swedberg M. D. B. and Järbe T. U. C. (1982) Morphine Cue Saliency: Limits of Discriminability and Third State Perception by Pigeons, in *Drug Discrimination: Applications in CNS Pharmacology* (Colpaert F. C.and Slangen J. L., eds.), Elsevier, Amsterdam.

Swedberg M. D. B., Loman P., and Järbe T. U. C. (1978) Effects of chlormethiazole (Heminevrin®) on drug discrimination and open-field behavior of gerbils. *Psychopharmacology* **59**, 165–170.

Valentino R. J., Herling S., and Woods J. H. (1983) Discriminative stimulus effects of naltrexone in narcotic-naive and morphine treated pigeons. *J. Pharmacol. Exp. Ther.* **224**, 307–313.

Weissman A. (1976) The discriminability of aspirin in arthritic and non-arthritic rats. *Pharmacol. Biochem. Behav.* **5**, 583–586.

White J. M. and Holtzman S. C. (1981) Three-choice drug discrimination in the rat: Morphine, cyclazocine and saline. *J. Pharmacol. Exp. Ther.* **217**, 254–262.

White J. M. and Holtzman S. G. (1983a) Further characterization of the three-choice morphine, cyclazocine and saline discrimination paradigm: Opioids with agonist and antagonist properties. *J. Pharmacol. Exp. Ther.* **224**, 95–99.

White J. M. and Holtzman S. G. (1983b) Three-choice drug discrimination: Phencyclidine-like stimulus effects of opiates. *Psychopharmacology* **80**, 1–9.

Winter J. C. (1978) Drug-Induced Stimulus Control, in *Contemporary Research in Behavioral Pharmacology* (Blackman D. E. and Sanger D. J., eds.), Plenum, New York.

Winter J. C. (1981) Drug induced stimulus control and the concept of breaking point: LSD and quipazine. *Psychopharmacology* **72**, 217–218.

York J. L. (1978) A comparison of the discriminative stimulus effects of ethanol, barbital and phenobarbital in rats. *Psychopharmacology* **60,** 19–23.

Young R. and Dewey W. L. (1982) Differentiation of the Behavioral Responses Produced by Barbiturates and Benzodiazepines by the Benzodiazepine Antagonist *Ro* 15-1788, in *Drug Discrimination: Applications in CNS Pharmacology* (Colpaert F. C. and Slangen J. L., eds.), Elsevier, Amsterdam.

Zenick H. and Goldsmith M. (1981) Drug discrimination learning in lead-exposed rats. *Science* **212,** 569–571.

Subject Index